Clinical Reasoning
Cases in Nursing

Clinical Reasoning Cases in Nursing

Mariann Harding, PhD, RN, CNE
Associate Professor
Department of Nursing
Kent State University at Tuscarawas
New Philadelphia, Ohio

Julie S. Snyder, MSN, RN-BC
Lecturer
School of Nursing
Regent University
Virginia Beach, Virginia

7th EDITION

ELSEVIER

CLINICAL REASONING CASES IN NURSING,
SEVENTH EDITION

ISBN: 978-0-323-52736-1

Library of Congress Control Number: 2018954100

Executive Content Strategist: Lee Henderson
Content Development Specialist: Laura Goodrich
Publishing Services Manager: Julie Eddy
Senior Project Manager: Tracey Schriefer
Design Direction: Margaret Reid

Printed in the United States of America
Last digit is the print number: 9 8 7 6 5 4 3 2 1

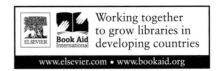

3251 Riverport Lane
St. Louis, Missouri 63043

Contributors

Meghan Davis, MSN-Ed, CCRN, RN
Registered Nurse
Virginia Beach, Virginia

Jatifha C. Felton, MSN-Ed, APRN, ACNCP-AG, CCRN
Critical Care Nurse Practitioner
Chesapeake Regional Healthcare
Chesapeake, Virginia

Sherry D. Ferki, RN, MSN
Adjunct Faculty
School of Nursing
Old Dominion University
Norfolk, Virginia

Joanna Van Sant, MSN, RN
Clinical Nurse Manager–Oncology Unit
Sentara Northern Virginia Medical Center
Woodbridge, Virginia

Reviewers

Heidi Matarasso Bakerman, RN, BA
Nursing, MscN
Nursing Instructor
Nursing
Vanier College
Montreal, Quebec, Canada

Beverly Banks, MSN, BSN, RN
Full Time Faculty
Nursing
Alpena Community College
Alpena, Michigan

Mitzi L. Bass, MPH, MSN, RN
Assistant Professor of Nursing
School of Nursing and Health Professions
Baltimore City Community College
Baltimore, Maryland

Michelle Bayard, BSN, RN
Teacher
Faculty of Careers and Technology: Nursing
Vanier College
Montreal, Quebec, Canada

Diana Lynne Burgess, MSN, RN
Nursing Faculty—ADN Program
St. Petersburg College of Nursing
St. Petersburg, Florida

Lacey M. Campbell, MSN, RN
Program Coordinator
Accelerated LPN to RN Program
Texas County Technical College
Houston, Missouri

Diane Cohen, MSN, RN
Professor—Nursing
MassBay Community College
Framingham, Massachusetts

Nicola Eynon-Brown, RN(EC), BNSc, MN,
NP, CPNP-PC
Professor
School of Baccalaureate Nursing
St. Lawrence College
Brockville, Ontario, Canada

Melissa Marie Fischer, MSN, RN
ADN Nursing Faculty
Nursing
Blackhawk Technical College
Janesville, Wisconsin

Victoria A. Greenwood, MSN, MSEd, RN-BC
Assistant Professor
Nursing
The Sage Colleges
Troy, New York

Rose A. Harding, MSN, RN
Coordinator, Standardized Test Evaluation
    Committee
JoAnne Gay Dishman School of Nursing
Lamar University
Beaumont, Texas

Antonea Jackson, PhD (c), MSN,
RN CNE
Clinical Assistant Professor
Nursing
Prairie View A&M University
Houston, Texas

Llynne C. Kiernan, DNP, MSN,
RN-BC
Assistant Professor of Nursing
Nursing
Norwich University
Northfield, Vermont

REVIEWERS

Introduction

To provide safe, quality care, nurses need to have well-developed clinical reasoning skills. As new graduates, you will make decisions and take actions of an increasingly sophisticated nature. You will encounter problems you have never seen or heard about during your classroom and clinical experiences. You will have to make complex decisions with little or no guidance and limited resources.

We want you to be exposed to as much as possible during your student days, but more importantly, we want you to learn to *think*. You cannot memorize your way out of any situation, but you can *think* your way out of any situation. We know that students often learn more and faster when they have the freedom to make mistakes. This book is designed to allow you to look at how to solve problems and find answers without the pressure of someone's life hanging in the balance. We want you to do well. We want you to be the best. It is our wish for you to grow into confident, competent nursing professionals. We want you to be very, very good at what you do!

What Is Clinical Reasoning?

Clinical reasoning is *not* memorizing lists of facts or the steps of procedures. Instead, clinical reasoning is an analytical process that can help you think about a patient care issue in an organized and efficient manner. Five steps are involved in clinical reasoning. Thinking about these steps may help you when you work through the questions in your cases. Here are the five steps with an explanation of what they mean.

1. *Recognize and define the problem by asking the right questions:* Exactly what is it you need to know? What is the question asking?

2. *Select the information or data necessary to solve the problem or answer the question:* First you have to ask whether all the necessary information is there. If not, how and where can you get the additional information? What other resources are available? This is one of the most difficult steps. In real clinical experiences, you rarely have all of the information, so you have to learn where you can get necessary data. For instance, patient and family interviews, nursing charting, the patient medical chart, laboratory data on your computer, your observations, and your own physical assessment can help you identify important clues. Of course, information can rapidly become outdated. To make sure you are accessing the most current and accurate information, you will occasionally need to use the Internet to answer a question.

3. *Recognize stated and unstated assumptions; that is, what do you think is or is not true?* Sometimes answers or solutions seem obvious; just because something seems obvious does not mean it is correct. You may need to consider several possible answers or solutions. Consider all clues carefully and *do not dismiss a possibility too quickly.* Remember, "*You never find an answer you don't think of.*"

4. *Formulate and select relevant and/or potential decisions:* Try to think of as many possibilities as you can. Consider the pros and cons of the consequences of making each decision. What is the best answer/solution? What could go wrong? This requires considering many different angles. In today's health care settings, decision making often requires balancing the well-being needs of the patient, the preferences and concerns of the patient and caregiver, and financial limitations imposed by the reimbursement system. In making decisions, you need to take into account all relevant factors. Remember, you may need to explain why you rejected other options.

5. *Draw a valid, informed conclusion:* Consider all data; then determine what is relevant and what makes the most sense. Only then should you draw your conclusion.

It may look as if this kind of reasoning comes naturally to your instructors and experienced nurses. You can be certain that even experienced nurses were once where you are now. The rapid and sound decision making that is essential to good nursing requires years of practice. The practice of good clinical reasoning leads to good thinking in clinical practice. This book will help you practice the important steps in making sound clinical judgments until the process starts to come naturally.

What Is New in This Edition

The conceptual approach to nursing education is a new way to manage information and help students develop clinical reasoning skills. In this edition, we chose to reorganize the cases in each section by health-illness concepts. Within each section, you will see the basic principles of that concept applied in exemplars, or models of that concept, that cross care settings, the life span, and the health-illness continuum. For example, you may be enrolled in a course that focuses on gas exchange, including risk factors, physiologic mechanisms, assessment, and interventions to promote optimal oxygenation. Based on prevalence and incidence, exemplars such as pneumonia, influenza, and asthma, are used to show how to apply principles across ages and care settings. To ensure that there are cases that cover common exemplars you may see in class, we added over 20 new cases. Like the existing cases, each of these are adaptations of actual scenarios encountered in the clinical setting—there is no better way to learn than from real patients!

Because nurses play a vital role in improving the safety and quality of patient care, you need to learn interventions you will use to deliver safe care and enhance patient outcomes. To help you learn key principles, you will note questions marked with a 🎯. These questions involve scenarios that typically include inherent risks, such as medication administration, fall and pressure injury reduction protocols, and preventing health care–associated infections.

The "How To" of Case Studies

When you begin each case, read through the whole story once, from start to finish, getting a general idea of what it is about. Write down things you have to look up. This will help you move through the case smoothly and get more out of it. How much you have to look up will depend on where you are in your program, what you know, and how much experience you already have. Preparing cases will become easier as you advance in your program.

Acknowledgments

We would like to express our appreciation to the editorial Elsevier staff, especially Laura Goodrich, Lee Henderson, and Tracey Schriefer for their professional support and contributions in guiding this text to publication. We extend a special thanks to our reviewers, who gave us helpful suggestions and insights as we developed this edition.

Mariann's gratitude goes to those she loves most—her husband, Jeff, and her daughters, Kate and Sarah. She gives a special thanks to her students, colleagues, and patients; each inspire her passion for nursing and education. Lastly, Mariann praises God, who has graciously bestowed more blessings than could ever be imagined.

Julie thanks her husband, Jonathan, for his love, support, and patience during this project. She is grateful for the encouragement from daughter Emily, son-in-law Randy, and parents Willis and Jean Simmons. Julie appreciates the hard work of colleagues Sherry Ferki, Jatifha Felton, Meghan Davis, Joanna Van Sant, Alicia Rose, and Alicia Powell as contributors and reviewers for this edition. She is especially thankful to the students, whose eagerness to learn is an inspiration. Most importantly, Julie gives thanks to God, our source of hope and strength.

Contents

Perfusion

Case Study 1

Name_____ Class/Group _____ Date _____

▶ Scenario

M.G., a "frequent flier," is admitted to the emergency department (ED) with a diagnosis of heart failure (HF). She was discharged from the hospital 10 days ago and comes in today stating, "I just had to come to the hospital today because I can't catch my breath and my legs are as big as tree trunks." After further questioning, you learn she is strictly following the fluid and salt restriction ordered during her last hospital admission. She reports gaining 1 to 2 pounds (0.5 to 1 kg) every day since her discharge.

1. What error in discharge teaching most likely occurred?

2. An echocardiogram revealed that her ejection fraction (EF) is 30%, but it was 40% a month ago. What is EF, and what does the decreased number indicate?

CASE STUDY PROGRESS

During the admission interview, the nurse makes a list of the medications M.G. took at home.

Chart View

Nursing Assessment: Medications Taken at Home

Enalapril (Vasotec)	5 mg PO bid
Pioglitazone (Actos)	45 mg PO every morning
Furosemide (Lasix)	40 mg/day PO
Potassium chloride (K-Dur)	20 mEq/day PO

3. Which of these medications may have contributed to M.G.'s HF? Explain.

4. How do angiotensin-converting enzyme (ACE) inhibitors, such as enalapril (Vasotec), work to reduce HF? Select all that apply.
   a. Cause systemic vasodilation
   b. Increase cardiac contractility
   c. Reduce preload and afterload
   d. Prevent the conversion of angiotensin I to angiotensin II
   e. Block sympathetic nervous system stimulation to the heart
   f. Promote the excretion of sodium and water in the renal tubules

CASE STUDY PROGRESS

After reviewing M.G.'s medications, the cardiologist writes the following medication orders.

Chart View

Medication Orders

Enalapril (Vasotec)	5 mg PO bid
Carvedilol (Coreg)	3.125 mg PO twice daily
Metformin (Glucophage)	500 mg twice daily
Furosemide (Lasix)	80 mg intravenous push (IVP) now, then 40 mg/day IVP
Potassium chloride (K-Dur)	20 mEq/day PO

5. What is the rationale for changing the route of the furosemide (Lasix)?

6. You give furosemide (Lasix) 80 mg IVP. Identify at least 4 parameters you would use to monitor the effectiveness of this medication.

7. What lab tests should be ordered for M.G. related to the order for furosemide (Lasix)? Select all that apply.
   a. Sodium level
   b. Potassium level
   c. Magnesium level
   d. Coagulation studies
   e. Serum glucose level
   f. Complete blood count

8. What is the reason for ordering the beta blocker carvedilol?
   a. Increase urine output
   b. Cause peripheral vasodilation
   c. Increase the contractility of the heart
   d. Reduce cardiac stimulation from catecholamines

 9. You assess M.G. for conditions that may be a contraindication to carvedilol. Which condition, if present, may cause serious problems if she takes this medication?
   a. Angina
   b. Asthma
   c. Glaucoma
   d. Hypertension

CASE STUDY PROGRESS

One day later, M.G. has shown only slight improvement, and digoxin (Lanoxin) 125 mcg PO daily is added to her orders.

10. What is the mechanism of action of digoxin?
   a. Causes systemic vasodilation
   b. Increases cardiac contractility and cardiac output
   c. Blocks sympathetic nervous system stimulation to the heart
   d. Promotes the excretion of sodium and water in the renal tubules

11. Which findings from M.G.'s assessment would indicate an increased possibility of digoxin toxicity? Explain your answer.
   a. Digoxin level 1.6 ng/mL (2.05 mmol/L)
   b. Serum sodium level of 139 mEq/L (138 mmol/L)
   c. Apical heart rate of 64
   d. Serum potassium level of 2.2 mEq/L (2.2 mmol/L)

 12. When preparing to give the digoxin, you notice that it is available in milligrams (mg) not micrograms (mcg). Convert 125 mcg to mg.

13. After 2 days, M.G.'s symptoms improve with intravenous diuretics and digoxin. She is placed back on oral furosemide (Lasix) once her weight loss is deemed adequate for achievement of a euvolemic state. What will determine whether the oral dose will be adequate for discharge to be considered?

14. M.G. is ready for discharge. According to the mnemonic *MAWDS,* what key management concepts should be taught to prevent relapse and another admission?

15. After the teaching session, the nurse asks M.G. to "teach back" one important concept of care at home. Which statement by M.G. indicates a need for further education? Explain your answer.
   a. "I will not add salt when I am cooking."
   b. "I will use a weekly pill calendar box to remind me to take my medicine."
   c. "I will weigh myself daily and tell the doctor at my next visit if I am gaining weight."
   d. "I will try to take a short walk around the block with my husband three times a week."

CASE STUDY OUTCOME

After M.G. has been at home for 2 days, the STOP Heart Failure Nurse Navigator calls to ask about her progress. M.G. reports that her weight has not increased since she has been home and she is breathing more easily.

Case Study **2**

Name _____   Class/Group _____   Date _____

▶ Scenario

M.P. is a 65-year-old African American woman who comes to the clinic for a follow-up visit. She was diagnosed with hypertension (HTN) 2 months ago and was given a prescription for a thiazide diuretic but stopped taking it 2 weeks ago because "it made me dizzy and I kept getting up during the night to empty my bladder." During today's clinic visit, she expresses fear because her mother died of a stroke (cerebrovascular accident [CVA]) at M.P.'s age, and M.P. is afraid she will suffer the same fate. She states, "I've never smoked and I don't drink, but I am so afraid of this high blood pressure." You review the data from her past clinic visits.

Chart View

Family History

> Mother, died at age 65 years of CVA
> Father, died at age 67 years of myocardial infarction (MI)
> Sister, alive and well, age 62 years
> Brother, alive, age 70 years, has coronary artery disease (CAD), HTN, type 2 diabetes mellitus (DM)

Patient Past History

> Married for 45 years, 2 children, alive and well, 6 grandchildren
> Cholecystectomy, age 42 years
> Hysterectomy, age 48 years

Blood Pressure Assessments

> January 2: 150/92
> January 31: 156/94 (given prescription for hydrochlorothiazide [HCTZ] 25 mg PO every
>   morning)
> February 28: 140/90

1. According to the most recent guidelines from the Joint National Committee on Prevention, Detection, Evaluation, and Treatment of High Blood Pressure, M.P.'s blood pressure (BP) falls under which classification?

2. What could M.P. be doing that is causing her nocturia?

CASE STUDY PROGRESS

During today's visit, M.P.'s vital signs are as follows: BP: 162/102; P: 78; R: 16; T: 98.2°F (36.8 °C). Her most recent basic metabolic panel (BMP) and fasting lipids are within normal limits. Her height is 5 ft, 4 in (163 cm), and she weighs 110 lb (50 kg). She tells you that she tries to go on walks but does not like to walk alone and so has done so only occasionally.

3. What risk factors does M.P. have that increase her risk for cardiovascular disease?

CASE STUDY PROGRESS

Because M.P.'s BP continues to be high, the provider decides to start another antihypertensive drug and recommends that she try again with the HCTZ, taken in the mornings.

4. According to the JNC 8 national guidelines, describe the drug therapy recommended for M.P. at this time.

5. M.P. goes on to ask whether there is anything else she should do to help with her HTN. She asks, "Do I need to lose weight?" Look up her height and weight for her age on a body mass index (BMI) chart. Is she considered overweight?

6. What nonpharmacologic lifestyle alteration measures might help M.P. control her BP? List 2 examples and explain.

The provider decreases M.P.'s HCTZ dose to 12.5 mg PO daily and adds a prescription for benazepril (Lotensin) 5 mg daily. M.P. is instructed to return to the clinic in 1 week to have her blood work checked. She is instructed to monitor her BP at least twice a week and return for a medication management appointment in 1 month with her list of BP readings.

7. Why did the provider decrease the dose of the HCTZ?

8. You provide M.P. with education about the common side effects of benazepril, which can include which of these? Select all that apply.
   a. Cough
   b. Dizziness
   c. Headache
   d. Constipation
   e. Shortness of breath

9. It is sometimes difficult to remember whether one has taken one's medication. What techniques might you teach M.P. to help her remember to take her medicines each day? Name at least 2.

10. After the teaching session about her medicines, which statement by M.P. indicates a need for further instructions?
   a. "I need to rise up slowly when I get out of bed or out of a chair."
   b. "I will leave the salt shaker off the table and not salt my food when I cook."
   c. "I will call if I feel very dizzy, weak, or short of breath while on this medicine."
   d. "It's okay to skip a few doses if I am feeling bad as long as it's just for a few days."

11. Describe 3 priority problems that will guide M.P.'s nursing care.

M.P. returns in 1 month for her medication management appointment. She tells you she is feeling fine and does not have any side effects from her new medication. Her BP, checked twice a week at the senior center, ranges from 132 to 136 systolic, and 78 to 82 diastolic.

12. When someone is taking HCTZ and an angiotensin-converting enzyme (ACE) inhibitor, such as benazepril, what lab test results would you expect to be monitored?

Chart View

Laboratory Test Results (Fasting)

Potassium	3.6 mEq/L (3.6 mmol/L)
Sodium	138 mEq/L (138 mmol/L)
Chloride	100 mEq/L (100 mmol/L)
CO_2	28 mEq/L (28 mmol/L)
Glucose	112 mEq/L (6.2 mmol/L)
Creatinine	0.7 mg/dL (61.9 mcmol/L)
Blood urea nitrogen (BUN)	18 mg/dL (6.4 mmol/L)
Magnesium	1.9 mEq/L (0.95 mmol/L)

13. What lab test results, if any, are of concern at this time?

14. You take M.P.'s BP and get 138/88. She asks whether these BP readings are okay. On what do you base your response?

15. List at least 3 important ways you might help M.P. maintain her success.

CASE STUDY PROGRESS

M.P. tells you she was recently at a luncheon with her garden club and that most of those women take BP pills different from the ones she does. She asks why their pills are different shapes and colors.

16. How can you explain the difference to M.P.?

17. During the visit, you ask M.P., "When was your last eye examination?" She answers, "I'm not sure, probably about 2 years ago. What does that have to do with my blood pressure?" What is your response?

CASE STUDY OUTCOME

M.P. comes in for a routine follow-up visit 3 months later. She continues to do well on her daily BP drug regimen, with average BP readings of 130/78. She participates in group walking program for senior citizens at the local mall. She admits she has not done as well with decreasing her salt intake but says she is trying. She visited an ophthalmologist last week and had no problems except for a slight cataract in one eye.

Case Study **3**

Name_____   Class/Group_____   Date_____

▶ Scenario

A.M. is a 52-year-old woman who has gained over 75 lbs (32 kg) over the past 30 years, after the birth of her 3 children. She has a sedentary job that requires sitting at a desk for most hours of the work day. When she is at home, she stays inside because she is afraid to walk by herself in her neighborhood. She lives alone, but her children live in the same city. She has a history of hypertension and states that she does not take her medications regularly. She came to the clinic today stating that she thinks she might have a urinary tract infection. Her weight is 255 lbs (102.5 kg). She is 5 feet, 4 inches tall (162.5 cm) and has a waist circumference of 41 inches (104 cm). Her abdomen is large, nontender, soft, and round. Her blood pressure is 160/104. You review fasting labs results that were drawn a week ago.

Chart View

Laboratory Results

Glucose	170 mg/dL (9.4 mmol/L)
Total cholesterol	215 mg/dL (5.6 mmol/L)
Triglycerides	267 mg/dL (3.0 mmol/L)
HDL	60 mg/dL (1.56 mmol/L)
LDL	116 mg/dL (3.0 mmol/L)
HbA_{1C}	5.9%

1. What is BMI? Calculate A.M.'s BMI and identify her classification based on the results.

2. Does A.M. have type 2 diabetes mellitus? Explain your answer.

A.M.'s urinalysis is clear, and upon examination she is diagnosed with a vaginal yeast infection. The health care provider discusses A.M.'s condition with her and tells her that in addition to the yeast infection, she has metabolic syndrome and reviews some treatment goals with her. In addition, the HCP reinforces the need for A.M. to take her blood pressure medication regularly. A.M. is visibly upset and has many questions.

3. What is metabolic syndrome?

4. Review A.M.'s history and assessment. What criteria for metabolic syndrome does A.M. have, if any?

5. What other lifestyle habits will you ask A.M. about during your assessment?

6. What health problems may result if metabolic syndrome remains untreated? Select all that apply.
   a. Stroke
   b. Diabetes
   c. Breast cancer
   d. Heart disease
   e. Renal disease

A.M. is given the following prescriptions:
   Metformin (Glucophage), 500 mg BID
   Atorvastatin (Lipitor), 10 mg PO at bedtime
   Lisinopril (Zestril) 5 mg PO, 1 tablet every morning
   Fluconazole (Diflucan) 150 mg tablet × 1 dose

7. Explain the purpose of each medication ordered.

8. Which are potential side effects of metformin? Select all that apply.
   a. Nausea
   b. Diarrhea
   c. Dizziness
   d. Constipation
   e. Abdominal bloating

CASE STUDY PROGRESS

You take the time to talk to A.M. about her concerns and provide health promotion teaching that includes increasing regular physical activity, weight reduction, and eating a diet low in saturated fats. A.M. tells you she is willing to make changes but that this is a lot of information to take in at this time.

9. She asks, "Why do I have to take a drug for diabetes if I don't have diabetes?" What is the **appropriate** answer?
   a. "Metformin will prevent you from ever developing diabetes."
   b. "Metformin provides the insulin your body is no longer making."
   c. "Metformin allows you to eat whatever you want and your glucose levels won't increase."
   d. "Metformin helps your cells to be less resistant to insulin, and, as a result, your glucose levels will decrease."

10. Explain the role of insulin resistance with metabolic syndrome and metformin's effect on insulin resistance.

11. Is A.M. at greater risk for coronary artery disease? Explain your answer.

12. A.M. asks you, "Won't all these pills help me? Why do I need to change how I eat and exercise?" Explain the role of reducing risk factors as part of the treatment for metabolic syndrome.

13. After visiting with the dietitian, you review what A.M. has learned. You ask her to tell you what food choices would be good for a low-fat diet. Which answer reflects a need for further education?
    a. "I will eat more fruits and vegetables."
    b. "I will try to eat more chicken and fish."
    c. "I can eat red meat as long as I don't fry it."
    d. "I will eat more whole grains, such as whole wheat bread."

A.M. is referred to a registered dietitian for nutrition education and decides to join the local YMCA for exercise. You teach her how to monitor blood glucose levels at home. She has an appointment to return to the clinic in one month. However, A.M. does not return to the clinic for her appointment. When you call to follow up with her, she agrees to come in a week later. At that time, she tells you that she did not do well with the exercise because it "hurts too much." She said she tried eating a low-fat diet but that it was difficult to stick to it. She did not check her blood glucose regularly, but told you that when she did check them, her fasting levels were in the "140s to 160s." Her weight is now 250 lbs (113 kg). She tells you that she feels so discouraged and that she will "never get better."

14. What resources do you suggest for A.M. at this time?

During the next year, A.M. continued to miss appointments, and her weight increased to 272 lbs (123 kg). She was eventually diagnosed with type 2 diabetes mellitus, and at her last visit she asked her HCP about having weight loss surgery.

Case Study 4

Name _____ Class/Group _____ Date _____

▶ Scenario

You are working in the internal medicine clinic of a large teaching hospital. Today your first patient is 70-year-old J.M., a man who has been coming to the clinic for several years for management of coronary artery disease (CAD) and hypertension (HTN). A cardiac catheterization done a year ago showed 50% stenosis of the circumflex coronary artery. He has had episodes of dizziness for the past 6 months and orthostatic hypotension, shoulder discomfort, and decreased exercise tolerance for the past 2 months. On his last clinic visit 3 weeks ago, a chest x-ray (CXR) examination revealed cardiomegaly and a 12-lead electrocardiogram (ECG) showed sinus tachycardia with left bundle branch block. You review J.M.'s morning blood work and initial assessment.

Chart View

Laboratory Results

Chemistry

Sodium	142 mEq/L (142 mmol/L)
Chloride	95 mEq/L (95 mmol/L)
Potassium	3.9 mEq/L (3.9 mmol/L)
Creatinine	0.8 mg/dL (70.7 mcmol/L)
Glucose	82 mg/dL (4.6 mmol/L)
BUN	19 mg/dL (6.8 mmol/L)

Complete Blood Count

WBC	5400/mm^3 (5.4 x 10^9/L)
Hgb	11.5 g/dL (115 g/L)
Hct	37%
Platelets	229,000/mm^3 (229 x 10^9/L)

Initial Assessment

J.M. reports increased fatigue and shortness of breath, especially with activity, and "waking up gasping for breath" at night, for the past 2 days.

Vital Signs

Temperature	97.9° F (36.6° C)
Blood pressure	142/83
Heart rate	105
Respiratory rate	18

1. As you review these results, which ones are of possible concern, and why?

2. Knowing his history and seeing his condition this morning, what further questions are you going to ask J.M. and his daughter?

CASE STUDY PROGRESS

J.M. tells you he becomes exhausted and has shortness of breath climbing the stairs to his bedroom and must lie down and rest ("put my feet up") at least an hour twice a day. He has been sleeping on 2 pillows for the past 2 weeks. He has not salted his food since the provider told him not to because of his high blood pressure, but he admits having had ham and a small bag of salted peanuts 3 days ago. He states that he stopped smoking 10 years ago. He denies having palpitations but has had a constant, irritating, nonproductive cough lately.

3. You think it's likely that J.M. has heart failure (HF). From his history, what do you identify as probable causes for his HF?

4. You are now ready to do your physical assessment. For each potential assessment finding for HF, indicate whether the finding indicates left-sided HF (L) or right-sided HF (R).
   1. Weakness
   2. Jugular (neck) vein distention
   3. Dependent edema (legs and sacrum)
   4. Hacking cough, worse at night
   5. Enlarged liver and spleen
   6. Exertional dyspnea
   7. Distended abdomen
   8. Weight gain
   9. S_3/S_4 gallop
   10. Crackles and wheezes in lungs

Chart View

Medication Orders

Enalapril (Vasotec) 10 mg PO twice a day
Furosemide (Lasix) 20 mg PO every morning
Carvedilol (Coreg) 6.25 mg PO twice a day
Digoxin (Lanoxin) 0.5 mg PO now, then 0.125 mg PO daily
Potassium chloride (K-Dur) 10 mEq tablet PO once a day

CASE STUDY PROGRESS

The provider confirms your suspicions and indicates that J.M. is experiencing symptoms of early left-sided heart failure. A two-dimensional (2D) echocardiogram is ordered. Medication orders are written.

5. For each medication listed, identify its class and describe its purpose in treating HF.

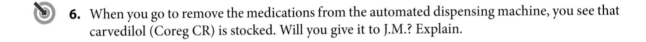

6. When you go to remove the medications from the automated dispensing machine, you see that carvedilol (Coreg CR) is stocked. Will you give it to J.M.? Explain.

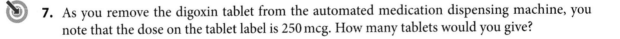

7. As you remove the digoxin tablet from the automated medication dispensing machine, you note that the dose on the tablet label is 250 mcg. How many tablets would you give?

8. Based on the new medication orders, which blood test or tests should be monitored carefully? Explain your answer.

9. When you give J.M. his medications, he looks at the potassium tablet, wrinkles his nose, and tells you he "hates those horse pills." He tells you a friend of his said he could eat bananas instead. He says he would rather eat a banana every day than take one of those pills. How will you respond?

10. The 2D echocardiogram shows that J.M.'s left ventricular ejection fraction (EF) is 49%. Explain what this test result means with regard to J.M.'s heart function.

CASE STUDY PROGRESS

This is J.M.'s first episode of significant HF. Before he leaves the clinic, you want to teach him about life-style modifications he can make and monitoring techniques he can use to prevent or minimize future problems.

11. List 5 suggestions you might make and the rationale for each.

12. You tell J.M. that the combination of high-sodium foods he had during the past several days might have contributed to his present episode of HF. He looks surprised. J.M. says, "But I didn't add any salt to them!" To what health care professional could J.M. be referred to help him understand how to prevent future crises? State your rationale.

13. After visiting with the cardiac dietitian, you review potential food choices with J.M. Which foods are high in sodium and must be avoided? Select all that apply.
   a. Canned soups
   b. Cheddar cheese
   c. Processed meats
   d. Whole wheat bread
   e. Fat-free fruit yogurt

14. You also include teaching about digoxin toxicity. When teaching J.M. about the signs and symptoms of digoxin toxicity, which should be included? Select all that apply.
a. Diarrhea
b. Visual changes
c. Increased urine output
d. Loss of appetite or nausea
e. Dizziness when standing up

CASE STUDY OUTCOME

J.M.'s condition improves after 5 days of treatment, and he is discharged to home. He has a follow-up appointment with a cardiologist in 2 weeks. He is enrolled in the clinic's STOP Heart Failure program, and a heart failure nurse navigator will contact him in a few days to check his progress.

Case Study **5**

Name _____ Class/Group _____ Date _____

▶ Scenario

It is midmorning on the cardiac unit where you work, and you are getting a new patient. G.P. is a 60-year-old retired businessman who is married and has 3 grown children. As you take his health history, he tells you that he began feeling changes in his chest about 10 days ago. He has hypertension (HTN) and a 3-year history of angina pectoris. During the past week, he has had frequent episodes of mid-chest discomfort. The chest pain responds to nitroglycerin (NTG), which he has taken sublingually about 8 to 10 times over the past week. During the week, he has also experienced increased fatigue. He states, "I just feel crappy all the time." A cardiac catheterization done several years ago revealed 50% stenosis of the right coronary artery and 50% stenosis of the left anterior descending coronary artery. He tells you that both his mother and his father had coronary artery disease (CAD). He is currently taking amlodipine (Norvasc), metoprolol (Lopressor), atorvastatin (Lipitor), and aspirin 81 mg/day. He is retired and says that he spends his days watching television, with some occasional yard work. He has gained 25 lb (11.3 kg) since retiring and admits that he is overweight.

1. What other information are you going to obtain about his episodes of chest pain?

2. What are common sites for radiation of ischemic cardiac pain?

3. There are several risk factors for coronary artery disease. For each risk factor listed, mark whether it is "M" modifiable or "N" nonmodifiable.
   a. ____ Age
   b. ____ Stress
   c. ____ Gender
   d. ____ Obesity
   e. ____ Smoking
   f. ____ Hypertension
   g. ____ Hyperlipidemia
   h. ____ Diabetes mellitus
   i. ____ Physical inactivity
   j. ____ Ethnic background
   k. ____ Excessive alcohol use
   l. ____ Family history of CAD

4. Based on the history you have so far, circle the modifiable and nonmodifiable risk factors in Question 3 that apply to G.P.

5. Although he has had a prescription for sublingual nitroglycerin (SL NTG) for a long time, you want to be certain he is using it correctly. Which actions are correct when taking SL NTG for chest pain? Select all that apply.
   a. Call 911 immediately.
   b. Stop the activity and lie or sit down.
   c. Chew the tablet slowly then swallow.
   d. Place the NTG tablet under the tongue.
   e. Call 911 if the pain is not relieved after taking 1 SL tablet.
   f. Call 911 if the pain is not relieved after taking 3 SL tablets, 5 minutes apart.

6. You review the use and storage of SL NTG with G.P. Which statement by G.P. indicates a need for further education? Explain your answer.
   a. "I carry the tablets with me at all times."
   b. "I will keep the pills in their original brown bottle."
   c. "I will not store other pills in the nitroglycerin bottle."
   d. "I will discard any open bottle of nitroglycerin after a year."

CASE STUDY PROGRESS

When you first admit G.P., you place him on telemetry and observe his cardiac rhythm.

7. Identify the rhythm:

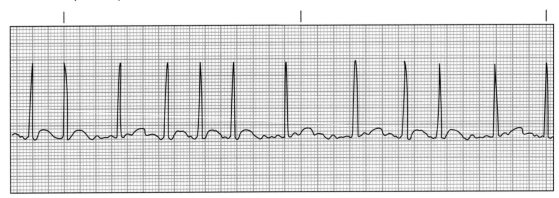

(From Ignatavicius DD, Workman ML. Medical-Surgical Nursing, ed. 6, St. Louis, MO: Saunders; 2010.)

8. Explain the primary complication that could occur if this heart rhythm were not treated.

9. Review G.P.'s history. What conditions may have contributed to the development of this dysrhythmia?

10. You review G.P.'s lab test results and note that all of them are within normal range, including troponin and creatinine phosphokinase levels. His potassium level is 4.7 mEq/L (4.7 mmol/L). Given this and his current dysrhythmia, what is the likely cause of the symptoms he has been experiencing this past week?

CASE STUDY PROGRESS

Within the hour, G.P. converts with intravenous diltiazem (Cardizem) to sick sinus syndrome with long sinus pauses that cause lightheadedness and hypotension.

11. What risks does the new rhythm pose for G.P.? Explain the reasons for your answers.

CASE STUDY PROGRESS

Because G.P.'s dysrhythmia is causing unacceptable symptoms, he is taken to surgery and a permanent DDDR pacemaker is placed and set at a rate of 70.

12. What does the code *DDDR* mean?

13. What is the purpose of DDDR pacing?

14. The pacemaker insertion surgery places G.P. at risk for several serious complications. List 3 potential problems you would monitor for as you care for him.

15. G.P. will need some education regarding his new pacemaker. What information will you give him before he leaves the hospital?

16. G.P. and his wife tell you they have heard that people with pacemakers can have their hearts stop because of microwave ovens and cell phones. Where can you help them find more information?

CASE STUDY PROGRESS

After discharge, G.P. is referred to a cardiac rehabilitation center to start an exercise program. He will be exercise tested, and an individualized exercise prescription will be developed for him, based on the results of the exercise test.

17. What information will be obtained from a graded exercise (stress) test?

18. What is included in an exercise prescription?

CASE STUDY OUTCOME

G.P. returns in 1 month for a pacemaker check. He reports that he and his wife go for a walk at least 3 times a week at the mall, and he is hoping to start volunteering soon. He has lost 8 lbs (3.6 kg).

Case Study **6**

Name _____ Class/Group _____ Date _____

▶ Scenario

S.P. is a 68-year-old retired painter who is experiencing right leg calf pain. The pain began approximately 2 years ago but has become significantly worse in the past 4 months. The pain is precipitated by exercise and is relieved with rest. Two years ago, S.P. could walk 2 city blocks before having to stop because of leg pain. Today, he can barely walk across the yard. S.P. has smoked 2 to 3 packs of cigarettes per day (PPD) for the past 45 years. He has a history of coronary artery disease (CAD), hypertension (HTN), peripheral artery disease (PAD), and osteoarthritis. Surgical history includes quadruple coronary artery bypass graft 3 years ago. He has had no further symptoms of cardiopulmonary disease since that time, even though he has not been compliant with the exercise regimen his cardiologist prescribed, continues to eat anything he wants, and continues to smoke 2 to 3 PPD. Other surgical history includes open reduction and internal fixation of a right femoral fracture 20 years ago.

S.P. is in the clinic today for a routine semiannual follow-up appointment with his primary care provider. As you take his vital signs, he tells you that in addition to the calf pain, he is experiencing right hip pain that gets worse with exercise, the pain does not go away promptly with rest, some days are worse than others, and his condition is not affected by a resting position.

Chart View

General Assessment

Weight	261 lb (118.4 kg)
Height	5 ft, 10 in (178 cm)
BP	163/91
Pulse	82
Respiratory rate	16
Temperature	98.4° F (36.9° C)

Laboratory Testing (Fasting)

Cholesterol	239 mg/dL (6.2 mmol/L)
Triglycerides	150 mg/dL (1.69 mmol/L)
HDL	28 mg/dL (0.73 mmol/L)
LDL	181 mg/dL (4.69 mmol/L)

Current Medications

Ramipril (Altace)	10 mg daily
Metoprolol (Lopressor)	25 mg twice a day
Aspirin	81 mg daily
Atorvastatin (Lipitor)	20 mg daily

1. What are the likely sources of his calf pain and hip pain?

2. S.P. has several risk factors for PAD. From his history, list 2 risk factors, and explain the reason they are risk factors.

3. You decide to look at S.P.'s lower extremities. What signs do you expect to find with PAD? Select all that apply.
   a. Ankle edema
   b. Thick, brittle nails
   c. Cool or cold extremity
   d. Thin, shiny, and taut skin
   e. Brown discoloration of the skin
   f. Decreased or absent pedal pulses

4. You ask further questions about the clinical manifestations of PAD. Which of these would you expect S.P. to have, given the diagnosis of PAD? Select all that apply.
   a. Paresthesia
   b. Elevation pallor
   c. Dependent rubor
   d. Rest pain at night
   e. Pruritus of the lower legs
   f. Constant, dull ache in his calf or thigh

5. What is the purpose of the daily aspirin listed in S.P.'s current medication?

CASE STUDY PROGRESS

S.P.'s primary care provider has seen him and wants you to schedule him for an ankle-brachial index (ABI) test to determine the presence of arterial blood flow obstruction. You confirm the time and date of the procedure and then call S.P. at home.

6. What will you tell S.P. to do to prepare for the tests?

CASE STUDY PROGRESS

S.P.'s ABI results showed 0.43 right (R) leg and 0.59 left (L) leg. His primary care provider discusses these results with him and decides to wait 2 months to see whether his symptoms improve with drug changes and risk factor modification before deciding about surgical intervention. S.P. receives a prescription for clopidogrel (Plavix) 75 mg daily and is told to discontinue the daily aspirin. In addition, S.P. receives a consultation for physical therapy.

7. What do these ABI results indicate?

8. You counsel S.P. on risk factor modification. What would you address, and why?

9. You provide teaching on proper care of his feet and lower extremities, then use "teach-back" to assess S.P.'s learning. Which statements by S.P. indicate a need for further instruction? Select all that apply.
   a. "I can go barefoot in the house, but not outside."
   b. "I will wear shoes that are roomy and protective."
   c. "I will avoid exposing my feet to extremes of heat and cold."
   d. "I will soak my feet in water once a day to make sure they are clean."
   e. "I will put lotion on my feet and lower legs, but not in between the toes."

10. How will the physical therapy help?

11. In addition to risk factor modification, what other measures to improve tissue perfusion or prevent skin damage should you recommend to S.P.?

12. S.P. tells you his neighbor told him to keep his legs elevated higher than his heart and asks for compression stockings to keep swelling down in his legs. How should you respond?

 13. S.P. has been on aspirin therapy but now will be taking clopidogrel instead. What is the most important aspect of patient teaching that you will emphasize with this drug?

CASE STUDY OUTCOME

S.P. asks for nicotine patches to assist with smoking cessation and makes an appointment for a physical therapy evaluation and a nutritional assessment. He assures you he does not want to lose his leg and will be more careful in the future.

Case Study **7**

Name _____ Class/Group _____ Date _____

▶ Scenario

You are the nurse working in an anticoagulation clinic. One of your patients is K.N., who has a long-standing history of an irregular heartbeat, known as *atrial fibrillation* or *A-fib,* for which he takes the oral anticoagulant warfarin (Coumadin). Recently K.N. had his mitral heart valve replaced with a mechanical valve.

1. How does atrial fibrillation differ from a normal heart rhythm?

2. What is the purpose of the warfarin (Coumadin) in K.N.'s case?

CASE STUDY PROGRESS

K.N. calls your anticoagulation clinic to report a nosebleed that is hard to stop. You ask him to come into the office to check his coagulation levels. The lab technician draws a PT/INR test.

3. What is a PT/INR test, and what are the expected levels for K.N.? What is the purpose of the INR?

4. When you get the results, his INR is critical at 7.2. What is the danger of this INR level?

CASE STUDY PROGRESS

The health care provider does a brief focused history and physical examination, orders additional lab tests, and determines there are no signs of bleeding other than the nosebleed, which has stopped. The provider discovers that K.N. recently started to take daily doses of an over-the-counter proton pump inhibitor (PPI), omeprazole (Prilosec OTC), for heartburn.

5. What happened when K.N. began taking the PPI?

6. What should K.N. have done to prevent this problem?

7. The provider gives K.N. a low dose of vitamin K orally, asks him to hold his warfarin dose that evening, and asks him to come back tomorrow for another prothrombin time (PT) and INR blood draw. Why is K.N. instructed to take the vitamin K?

8. You want to make certain K.N. knows what "hold the next dose" means. What should you tell him?

9. K.N. asks you why his PT/INR has to be checked so soon. How will you respond?

CASE STUDY PROGRESS

K.N.'s INR the next day is 3.7, and the health care provider makes no further medication changes. K.N. is instructed to return again in 7 days to have another PT/INR drawn.

10. Why should the INR be checked again so soon instead of the usual monthly follow-up?

11. K.N. grumbles about all of the lab tests but agrees to follow through. You provide patient education to K.N. and start with reviewing the signs and symptoms (S/S) of bleeding. What are potential S/S of bleeding that should be taught to K.N.? Select all that apply.
   a. Insomnia
   b. Black, tarry stool
   c. New onset of dizziness
   d. Stool that is pale in color
   e. New joint pain or swelling
   f. Unexplained abdominal pain

12. Identify 2 other patient education needs you will stress at this time.

13. K.N. tells you that he has had a lot of pain in his knee and wants to take ibuprofen (Advil) because it is an over-the-counter product. How do you reply to his request?

14. Four months later, K.N. informs you that he is going to have a knee replacement next month. What will you do with this information?

CASE STUDY PROGRESS

You know that sometimes the only needed action is to stop the warfarin (Coumadin) several days before the surgery. Other times, the provider initiates "bridging therapy," or stops the warfarin and provides anti-coagulation protection by initiating low-molecular-weight heparin. After reviewing all of his anticoagulation information, the provider decides that K.N. will need to stop the warfarin (Coumadin) 1 week before the surgery and in its place be started on enoxaparin (Lovenox) therapy.

15. Compare the duration of action of warfarin (Coumadin) and enoxaparin (Lovenox) and explain the reason the provider switched to enoxaparin at this time.

CASE STUDY PROGRESS

K.N. is in the office and ready for his first enoxaparin (Lovenox) injection.

16. Which nursing interventions are appropriate when administering enoxaparin? Select all that apply.
a. Massage the area after the injection has been given.
b. Hold extra pressure over the site after the injection.
c. Monitor activated partial thromboplastin time (aPTT) levels.
d. The preferred site of injection is the lateral abdominal fatty tissue.
e. Administer via intramuscular (IM) injection into the deltoid muscle.

CASE STUDY PROGRESS

K.N. undergoes knee surgery without complications. Just before his discharge, his physician reviews the instructions and gives him a new prescription for warfarin (Coumadin). K.N. tells his doctor, "I saw this commercial for a new blood thinner called Xarelto. I'd like to take that instead because I wouldn't need to have all this blood work done."

17. How do you expect the physician to respond?

CASE STUDY OUTCOME

K.N. is discharged to a rehabilitation facility, where he makes a quick recovery from the knee replacement surgery. He does not experience any thrombotic events or bleeding episodes during his recovery.

Case Study **8**

Name _____ Class/Group _____ Date _____

▶ Scenario

You are assigned to care for L.J., a 70-year-old retired bus driver who has just been admitted to your medical floor with right leg deep vein thrombosis (DVT). L.J. has a 48–pack-year smoking history, although he states he quit 2 years ago. He has had pneumonia several times and frequent episodes of atrial flutter or fibrillation. He has had 2 previous episodes of DVT and was diagnosed with rheumatoid arthritis 3 years ago. Two months ago he began experiencing shortness of breath on exertion and noticed increasing swelling of his right lower leg that became progressively worse until it extended up to his groin. His wife brought him to the hospital when the pain in his leg became increasingly severe. After a Doppler study showed a probable thrombus of the external iliac vein extending distally to the lower leg, he was admitted for bed rest and to initiate heparin therapy. His basic metabolic panel was normal; other lab results were as follows.

Chart View

Laboratory Testing	
PT	12.4 seconds
INR	1.11
aPTT	25 seconds
Hgb	13.3 g/dL (133 g/L)
Hct	38.9%
Cholesterol	206 mg/dL (5.34 mmol/L)

1. List 6 risk factors for DVT.

2. Identify at least 5 risk factors from L.J.'s history.

3. Something is missing from the scenario. Based on his history, L.J. should have been taking an important medication. What is it, and why should he be taking it?

4. Keeping in mind L.J.'s health history and admitting diagnosis, outline the most important assessments you will make during your physical examination.

5. What is the most serious complication of DVT?

6. List at least 8 assessment findings you should monitor closely for in the development of the complication identified in Question 5.

7. You review the literature for DVT and see the abbreviation *VTE*. What does VTE mean?

CASE STUDY PROGRESS

Your assessment of L.J. reveals bibasilar crackles with moist cough, normal heart sounds, BP 138/88, pulse 104, 4+ pitting edema of right lower extremity, mild erythema of right foot and calf, and severe right calf pain. He is awake, alert, and oriented but a little restless. His Spo_2 is 92% on room air. He denies chest pain but does have shortness of breath with exertion. He states he is anxious about missing his grandson's wedding. He denies any voiding problems.

8. Your institution uses electronic charting. Based on the assessment noted previously, which of the following systems would you mark as "abnormal" as you document your findings? For abnormal findings provide a brief narrative note.

☐ Neurologic:

☐ Respiratory:

☐ Cardiovascular:

☐ Genitourinary:

☐ Skin:

☐ Psychosocial:

☐ Pain:

CASE STUDY PROGRESS

L.J. is placed on 72-hour bed rest with bathroom privileges and given acetaminophen (Tylenol) for pain. The physician writes orders for enoxaparin (Lovenox) injections.

9. L.J. asks, "Why do I have to get these shots? Why can't I just get a Coumadin pill to thin my blood?" What would be your response?" Explain your answer.
a. "Your physician prefers the injections over the pills."
b. "The enoxaparin will work to dissolve the blood clot in your leg."
c. "It would take the Coumadin pills several days to become effective."
d. "Good idea! I will call and ask your physician to switch medications."

 10. The order for the enoxaparin reads: Enoxaparin 70 mg every 12 hours subQ. L.J. is 5 ft, 6 in tall and weighs 156 lb. Is this dose appropriate?

11. What special techniques do you use when giving the subcutaneous injection of enoxaparin? Select all that apply.
a. Rotate injection sites.
b. Give the injection near the umbilicus.
c. Massage the injection site gently after the injection is given.
d. After inserting the needle, do not aspirate before giving the injection.
e. Expel the bubble from the prefilled syringe before giving the injection.

12. True or False? Enoxaparin dosage is directed by monitoring aPTT levels. Explain your answer.

13. L.J. asks you how long it will take for the Lovenox injections to dissolve his blood clot. What is your response to him?

14. After providing teaching about anticoagulant therapy, you ask L.J. to teach back to you what he has learned. Which statements indicate a need for further education? Select all that apply.
a. "I will not blow my nose really hard."
b. "I will brush my teeth gently with a soft toothbrush."
c. "I will take aspirin or ibuprofen if I have a headache."
d. "I will shave very carefully with my disposable razor."
e. "I will put lotion on my skin to keep it from getting to dry."
f. "I will purchase and wear a medical alert necklace for blood thinners."
g. "I will get help right away if I notice bleeding in my stools or urine or if I have a bad headache or stomach pain."

15. You identify pain as a key issue in the care of L.J. List 4 interventions you will choose for L.J. to address his pain.

16. What pertinent lab values and measurements would you expect the physician to order and the results of which you will monitor? Explain the reason for each test.

17. You evaluate L.J.'s electrocardiogram (ECG) strip. Name this rhythm, and explain what consequences it could have for L.J.

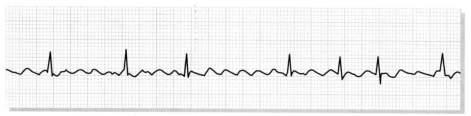

(Modified from Lilley LL, Rainforth Collins S, Harrington S, et al: Pharmacology and the Nursing Process, *ed. 8, St. Louis, MO: Mosby; 2017.)*

CASE STUDY PROGRESS

A week has passed. L.J. responded to heparin therapy and was bridged to oral warfarin therapy. His heart dysrhythmia converted to sinus rhythm after he started taking cardiac medications, and he is being discharged to home with home care follow-up. "Good," he says, "just in time to fly out west for my grandson's wedding. His wife, who has come to pick him up, rolls her eyes and looks at the ceiling.

18. Although you are surprised at his comment, you realize he is serious about going to the wedding. What are you going to tell him?

19. What discharge instructions about activity will you give L.J.?

CASE STUDY OUTCOME

L.J. listens to you, and his wife is quite relieved. They were able to watch the wedding ceremony via a live-stream connection, and he watches the recording daily and points out his favorite parts to the home care nurse every time she visits.

Case Study 9

Name _____ Class/Group _____ Date _____

▶ Scenario

You are working at the local cardiac rehabilitation center, and R.M. is walking around the track. He summons you and asks if you could help him understand his recent lab report. He admits to being confused by the overwhelming data on the test and does not understand how the results relate to his recent heart attack and need for a stent. You take a moment to locate his lab reports and review his history. The findings are as follows.

R.M. is an active 61-year-old married man who works full time for the postal service. He spends most of his day in a mail truck, and admits he does not eat a "perfect diet." He enjoys 2 or 3 beers every night, uses stick margarine, eats red meat 2 or 3 times per week, and is a self-professed "sweet eater." He has tried to quit smoking and is down to 1 pack per day. Cardiac history includes a recent inferior myocardial infarction (MI) and a heart catheterization revealing three-vessel disease: in the left anterior descending (LAD) coronary artery, a proximal 60% lesion; in the right coronary artery (RCA), proximal 100% occlusion with thrombus; and a circumflex artery with 40% to 60% diffuse dilated lesions. A stent was deployed to the RCA and reduced the lesion to 0% residual stenosis. He has had no need for sublingual nitroglycerin (NTG). He was discharged on enteric-coated aspirin 325 mg daily, clopidogrel (Plavix) 75 mg daily, atorvastatin (Lipitor) 10 mg at bedtime, and ramipril (Altace) 10 mg/day. Six weeks after his MI and stent placement, he had a fasting advanced lipid profile with other blood work.

Chart View

Six-Week Postprocedure Laboratory Work (Fasting)

Total cholesterol	188 mg/dL (4.87 mmol/L)
HDL	34 mg/dL (0.88 mmol/L)
LDL	98 mg/dL (2.54 mmol/L)
Triglycerides	176 mg/dL (1.99 mmol/L)
Homocysteine	18 mmol/L
C-reactive protein (CRP)	8 mg/dL (80 mg/L)
FBG	99 mg/dL (5.5 mmol/L)
TSH	1.04 mU/L

1. When you start to discuss R.M.'s lab values with him, he is pleased about his results. "My cholesterol level is below 200!—and my 'bad cholesterol' is good! That's good news, right?" What would you say to him?

2. Which lab test is considered the "good cholesterol," and why?

3. Discuss the significance of R.M.'s CRP level.

4. Discuss the significance of the homocysteine test and R.M.'s results.

5. What else in R.M.'s history might be contributing to his elevated homocysteine levels?

6. Identify R.M.'s health-related problems. List the problem that is potentially life-threatening first.

CASE STUDY PROGRESS

7. R.M.'s physician adds niacin, a vitamin preparation (folic acid, vitamin B_6, and vitamin B_{12} [Foltx]) daily with food, and omega-3 fatty acids to his list of medications. How do these medications affect lipids? R.M. states, "But I already take Lipitor. What do all these medications do?" How do you answer him?

8. You are teaching R.M. about the side effects of niacin. Which effects will you include in your teaching? Select all that apply.
   a. Pruritus
   b. Dizziness
   c. Headache
   d. Flushed skin
   e. Gastrointestinal distress

9. R.M. tells you that he really does not want to "put up with" the side effects of the niacin. Is there an alternative to niacin?

10. You review his other medications, including atorvastatin (Lipitor). Which statement by R.M. indicates a need for further teaching about atorvastatin?
    a. "I will take this drug at night."
    b. "I will try to exercise more each week."
    c. "I like to take my medicines with grapefruit juice."
    d. "I will call my doctor right away if I experience muscle pain."

CASE STUDY PROGRESS

You enter R.M.'s room and hear the physician say, "There are many options for changing your LDL and triglyceride levels. You need to continue modifying your diet and exercise to enhance your medication regimen. And stop smoking!" The physician asks R.M. whether he has any questions, and he responds, "No."

11. After the physician leaves the room, R.M. tells you he really did not understand what the physician said. Explain the need for lifestyle changes to R.M.

12. You review the DASH diet with R.M. and his wife. Which food choices would follow the DASH diet? Select all that apply.
    a. Fish and chips
    b. Fresh fruit salad
    c. Apples fried in butter and brown sugar
    d. Fat-free yogurt with tablespoon of almonds
    e. Grilled chicken sandwich on whole wheat bun

13. R.M. tells you that he knows exercise will help him to lose weight, which is good, but he does not understand how exercise helps his cholesterol levels. How do you answer him?

 14. Of all of R.M.'s behaviors, which one is the most significant in promoting cardiac disease and why?

15. Develop a comprehensive teaching plan directed toward helping R.M. with addressing this behavior.

CASE STUDY OUTCOME

R.M. tells you that he is determined to stop smoking. At his next checkup 3 months later, he proudly shows off his 15 lb (6.8 kg) weight loss and tells you that he has not had a cigarette for 10 weeks.

Case Study 10

Name _____ Class/Group _____ Date _____

▶ Scenario

The wife of C.W., a 70-year-old man, brought him to the emergency department (ED) at 0430. She told the ED triage nurse that he had diarrhea for the past 2 days and that last night he had a lot of "dark red" diarrhea. When he became very dizzy, disoriented, and weak this morning, she decided to bring him to the hospital. C.W.'s vital signs (VS) in the ED were 70/– (systolic blood pressure [SBP] 70, diastolic blood pressure [DBP] inaudible), pulse rate 110, respirations 22, oral temperature 99.1° F (37.3° C). A 16-gauge IV catheter was inserted and a lactated Ringer's infusion was started. The triage nurse learned C.W. has had idiopathic dilated cardiomyopathy for several years. The onset was insidious, but the cardiomyopathy is now severe. His last cardiac catheterization showed an ejection fraction of 13%. He has frequent problems with heart failure (HF) because of the cardiomyopathy. Two years ago, he had a cardiac arrest that was attributed to hypokalemia. He has a long history of hypertension and arthritis. He had atrial fibrillation in the past, but it has been under control recently. Fifteen years ago he had a peptic ulcer.

Endoscopy showed a 25- × 15-mm duodenal ulcer with adherent clot. The ulcer was cauterized, and C.W. was admitted to the medical intensive care unit (MICU) for treatment of his volume deficit. You are his admitting nurse. As you are making him comfortable, Mrs. W. gives you a paper sack filled with the bottles of medications he has been taking: enalapril (Vasotec) 5 mg PO bid, warfarin (Coumadin) 5 mg/day PO, digoxin (Lanoxin) 0.125 mg/day PO, potassium chloride 20 mEq PO bid, and diclofenac (Voltaren) 50 mg PO tid. As you connect him to the cardiac monitor, you note he is in sinus tachycardia. Doing a quick assessment, you find a pale man who is sleepy but arousable and slightly disoriented. He states he is still dizzy and feels weak and anxious overall. His BP is 98/52, pulse is 118, and respiratory rate 26. You hear S_3 and S_4 heart sounds and a grade II/VI systolic murmur. Peripheral pulses are all 2+, and trace pedal edema is present. Capillary refill is slightly prolonged. Lungs are clear. Bowel sounds are present, mid-epigastric tenderness is noted, and the liver margin is 4 cm below the costal margin. Has not yet voided since admission. Rates his pain level as "2." A Swan-Ganz pulmonary artery catheter and a peripheral arterial line are inserted.

1. What may have precipitated C.W.'s gastrointestinal (GI) bleeding?

2. From his history and assessment, identify 5 signs and symptoms of GI bleeding and loss of blood volume, and explain the pathophysiology for each one listed.

3. What is the most serious potential complication of C.W.'s bleeding?

4. Your institution uses electronic charting. Based on the assessment just described, which of the following systems would you mark as "abnormal" as you document your findings? Mark abnormal findings with an X and provide a brief narrative note.
☐ Neurologic:

☐ Respiratory:

☐ Cardiovascular:

☐ GI:

☐ Genitourinary:

☐ Musculoskeletal:

☐ Skin:

☐ Psychosocial:

☐ Pain:

5. What intervention is required to assess his renal function?

6. Calculate C.W.'s mean arterial pressure (MAP) and explain why this measure is important.

CASE STUDY PROGRESS

As soon as you get a chance, you review C.W.'s admission lab results.

Chart View

Laboratory Results

Sodium	138 mEq/L (138 mmol/L)
Potassium	6.9 mEq/L (6.9 mmol/L)
BUN	90 mg/dL (32.1 mmol/L)
Creatinine	2.1 mg/dL (185.6 mcmol/L)
WBC	16,000/mm³ (16 x 10⁹/L)
Hgb	8.4 g/dL (84 g/L)
Hct	25%
PT	23.4 seconds
INR	4.8

7. After examination of the lab results, do you have any concerns with C.W.'s electrolyte levels? Explain your answer.

8. In view of the previous lab results, what diagnostic test will be performed and why?

9. Evaluate this electrocardiogram (ECG) strip and note the effect of any electrolyte imbalances.

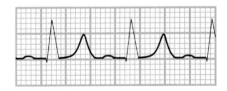

10. Why do you think the BUN and creatinine are elevated?

11. What do the low Hgb and Hct levels indicate about the rapidity of C.W.'s blood loss?

12. What is the explanation for the prolonged PT/INR?

13. What will be your response to the prolonged PT/INR? Select all that apply.
  a. Hold the warfarin dose.
  b. Avoid injections as much as possible.
  c. Obtain an order for aspirin if needed for pain.
  d. Monitor C.W. for signs and symptoms of bleeding.
  e. Prepare to administer a STAT dose of protamine sulfate.

 14. What safety precautions should you initiate in light of his prolonged PT and INR?

15. How do you explain the elevated WBC count?

CASE STUDY PROGRESS

C.W. receives a total of 4 units of packed red blood cells (PRBCs), 5 units of fresh frozen plasma (FFP), and several liters of crystalloids to keep his mean BP above 60. On the second day in the MICU, his total fluid intake is 8.498 L and output is 3.66 L. His hemodynamic parameters after fluid resuscitation are pulmonary capillary wedge pressure (PCWP) 30 mm Hg and cardiac output (CO) 4.5 L/min.

16. Calculate his fluid balance and identify whether it is positive or negative.

17. Why will you want to monitor his fluid status very carefully?

18. List at least 6 things you will monitor to assess C.W.'s fluid balance.

19. Explain the purpose of the FFP for C.W.

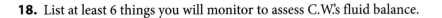 **CASE STUDY PROGRESS**

Mrs. W. has been with her husband since he arrived at the emergency department and is worried about his condition and his care.

20. List 5 things you might do to make her more comfortable while her husband is in the MICU.

CASE STUDY OUTCOME

After the transfusions, C.W.'s BP is 110/78, his pulse is 94, and his respirations are 18. His urine output is now 60 mL/hour. He seems more alert and asks you, "What happened?" He is transferred to a step-down unit the next day and is eventually transferred to a rehabilitation facility for a week of physical therapy before returning home.

Case Study **11**

Name _____ Class/Group _____ Date _____

▶ Scenario

J.F. is a 50-year-old married woman with a genetic autoimmune deficiency; she has had recurrent infective endocarditis. The most recent episodes were a *Staphylococcus aureus* infection of the mitral valve 16 months ago and a *Streptococcus viridans* infection of the aortic valve 1 month ago. During the latter hospitalization, an echocardiogram showed moderate aortic stenosis, moderate aortic insufficiency, chronic valvular vegetations, and moderate left atrial enlargement. Two years ago, J.F. received an 18-month course of parenteral nutrition (PN) for malnutrition caused by idiopathic, relentless nausea and vomiting (N/V). She has had coronary artery disease (CAD) for several years and 2 years ago had an acute anterior wall myocardial infarction (MI). In addition, she has a history of chronic joint pain.

Now, after having been home for only a week, J.F. has been readmitted to your floor with infective endocarditis (IE), N/V, and renal failure. Since yesterday, she has been vomiting and retching constantly. She also

Chart View

Admission Orders

> STAT blood cultures (aerobic and anaerobic) × 2, 30 minutes apart
> STAT CMP & CBC
> Begin PN at 85 mL/hr
> Piperacillin sodium/tazobactam sodium (Zosyn) 2.25 g q6hr
> Vancomycin (Vancocin), renal dosing per pharmacy, IVPB q12hr
> Furosemide (Lasix) 80 mg PO daily
> Amlodipine (Norvasc) 5 mg PO daily
> Potassium chloride (K-Dur) 40 mEq PO daily
> Metoprolol (Lopressor) 25 mg PO bid
> Ondansetron 4 mg IV every 6 hours PRN
> Transesophageal echocardiogram ASAP

Admission Assessment

Blood pressure	152/48 (supine) and 100/40 (sitting)
Pulse rate	116
Respiratory rate	22
Temperature	100.2° F (37.9° C)

> Oriented × 3 to person, place, and time, but drowsy
> Grade II/VI holosystolic murmur and a grade III/VI diastolic murmur
> Lungs clear bilaterally
> Abdomen soft with slight left upper quadrant tenderness
> Multiple petechiae on skin of arms, legs, and chest; splinter hemorrhages under the fingernails; hematuria noted in voided urine

has had chills, fever, fatigue, joint pain, and headache. As you go through the admission process with her, you note that she wears glasses and has dentures. Intravenous (IV) access is obtained with a double-lumen peripherally inserted central catheter (PICC) line. Other orders and your assessment are shown in the box.

1. Which of these statements about IE are true? Select all that apply.
   a. IE may affect the heart valves.
   b. IE is an inflammation of the pericardial sac.
   c. IE is an infection of the innermost layer of the heart.
   d. Cardiac tamponade is a common complication of IE.
   e. Heart failure, sepsis, and dysrhythmias may occur with IE.

2. What is the significance of the orthostatic hypotension and tachycardia?

3. What is the significance of the abdominal tenderness, hematuria, joint pain, and petechiae?

4. What are splinter hemorrhages, and how are they related to IE?

5. Mark the area on the accompanying diagram where you would place the stethoscope to auscultate an aortic valve murmur.

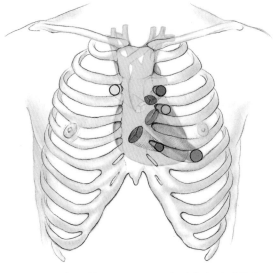

(From Jarvis C. Physical Examination and Health Assessment. 6th ed. St. Louis, MO: Saunders; 2012.)

6. As you monitor J.F. throughout the day, what other signs and symptoms of embolization will you watch for?

7. Explain the diagnostic criteria for infectious endocarditis.

CASE STUDY PROGRESS

The next day, you review J.F.'s lab test results.

Chart View

Laboratory Test Results	
Na	138 mEq/L (138 mmol/L)
K	3.9 mEq/L (3.9 mmol/L)
Cl	103 mEq/L (103 mmol/L)
BUN	85 mg/dL (30.3 mmol/L)
Creatinine	3.9 mg/dL (345 mcmol/L)
Glucose	165 mg/dL (9.2 mmol/L)
WBC	6700/mm³ (6.7 x 10⁹/L)
Hct	27%
Hgb	9.0 g/dL (90 g/L)

8. Identify the values that are not within normal ranges and explain the reason for each abnormality.

9. You note that a new intern writes an order for "Fasting blood glucose levels daily." Is this order appropriate for J.F.? Explain.

 10. What is the greatest risk for J.F. during the process of rehydration, and what would you monitor to detect its development?

CASE STUDY PROGRESS

You were aware that as soon as J.F. became stable, she would be going home on parenteral nutrition (PN) and IV antibiotics. As part of the discharge preparations, you contact the home care agency that will be providing her care

11. List 5 important questions in assessing her home health care needs.

CASE STUDY PROGRESS

Fortunately, J.F. has a supportive husband and 2 daughters who live nearby who can function as caregivers when J.F. is discharged. They, along with J.F., will need teaching about endocarditis. Although J.F. has been ill for several years, you discover that she and her family have received little education about the disease. You prepare a teaching plan for the family.

12. Develop a teaching plan for J.F. and her family.

13. J.F.'s daughter tells you that she thinks her mother will have to stay in bed until the infection is cured. How will you respond, and what measures can be implemented to prevent problems related to decreased mobility?

14. After you have taught J.F. about oral hygiene, which statement by J.F. reflects a need for further education?
   a. "I will use a soft toothbrush to brush my teeth."
   b. "I will use a water irrigation device to clean my teeth and gums."
   c. "I will rinse my mouth thoroughly with water after brushing my teeth."
   d. "I will remove my dentures after every meal and clean them thoroughly before replacing them."

CASE STUDY PROGRESS

Your hospital discharge planner facilitates J.F.'s transition to home care. During the initial home visit, the home health nurse evaluates J.F.'s IV site for implementation of the IV therapy program. The nurse interviews the family members to determine their willingness to be caregivers and their level of understanding and enlists the patient's and family's assistance to identify goals.

15. The home health nurse also writes short- and long-term goals for J.F. and her family. Identify 2 short-term and 3 long-term goals.

CASE STUDY OUTCOME

Mr. F. and his 2 daughters learned to administer J.F.'s antibiotic and 8-month treatment of PN. J.F.'s endocarditis eventually resolves with no worsening of her cardiac condition.

Case Study 12

Name _____ Class/Group _____ Date _____

▶ Scenario

Your patient, 58-year-old K.Z., has a significant cardiac history. He has long-standing coronary artery disease (CAD) with occasional episodes of heart failure (HF). One year ago, he had an apical myocardial infarction (MI). In addition, he has chronic anemia, hypertension, chronic renal insufficiency, and a recently diagnosed 4-cm suprarenal abdominal aortic aneurysm. Because of his severe CAD, he had to retire from his job as a railroad engineer about 6 months ago. This morning, he is being admitted to your telemetry unit for a same-day cardiac catheterization. As you take his health history, you note that his wife died a year ago (at about the same time he had his MI) and he does not have any children. He is a current cigarette smoker with a 50-pack-year smoking history. His vital signs are 158/94, 88, 20, and 97.2° F (36.2° C). As you talk with him, you realize he has only a minimal understanding of the catheterization procedure.

1. Before he leaves for the cath lab, you briefly teach him the important things he needs to know before having the procedure. List 5 priority topics you will address.

2. Look at his past history. What other factors are present that could contribute to his risk for cardiac ischemia?

CASE STUDY PROGRESS

Several hours later, K.Z. returns from his catheterization. The catheterization report shows 90% occlusion of the proximal left anterior descending (LAD) coronary artery, 90% occlusion of the distal LAD, 70% to 80% occlusion of the distal right coronary artery (RCA), an old apical infarct, and an ejection fraction (EF) of 37%. About an hour after the procedure is finished, you perform a brief physical assessment and note a grade III/VI systolic ejection murmur at the cardiac apex, crackles bilaterally in the lung bases, and trace pitting edema of his feet and ankles. Except for the soft systolic murmur, these findings were not present before the catheterization.

3. Using the following diagram, identify the superior vena cava, the aorta, and the left and right ventricles. Identify the main coronary arteries and circle the areas of the LAD and RCA that have significant occlusion, as identified in the previous report. Lightly shade the area of the heart where K.Z. had the earlier infarct.

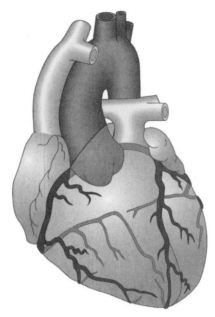

(Modified from Fuller JK. Surgical Technology: Principles and Practice. 5th ed. St. Louis, MO: Saunders; 2010.)

4. What is your evaluation of the catheterization results?

5. Explain the significance of having an EF of 37%.

6. What problem(s) do(es) the changes in assessment findings suggest to you? What led you to your conclusion?

7. List 5 actions you should take as a result of your evaluation of the assessment and state your rationale for each.

8. You decide to notify the physician of K.Z.'s condition. Using SBAR (*Situation*, *Background*, *Assessment*, *Recommendation*), what information would you provide to the physician when you call?

CASE STUDY PROGRESS

After assessing K.Z., the physician admits him with a diagnosis of CAD and HF and plans coronary artery bypass graft (CABG) surgery. Results of significant lab tests performed at this time are Hct 25.3%, Hgb 8.8 g/dL (88 g/L), BUN 33 mg/dL (11.8 mmol/L), and creatinine 3.1 mg/dL (274 mcmol/L). K.Z. is given furosemide (Lasix) and 2 units of packed red blood cells (PRBCs).

9. Review K.Z.'s health history. Can you identify a probable explanation for his chronic renal insufficiency and anemia?

10. Why is he receiving 2 units of PRBCs? What is the purpose of the furosemide?

CASE STUDY PROGRESS

Two days later, after his condition is stabilized, K.Z. is taken to surgery for a three-vessel coronary artery bypass graft (CABG × 3 V). When he arrives in the surgical intensive care unit, he has a Swan-Ganz catheter in place for hemodynamic monitoring and is intubated. He is put on a ventilator at Fio_2 0.70 and positive end-expiratory pressure (PEEP) at 5 cm H_2O. His latest Hgb is 10.3 mg/dL (103 g/L). You review his first hemodynamic readings and arterial blood gases.

Chart View

Hemodynamic Readings

Pulmonary artery pressure (PAP)	38/23 mm Hg
Central venous pressure (CVP)	14 mm Hg
Pulmonary artery wedge pressure (PAWP)	18 mm Hg
Cardiac index (CI)	1.88 L/min/mm^2

Arterial Blood Gases

pH	7.37
Paco$_2$	46 mm Hg
Pao$_2$	61 mm Hg
Sao$_2$	85%

11. Why are ABG values necessary in K.Z.'s case? Explain why it would be inappropriate to use pulse oximetry to assess his O$_2$ saturation status.

12. What is your interpretation of his ABG values on 70% oxygen?

13. What is your evaluation of K.Z.'s hemodynamic status, based on the results displayed?

14. Do you think the hemodynamic values reported previously reflect poor left ventricular function or fluid overload? Defend your answer.

15. K.Z. is receiving continuous IV infusions of norepinephrine (Levophed) and dobutamine. Why is K.Z. receiving these medications?

16. What assessment findings would indicate that these drugs are having a therapeutic effect?

17. What are the major side effects of norepinephrine and dobutamine, and what do you monitor while these drugs are infusing?

18. K.Z. states that he is feeling more "skipping beats," even while lying quietly in the bed. What will you do next?
a. Stop the dobutamine immediately.
b. Assess his vital signs and cardiac rhythm.
c. This is a normal side effect; no interventions are needed.
d. Titrate the dobutamine to a higher dose to reduce the palpitations.

After 3 days in the SICU, K.Z.'s condition was stable and he was returned to your telemetry floor. Now, 5 days later, he is ready to go home and you are preparing him for discharge.

19. List at least 4 general areas related to his CABG surgery in which he should receive instruction before he goes home.

CASE STUDY OUTCOME

K.Z. decided to sell his home and move to a seniors' apartment complex. He completed the cardiac rehabilitation program and became a volunteer to support others who have had heart surgery. He has not had a cigarette since his surgery.

1 Perfusion

Case Study 13

Name _____ Class/Group _____ Date _____

▶ Scenario

R.K. is an 85-year-old woman who lives with her husband, who is 87. Two nights before her admission to your cardiac unit, she awoke with heavy substernal pressure accompanied by epigastric distress. The pain was reduced somewhat when she rolled onto her side but did not completely subside for about 6 hours. The next night, she experienced the same chest pressure. The following morning, R.K.'s husband took her to the physician, and she was subsequently hospitalized to rule out myocardial infarction (MI). Lab specimens were drawn in the emergency department. She was given 325 mg chewable, non–enteric-coated aspirin, and an IV line was started. She was placed on oxygen (O_2) at 2 L via nasal cannula.

You obtain the following information from your history and physical examination: R.K. has no history of smoking or alcohol use, and she has been in good general health, with the exception of osteoarthritis of her hands and knees and some osteoarthritis of the spine. Her only medications are simvastatin (Zocor), ibuprofen as needed for bone and joint pain, and "herbs." Her admission vital signs (VS) are blood pressure 132/84, pulse 88, respirations 18, and oral temperature 99° F (37.2° C). Her weight is 114 lbs (51.7 kg) and height is 5 ft, 4 in (163 cm). Moderate edema of both ankles is present; capillary refill is brisk, and peripheral pulses are 1+. You hear a soft systolic murmur. She denies any discomfort at present. You place her on telemetry, which shows the rhythm in the following figure.

1. Identify her cardiac rhythm.

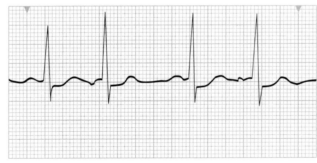

(Modified from Huszar R. Basic Dysrhythmias: Interpretation and Management—Revised Reprint. ed. 3, St. Louis, MO: Mosby; 2007.)

2. Give at least 2 reasons for inserting an IV line.

3. Explain the purpose of the aspirin tablet. Why is "non–enteric-coated" aspirin specified? What would be a contraindication to administering aspirin?

4. What additional history and physical information should you obtain related to her admitting diagnosis? Name at least 4 for each.

5. List 7 lab or diagnostic tests you would expect to be performed; suggest what each might contribute.

6. What other sources, in addition to cardiac ischemia, might be responsible for her chest and abdominal discomfort?

7. Define the concept of *differential diagnosis* and explain how the concept applies to R.K.'s symptoms.

CASE STUDY PROGRESS

After some rest, R.K.'s chest pain has subsided, and she tells you she feels much better now. You review her lab results.

Chart View

Laboratory Results

12-Lead ECG: Light left-axis deviation, normal sinus rhythm, with no ventricular ectopy

Cardiac troponin T is less than 0.01 ng/mL (0.01 mcg/L) (at admission) and same result 4 hours after admission

Cardiac troponin T is less than 0.03 ng/mL (0.03 mcg/L) (at admission) and the same 4 hours after admission

Serial CPK tests are 30 units/L at admission, 32 units/L 4 hours after admission

Copeptin 5 pmol/L at admission, 5.1 pmol/L 4 hours after admission

d-Dimer test result less than 250 ng/mL (250 mcg/L)

---

8. On the basis of the information presented so far, do you believe she had an MI? What is your rationale?

9. Do you think she may have a pulmonary embolus?

10. While you care for R.K., you carefully observe her. Identify 2 possible complications of coronary artery disease (CAD) and the signs and symptoms associated with each.

11. R.K. rings her call bell. When you arrive, she has her hand placed over her heart and tells you she is "having that heavy feeling again." She is not diaphoretic or nauseated, but states she is short of breath. Use the PQRST Assessment of Angina to assess her episode of chest pain. What questions would you ask for each factor?

12. What else do you assess, and what priority actions does the nurse need to take right now?

CASE STUDY PROGRESS

During the episode of chest pain, R.K.'s vital signs were as follows: BP 140/92, P 110, R 20. The rhythm strip shows sinus tachycardia, and she was very anxious. Her chest discomfort subsided in 3 minutes after 1 nitroglycerin (NTG) dose, and she is resting quietly with O_2 per nasal cannula at 2 L/min. R.K.'s physician is making rounds.

13. Using SBAR (*Situation*, *Background*, *Assessment*, *Recommendation*), how would you communicate this episode to R.K.'s physician?

R.K.'s husband is upset. He tells you they have been married for 62 years and he does not know what he would do without his wife. One way to help people deal with their anxieties is to help them focus on concrete issues.

14. What information would be useful to get from him? What other health care professional might be able to help with some of these issues?

The cardiologist diagnosed R.K. with angina associated with coronary artery disease. She has had no further episodes of chest pain and is discharged to home the next day. She is to see a cardiologist this week and set up an appointment for outpatient testing. As you present the discharge instructions, you review the proper technique for taking sublingual NTG for chest pain.

15. Using the teach-back method, you ask R.K. what to do if she experiences chest pain. Which statement by R.K. indicates that further teaching is needed? Explain your answer.
   a. "If I have chest pain, I will place 1 nitroglycerin tablet under my tongue."
   b. "At the first sign of chest discomfort, I will stop what I'm doing and sit down."
   c. "If the chest pain does not stop or ease up, I can take another tablet in 5 minutes."
   d. "My husband will need to call 911 if the chest pain does not stop after 3 nitroglycerin tablets."

16. R.K. tells you that she hates the headache that happens after she takes a nitroglycerin tablet. What can you suggest to her for this problem?

17. What essential safety point will you emphasize when discussing sublingual nitroglycerin with R.K.?

R.K.'s outpatient testing showed coronary artery disease, and the cardiologist recommended medical treatment at this time. She has not experienced an increased number of episodes of angina.

Case Study **14**

Name _____ Class/Group _____ Date _____

▶ **Scenario**

The time is 1900. You are working in a small, rural hospital. It has been snowing heavily all day, and the medical helicopters at the large regional medical center, 4 hours away by car (in good weather), have been grounded by the weather until morning. The roads are barely passable. W.R., a 48-year-old plumber with a 36-pack-year smoking history, is admitted to your floor with a diagnosis of rule out myocardial infarction (R/O MI). He has significant male-pattern obesity ("beer belly," large waist circumference) and a barrel chest and reports a dietary history of high-fat food. His wife brought him to the emergency department after he complained of unrelieved "indigestion." His admission vital signs (VS) were BP 202/124, pulse 106, respirations 18, and oral temperature 98.2° F (36.8° C). W.R. was put on oxygen (O_2) by nasal cannula (NC) titrated to maintain Spo_2 over 92% and started on an IV nitroglycerin (NTG) infusion. He was given aspirin 325 mg to chew and swallow and was admitted to Dr. A.'s service. There are plans to transfer him by helicopter to the regional medical center for a cardiac catheterization in the morning when the weather clears. Meanwhile, you have to deal with limited lab and pharmacy resources. The minute W.R. comes through the door of your unit, he announces he's "just fine" in a loud and angry voice and demands a cigarette. He also says he has no time to fool around with hospitals.

1. What is the first priority in his care?

2. Are these VS typical for a man of his age? If not, which one(s) concern(s) you? Explain why or why not.

3. Identify 5 priority problems associated with the care of a patient such as W.R.

4. Which lab tests might be ordered to investigate W.R.'s condition? If the order is appropriate, place an *A* in the space provided. If inappropriate, mark with an *I*. Provide rationales for your decisions.

_____ 1. Complete blood count (CBC)
_____ 2. Electroencephalogram (EEG) in the morning
_____ 3. Basal metabolic panel (BMP)
_____ 4. Prothrombin time (PT) and partial thromboplastin time (PTT)
_____ 5. Bilirubin
_____ 6. Urinalysis (UA)
_____ 7. STAT 12-lead electrocardiogram (ECG) and repeat in the morning
_____ 8. Type and crossmatch for 2 units of packed red blood cells (PRBCs)
_____ 9. Chest x-ray on admission and in the morning

5. What significant lab tests are missing from the previous list?

6. How are you going to respond to W.R.'s angry demands for a cigarette? He also requests something for his "heartburn." How will you respond?

7. Mrs. R. asks you, "If he can't smoke, why can't you give him one of those nicotine patches or some nicotine gum?" How will you respond?

8. Are there any alternatives to help him with his nicotine cravings? Would they be helpful now?

CASE STUDY PROGRESS

At 2000, you phone Dr. A.'s partner, who is on call. She prescribes morphine sulfate 4 mg STAT IV push (IVP), then 2 to 4 mg IVP q1hr prn for pain (burning, pressure, and angina).

9. Explain 2 reasons for this order.

10. What special precautions should you follow when administering morphine sulfate via IVP?

11. The pharmacy supplies morphine for injection in vials of 5 mg/mL only. For the first dose, you will be giving 4 mg of morphine. How many milliliters will you give for this dose? Mark the syringe with your answer.

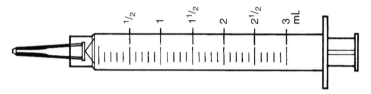

(From Gray Morris D. Calculate with Confidence. 5th ed. St. Louis, MO: Mosby; 2010.)

12. What will you do with the rest of the morphine in the vial?
    a. Discard it
    b. Save it for the next dose
    c. Return it to the pharmacy
    d. Discard it with a second witness

13. Angina is not always experienced as "pain" as many people understand pain. How would you describe symptoms you want him to warn you about? Why is this important?

14. What safety measures or instructions would you give W.R. before you leave his room?

15. Mrs. R. is unable to leave the hospital because of the bad weather. She approaches you and asks, "Did my husband have a heart attack? I'm really scared. His father died of one when he was 51." How are you going to respond to her question?

CASE STUDY PROGRESS

When you come into W.R.'s room at 2230 hours to answer his call light, you see he is holding his left arm and complaining about aching in his left shoulder and arm.

16. What information will you gather? What questions will you ask him?

CASE STUDY PROGRESS

You titrate the NTG drip up, assess whether he is using the oxygen cannula, and assess his vital signs. In addition, you administer a dose of morphine, but his pain is not relieved. Based on your assessment findings, you decide to call the physician.

17. Using SBAR (*Situation*, *Background*, *Assessment*, *Recommendation*), what information would you provide to the physician when you call?

18. W.R.'s chest pain subsides after the dose of morphine and he settles down for the night. You monitor him closely and watch for side effects of the NTG infusion. Side effects of NTG include which of these? Select all that apply.
   a. Headache
   b. Tachycardia
   c. Constipation
   d. Postural hypotension
   e. Decreased respirations

CASE STUDY PROGRESS

In the morning, W.R. is transferred by helicopter to the medical center, and a cardiac catheterization is performed. It is determined that W.R. has coronary artery disease (CAD) but has not had an MI. The cardiologist suggests it would be best to treat him medically for now.

19. What does it mean to treat him "medically"? What other approaches might be used to treat CAD?

20. A new order for atenolol (Tenormin) is added to his medication list. Which is/are a rationale for starting a beta blocker at this time? Select all that apply.
   a. Reduction of myocardial stimulation
   b. Increased force of cardiac contractions
   c. Decreased myocardial oxygen demand
   d. Prolonged sinoatrial (SA) node recovery
   e. Increased conduction through the atrioventricular (AV) node

CASE STUDY OUTCOME

The physician orders follow-up counseling regarding risk factor modification, especially smoking cessation, hypertension management, weight loss, and lipid (cholesterol) management. W.R. is discharged with a referral for a follow-up visit to his local internist in 1 week.

Case Study **15**

Name _____ Class/Group _____ Date _____

▶ **Scenario**

You are just getting caught up with your work when you receive the following phone call: "Hi, this is Deb in the emergency department (ED). We're sending you M.M., a 63-year-old Hispanic woman with a past medical history of coronary artery disease (CAD). Her daughter reports that her mom has become increasingly weak over the past couple of weeks and has been unable to do her housework. Apparently, she has had swelling in her ankles and feet by late afternoon so much that she could not wear her shoes and has nocturnal diuresis × 4. Her daughter brought her in because she has had heaviness in her chest off and on over the past few days but denies any discomfort at this time. She says that the chest heaviness is not related to activity and has become increasingly more frequent over the past few days, sometimes lasting up to 10 minutes at a time. The daughter took her to see her family physician, who immediately sent her here. Vital signs are 146/92, 96, 24, 99° F (37.2° C). She has an IV of D_5W at 50 mL/hr in her right forearm. Her lab results are as follows: Na 134 mEq/L (134 mmol/L), K 3.5 mEq/L (3.5 mmol/L), Cl 103 mEq/L (103 mmol/L), HCO_3 23 mEq/L (23 mmol/L), BUN 13 mg/dL (4.6 mmol/L), creatinine 1.3 mg/dL (115 mmol/L), glucose 153 mg/dL (8.5 mmol/L), WBC 8300/mm³ (8.3 × 10⁹/L), Hct 33.9%, Hgb 11.7 g/dL (117 g/L), platelets 162,000/mm³ (162 × 10⁹/L), PT/INR/PTT, and urinalysis are pending. She has had her chest x-ray and ECG, and her orders have been written."

1. What additional information do you need from the emergency department nurse?

2. How are you going to prepare for this patient?

3. M.M. arrives by wheelchair. As she transfers to the bed, what observations will you make? Why?

4. With the interpreter phone, M.M. tells you that she feels very tired. Is this symptom significant? Explain your answer.

5. Based on M.M.'s history, you suspect that she is experiencing angina. Which type of angina do you think she has? Explain your answer.

6. Given the previous information, you expect orders for M.M. Carefully review each to determine whether it is appropriate or inappropriate as written. If the order is appropriate, mark it as *A*; if the order is inappropriate, mark it as *I* and change the order to make it appropriate. Provide any other orders that might be appropriate for M.M.

_____   1. VS once per shift
_____   2. Serum magnesium (Mg) STAT
_____   3. Up ad lib
_____   4. 10 g sodium (Na), low-fat diet
_____   5. Change IV to a saline lock
_____   6. Cardiac enzymes on admission and q8hr × 24 hr, then daily every morning
_____   7. CBC, BMP, and fasting lipid profile in morning
_____   8. Schedule for abdominal CT scan for morning
_____   9. Heparin 10,000 units subQ q8hr
_____ 10. Docusate sodium (Colace) 100 mg PO daily
_____ 11. Ampicillin 250 mg IV piggyback q6hr
_____ 12. Furosemide (Lasix) 200 mg IV push STAT
_____ 13. Nitroglycerin (NTG) 0.4 mg 1 SL q4hr prn for chest pain
_____ 14. Schedule echocardiogram

7. Which interventions are appropriate for administering subcutaneous heparin? Select all that apply.
   a. Massage the area after the injection.
   b. Rotate injection sites with each dose.
   c. Do not aspirate the syringe before injecting the heparin.
   d. Give the injection at least 2 inches (5 cm) away from the umbilicus.
   e. Monitor activated partial thromboplastin time (aPTT) levels daily.

CASE STUDY PROGRESS

Shortly after admission, M.M.'s call light comes on. When you respond to M.M.'s call light, you observe she is talking rapidly in Spanish and pointing to the bathroom. Her speech pattern indicates she is short of breath; she is having trouble completing a sentence without taking a labored breath. You help her use a bedpan and note that her skin feels clammy. While sitting on the bedpan, she vomits.

8. On a scale of 0 to 10 (0 being no problem, 10 being a code-level emergency), how would you rate this situation, and why?

9. Identify at least 4 actions you should take next and state your rationale.

10. M.M.'s physician calls your unit to find out what is happening. Using SBAR, what information would you need to convey at this time?

11. The hospital's staff physician is coming to the floor immediately to evaluate the patient. In the meantime, she orders furosemide (Lasix) 40 mg IV push STAT. You have only 20 mg in stock. Should you give the 20 mg now, and then give the additional 20 mg when it comes up from the pharmacy? Explain your answer.

12. M.M. continues to experience vomiting and diaphoresis that are unrelieved by medication and comfort measures. A STAT 12-lead ECG reveals ischemic changes, and she is transferred to the coronary care unit. As you give the report to the receiving registered nurse, what lab value is the most important to report, and why?

13. You are observing while a new nurse prepares to administer IV potassium to M.M. Which technique is correct? Explain why the other answers are incorrect.
a. Give the IV potassium by slow IV push.
b. Administer the IV potassium by gravity drip.
c. Add potassium to a hanging IV bag as needed.
d. The rate of IV administration should not exceed 10 mEq/hr (10 mmol/L).

CASE STUDY PROGRESS

A case manager has been asked to evaluate M.M.'s home to see whether she can be discharged to her own home or will need to stay in a long-term care facility.

14. Identify at least 8 things that the case manager would assess.

15. M.M.'s nutritional intake over the past few weeks has been poor. What are some of the nutritional needs that should be met? What would you recommend to help her with this?

CASE STUDY PROGRESS

Because the case manager determined that M.M. lived in an apartment with poor access, M.M. elects to stay with her daughter and 5 grandchildren in their small home. A home care nurse comes 3 times a week to check on her. M.M. is easily fatigued, and the children are quite lively. School is out for the summer.

16. Suggest some ways for M.M.'s daughter to ensure that her mother is not overwhelmed and does not become exhausted in this situation.

CASE STUDY OUTCOME

M.M. stays with her daughter for 2 weeks, but the active children are too much for her and she moves back to her apartment. Her daughter checks on her there daily and brings her meals.

Case Study 16

Name _____ Class/Group _____ Date _____

▶ Scenario

You are in the middle of your shift in the coronary care unit (CCU) of a large urban medical center. Your new admission, C.B., a 47-year-old woman, was just flown to your institution from a small, rural community more than 100 miles away. She had a STEMI (ST-segment-elevation myocardial infarction) last evening. Her current vital signs (VS) are 100/60, 86, 14. After you make C.B. comfortable, you receive this report from the flight nurse: "C.B. is a full-time homemaker with 4 children. She has had episodes of "chest tightness" with exertion for the past year, but this is her first known myocardial infarction (MI). She has a history of hyperlipidemia and has smoked 1 pack of cigarettes daily for 30 years. Surgical history consists of total abdominal hysterectomy 10 years ago after the birth of her last child. She has no other known medical problems. Yesterday at 8 p.m. she began to have severe substernal chest pain that referred into her neck and down both arms. She rated the pain as 9 or 10 on a scale of 0 to 10. She thought it was severe indigestion and began taking Maalox with no relief. Her husband then took her to the local emergency department, where a 12-lead electrocardiogram (ECG) showed hyperacute ST elevation in the inferior leads II, III, aV_F, and V5 to V6. Before any interventions could be started, she went into ventricular fibrillation (V-fib). CPR was started and when the code team arrived, she was successfully defibrillated after 2 shocks. She then was started on nitroglycerin (NTG), heparin, and amiodarone drips. She was given IV metoprolol (5 mg every 2 minutes for a total of 3 doses) and aspirin 325 mg to chew and swallow. This morning her systolic pressure dropped into the 80s, and she was placed on a low-dose norepinephrine drip and urgently flown to your institution for coronary angiography and possible percutaneous transluminal coronary angioplasty. Currently, she has amiodarone infusing at 1 mg/min, heparin at 18 units/kg/minute, and norepinephrine at 0.5 mcg/kg/min. The NTG has been stopped because of low blood pressure. Lab work that was done yesterday showed Na 145 mEq/L (145 mmol/L), K 3.6 mEq/L (3.6 mmol/L), HCO_3 19 mEq/L (19 mmol/L), BUN 9 mg/dL (3.2 mmol/L), creatinine 0.8 mg/dL (70 mcmol/L), WBC 14,500/mm_3 (14.5 x 10^9/L), Hct 44.3%, and Hgb 14.5 g/dL (145 g/L)."

1. Because the 12-lead ECG can tell you the location of the infarction, evaluate the leads that showed ST elevation. What areas of C.B.'s heart have been damaged?

2. Given the diagnosis of acute ST-segment–elevation myocardial infarction (STEMI), what other lab results are you going to review?

3. For each of the characteristics listed below, specify whether they are associated with a STEMI or an NSTEMI (non-ST-segment–elevation MI).
   ____a. Caused by a nonocclusive thrombus.
   ____b. Caused by an occlusive thrombus.
   ____c. An emergency situation; the artery must be opened within 90 minutes of presentation.
   ____d. Patients usually undergo catheterization within 12 to 72 hours of presentation.
   ____e. A 12-lead ECG will show ST segment elevation.
   ____ f. The patient will not need thrombolytic therapy.
   ____g. Percutaneous coronary intervention (PCI) is the first-line treatment.

4. Indicate the expected outcome for C.B. associated with each medication she is receiving. For each drug listed, state the purpose.
   a. IV heparin
   b. IV amiodarone
   c. IV metoprolol
   d. Aspirin, chewed and swallowed
   e. IV norepinephrine

Chart View

Laboratory Test Results

Creatine Phosphokinase (CPK) Levels

On ED admission	95 units/L
4 hours	1931 units/L
8 hours	4175 units/L

Creatine Kinase–Myocardial Bound (CK-MB) Isoenzymes

On ED admission	5%
4 hours	79%
8 hours	216%

Troponin T

On ED admission	11 ng/mL (11 mcg/L)
6 hours	30 ng/mL (30 mcg/L)

Troponin I

On ED admission	3.9 ng/mL (3.9 mcg/L)
6 hours	9 ng/mL (9 mcg/L)
LDL	160 mg/dL (4.1 mmol/L)
PT	11.9 sec
INR	1.02
aPTT (before heparin)	26.9 sec
Mg	2.2 mg/dL (0.9 mmol/L)
K	3.3 mEq/L (3.3 mmol/L)

5. You review the lab work on her chart. For each lab value listed previously, interpret the result and evaluate the meaning for C.B.

6. List the 2 primary complications C.B. is at risk for at this time and the assessments that are needed to identify these risks.

7. You note that C.B.'s Spo$_2$ on oxygen at 6 L/min by nasal cannula is 92%. How do you interpret this result?

8. What can be done to promote her oxygenation at this time?

9. An hour after her admission, you are preparing C.B. for her coronary intervention. Evaluate her readiness for teaching and her learning needs. What would you tell her?

CASE STUDY PROGRESS

The following day, you care for C.B. again. She is now on oral metoprolol, amiodarone, aspirin, and clopidogrel (Plavix). The norepinephrine and heparin have been discontinued. VS are stable.

10. Which lab test result should you check before beginning the clopidogrel therapy?
   a. aPTT
   b. PT/INR
   c. Potassium
   d. Platelet count

CASE STUDY PROGRESS

As you work with C.B., you notice that she is extremely anxious. You had observed some anxiety yesterday, which you had attributed to the strange CCU environment, pain, and anticipation of the stenting procedure. The postprocedure test results showed that the stent was performing appropriately. You wonder what is wrong. She tells you that her heart attack occurred right in the middle of a move with her family from her rural community to an even smaller and unfamiliar town some 500 miles away in a neighboring state. She is dreading the move. Her husband "becomes angry easily and starts lashing out" toward her and the children. She is afraid to move to a community where she will have no friends and family to support her.

11. How can you help your patient? Evaluate the situation and describe possible interventions.

CASE STUDY OUTCOME

C.B. agrees to speak with a social worker, and you set up the meeting before she is discharged. As a result, C.B. decides to postpone the move and stay with the children at her sister's home while she recuperates and seeks counseling at a women's support shelter. She tells you she will keep her appointment with the internist in 2 weeks.

Case Study **17**

Name _____ Class/Group _____ Date _____

▶ **Scenario**

A.H. is a 70-year-old retired construction worker who has experienced lumbosacral pain, nausea, and upset stomach for the past 6 months. He has a history of heart failure, high cholesterol, hypertension (HTN), sleep apnea, and depression. His chronic medical problems have been managed over the years with benazepril (Lotensin) 5 mg/day, fluoxetine (Prozac) 40 mg/day, furosemide (Lasix) 20 mg/day, potassium chloride (KCl) 20 mEq (20 mmol) bid, and atorvastatin 40 mg each evening.

A.H. has just been admitted to the hospital for surgical repair of a 6.2-cm abdominal aortic aneurysm (AAA) that is now causing him constant pain. On arrival to your floor, his vital signs (VS) are 109/81, 61, 16, and 98.3° F (36.8° C). When you perform your assessment, you find that his apical heart rhythm is regular, and his peripheral pulses are all 2+. His lungs are clear, and he is awake, alert, and oriented. There are no abnormal physical findings; however, he has not had a bowel movement for 3 days. His electrolytes, blood chemistries, and clotting studies are within normal range, except his hematocrit is 30.1%, and hemoglobin is 9 g/dL (90 g/L).

1. A.H. has several common risk factors for AAA in his health history. Name and explain 3 factors.

2. How is testing used to diagnose an AAA?

3. A.H.'s aneurysm has the shape as in the accompanying illustration. What type of aneurysm is this?
   a. Aortic dissection
   b. False aortic aneurysm
   c. Saccular aortic aneurysm
   d. Fusiform aortic aneurysm

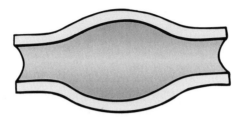

(From Lewis SL, Dirksen SR, Heitkemper MM, et al. Medical-Surgical Nursing: Assessment and Management of Clinical Problems. 8th ed. St. Louis, MO: Mosby; 2011.)

CASE STUDY PROGRESS

While A.H. awaits his surgery, it is important that you monitor him carefully for decreased tissue perfusion.

4. Name 5 things you would assess for, stating your rationale for each.

5. What is the most serious, life-threatening complication of AAA and why?

6. What single problem mentioned at the beginning of this case study is a risk for this complication? Why?

7. During your assessment, you note a pulsation in A.H.'s upper abdomen, slightly left of the midline, between the umbilicus and the xiphoid process. True or False: You must palpate this mass as part of your physical assessment. Explain your answer.

8. What common complications may occur after a AAA repair?

CASE STUDY PROGRESS

A.H.'s aneurysm resection is successful, and he maintains normal leg movement and sensation. However, for the first 2 postoperative days he is delirious and needs one-to-one nursing care in the intensive care unit. After he becomes coherent and oriented again, he is transferred back to your floor.

9. What assessments do you need to make specific to his postoperative care?

10. List 6 problems that are high priorities in A.H.'s postoperative care.

11. When you perform A.H.'s abdominal assessment, you do not hear any bowel sounds when auscultating his abdomen. What should you do?

12. Which interventions would you implement after an abdominal aortic aneurysm repair? Select all that apply.
   a. Keep the head of the bed elevated at 60 degrees.
   b. Assess peripheral pulses of both lower extremities.
   c. Change dressings as ordered with aseptic technique.
   d. Use the bed's knee gatch to allow for knee flexion during bed rest.
   e. Keep firm pressure on the abdominal incision during coughing exercises.

CASE STUDY PROGRESS

A.H.'s recovery is uneventful. While preparing him for discharge, you talk to him about health promotion and lifestyle change issues that are pertinent to his health problems.

13. Name 4 health-related issues you might discuss with him and what you would teach in each area.

14. A.H. will be receiving follow-up visits from the home health care nurse to change his dressing and evaluate his incision. What can you discuss with A.H. before discharge that will help him understand what the nurse will be doing?

15. Which statement by A.H. indicates a need for further education?
    a. "I will report any fever greater than 100 ° F."
    b. "I will avoid heavy lifting for 3 more weeks."
    c. "I will look for color changes in my feet and lower legs."
    d. "I will call the surgeon if I notice redness or swelling at the incision."

CASE STUDY OUTCOME

After a few more days in the hospital receiving physical therapy, A.H. could ambulate on his own. He was discharged from the hospital after a 9-day stay. Since discharge, he has not experienced any further problems and has not needed to return.

Case Study 18

Name _____ Class/Group _____ Date _____

▶ Scenario

Three-week-old J.T. and her parents arrive at the cardiac cath lab for her cardiac catheterization. She was born at term with Down syndrome, and her pediatrician is concerned because of lack of weight gain and poor feeding. You are getting her and her parents prepared for the procedure.

1. As you obtain her history and take vital signs, which statements or findings would be concerning and suggestive of heart failure (HF)? Select all that apply and explain your answers.
   a. Peripheral pulses +3
   b. Heart rate: 195 at rest
   c. Rectal temperature: 36.6° C (97.8° F)
   d. "J. gets damp and sweaty when she feeds."
   e. "J. takes 30 to 40 minutes to take 2 to 3 ounces (60 to 90 mL) of formula."
   f. "J. seems to have fewer wet diapers than when we brought her home from the hospital."

2. You are preparing J.T.'s parents for the procedure. Describe the points you would address in your teaching.

CASE STUDY PROGRESS

After the catheterization, J.T. returns to the unit in a crib. The orders shown in the chart have been written.

Chart View

Physician's Orders

> Daily weights: Current weight 8.8 lbs (4 kg)
> Strict intake and output
> O$_2$ per nasal cannula as needed to maintain O$_2$ saturation greater than 93%
> VS every 15 minutes × 4, then every 1 hour × 4, then every 4 hours
> Digoxin (Lanoxin) 70 mcg PO now, then 35 mcg PO every 6 hours for 2 doses
> Furosemide (Lasix) 4 mg PO now, then 4 mg PO every 12 hours

3. What will you document in your postprocedure assessment? Include rationale.

4. You are reviewing J.T.'s medications. J.T.'s mother states the following rationale for starting J.T. on digoxin (Lanoxin): "I need to give this to J. to decrease her blood pressure so her heart doesn't have to work so hard." Is this true or false? Explain your answer.

5. You have a student nurse working with you, and the student asks why the first ordered doses are high. What would be a possible explanation for this?

6. The student nurse asks whether there are any precautions to observe when giving digoxin to a neonate. Describe medication safety precautions that should be observed when giving this medication.

7. Which of these are potential signs of digoxin toxicity in an infant? Select all that apply.
   a. Vomiting
   b. Bradycardia
   c. Tachycardia
   d. Decreased blood pressure
   e. Lack of interest in feeding

CASE STUDY PROGRESS

You administer the ordered medication and proceed with your assessment.

8. Which of these are possible complications to monitor for after a cardiac catheterization? Select all that apply.
   a. Hematoma
   b. Vasospasm
   c. Hemorrhage
   d. Hyperglycemia
   e. Transient dysrhythmia
   f. Decreased pulse in unaffected leg

9. You are preparing to administer J.T.'s furosemide. Your drug reference gives the following therapeutic dose for edema in a neonate: 1 mg/kg per dose every 12 to 24 hours. Is the ordered dose of 4 mg a safe dose for J.T?

CASE STUDY PROGRESS

You note the following serum metabolic panel results for J.T.

Chart View

Laboratory Results

Glucose	85 mg/dL (4.7 mmol/L)
Calcium	9.1 mg/dL (2.28 mmol/L)
Sodium	142 mEq/L (142 mmol/L)
Potassium	3.3 mEq/L (3.3 mmol/L)
Chloride	101 mEq/L (101 mmol/L)

10. Which lab finding would concern you, and why?

11. The cardiologist tells J.T.'s parents that J.T. has a ventricular septal defect (VSD). On the diagram, circle the area affected by this defect.

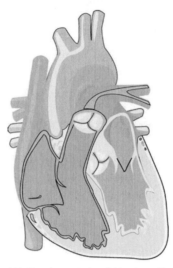

(Modified from Harkreader H, Hogan MA. Fundamentals of Nursing: Caring and Clinical Judgment. *2nd ed. St. Louis, MO: Saunders; 2004.)*

12. True or False? This defect would create decreased pulmonary flow. Explain your answer.

CASE STUDY PROGRESS

The cardiologist consults with the family, and it is decided that J.T. will be discharged to home the following day with medications and close monitoring. J.T. will return in several months for surgical repair of the VSD.

13. You begin your discharge teaching. Describe the information you will include in teaching.

CASE STUDY OUTCOME

J.T. undergoes surgical repair of the VSD 3 months later, and her recovery goes well. She continues to grow without further cardiac issues.

Case Study 19

Name _____ Class/Group _____ Date _____

▶ Scenario

J.E. is a 34-year-old Filipino man who presents to the emergency department reporting shortness of breath, dizziness, and a rapid fluttering in his chest. He states that he occasionally has had the same symptoms but they usually pass if he sits or lies down to rest. But this time resting has not helped the symptoms to subside. J.E. has a past medical history of an appendectomy and rheumatic fever as a child. His current vital signs are BP 164/78, P 160, R 28, T 98.1° F (36.7° C). His oxygen saturation is 94% on room air.

1. What further assessment and testing are needed at this time? Based on his vital signs and symptoms, what might the results be?

2. The echocardiogram reveals mitral valve stenosis. Describe mitral valve stenosis.

3. What typical heart sounds are heard with mitral stenosis, and where is the best place to listen?

4. What from J.E.'s past medical history could be the cause of mitral stenosis, given his young age? Explain your answer.

5. Locate the mitral valve on this diagram of the heart.

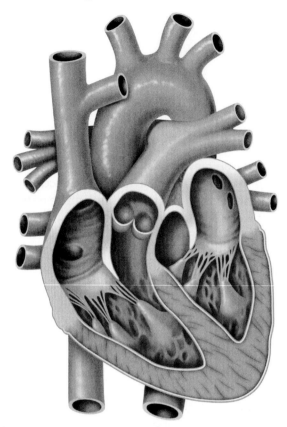

(From Solomon EP. Introduction to Human Anatomy and Physiology. *4th ed. Philadelphia, PA: Saunders; 2016.)*

CASE STUDY PROGRESS

J.E. is referred to a cardiothoracic surgeon to decide the best course of action for treating his mitral valve stenosis. At this time, he is still experiencing atrial fibrillation, with a heart rate in the 160s.

6. Which drugs do you expect to be started at this time? Explain your rationale.
   a. Amiodarone infusion and a heparin infusion
   b. IV push metoprolol and enoxaparin (Lovenox) subcutaneous injections
   c. A one-time oral dose of diltiazem (Cardizem) and subcutaneous heparin
   d. Lidocaine bolus, followed by an infusion, and subcutaneous heparin injections

CASE STUDY PROGRESS

The cardiothoracic surgeon determines that J.E. must have valve replacement surgery because of the severity of the mitral valve stenosis. The surgeon discusses valve surgery with J.E. and answers questions.

7. There are 2 types of valves used for valve replacement. Identify the types and discuss the advantages and disadvantages of each type.

8. Discuss why the surgeon might pick one valve over the other for J.E.

CASE STUDY PROGRESS

J.E. had successful mitral valve replacement surgery and is now recovering in the cardiac surgery intensive care unit. He is on a ventilator and has a chest tube but is awake and able to follow commands.

9. List 5 things the nurse will assess and monitor during the first 12 hours postoperatively.

CASE STUDY PROGRESS

Twenty-four hours after J.E.'s surgery, he has been successfully extubated, and is transferred to the cardiac surgery step-down unit.

10. What teaching will you provide to prevent respiratory complications?

11. You are teaching J.E. about care of the sternal incision. Which statement by J.E. indicates a need for further education?
    a. "I will call my doctor if I develop a fever."
    b. "I will report any bleeding that occurs from the incision."
    c. "I will wash the incision with soap and water when I get home."
    d. "If the incision looks red or has drainage, I will call my doctor right away."

CASE STUDY PROGRESS

J.E. is eager to go home. He has been started on warfarin (Coumadin) therapy and knows that he will need to be on anticoagulation for life.

12. What education about anticoagulation do you need to provide?

13. Which lab result reflects an appropriate goal for a patient who is on warfarin after heart valve surgery? Explain your answer.
a. INR 3.2
b. PT 12.5 seconds
c. aPTT 40 seconds
d. Bleeding time 9 minutes

14. J.E. has many questions about returning to work, driving, and exercise. What will you tell him?

15. True or False? There is no need for J.E. to inform health care providers about his valvular heart surgery because he has a mechanical valve. If false, correct the statement.

16. J.E. asks you, "What is a good way to let someone know that I have an artificial heart valve? Do I have to carry paperwork with me at all times?" How will you answer him?

CASE STUDY OUTCOME

J.E. returns to work after 6 weeks and becomes an active member of the local American Heart Association Mended Hearts community support group.

Case Study **20**

Name _____ Class/Group _____ Date _____

▶ Scenario

You are the 1900- 0700 charge nurse on the intermediate cardiac care unit in a large hospital. One of the patients, R.J., is being cared for by a new graduate nurse under your supervision. R.J. was admitted at 1300 after an auto accident in which he sustained a chest contusion and fractures of the fourth and fifth ribs on his left side. At about 2000 hours, his wife runs up to you at the nurses' station and says, "I think my husband just had a heart attack. Come quick!" She follows you into his room, where you find him still in bed. He is breathing and is cyanotic from the neck up. His pulse is rapid but very weak.

1. What will your first action be?

2. What immediate care will you provide to R.J.?

3. Given R.J.'s admitting diagnosis, what differential diagnoses do you consider?

4. What immediate information do you need to obtain from the nurse who is caring for R.J.?

5. Suddenly you remember R.J.'s wife, who is anxiously hovering over you in the room. What are you going to do?

CASE STUDY PROGRESS

The code team arrives. R.J.'s trauma surgeon is making rounds on your unit when the code is called, and he runs into the room. R.J. is intubated, and the normal saline lock is changed to an IV of lactated Ringer's solution at "wide open." The trauma surgeon recognizes Beck's triad associated with cardiac tamponade and calls for a cardiac needle and syringe. He inserts the needle below the xiphoid process and aspirates 75 mL of unclotted blood.

6. What is Beck's triad?

7. Describe cardiac tamponade.

8. What is the most likely reason R.J. developed cardiac tamponade?

9. Explain why the surgeon performed a pericardiocentesis.

10. What is the significance of the surgeon aspirating unclotted blood?

11. The surgeon orders IV dopamine to "begin at 4 mcg/kg/min and titrate to maintain a systolic BP over 100." What is the reason for this order?

12. The stock dopamine solution contains 320 mg dopamine in 100 mL of 5% dextrose. R.J. weighs 240 lb. How many micrograms should R.J. receive per minute? How many total milligrams of dopamine should R.J. initially receive per hour? (Round to the hundredth.) At how many milliliters per hour would you set the infusion pump? (Round to the tenth.)

13. Describe how you titrate a dopamine infusion.

14. Since R.J. underwent an emergency pericardiocentesis, which nursing interventions should you include in his immediate postprocedural care? Select all that apply.
   a. Maintain continuous ECG monitoring
   b. Closely assess for further cardiac tamponade
   c. Obtain blood cultures at 2 sites and send to the lab
   d. Be prepared for an emergency thoracotomy if tamponade recurs
   e. Observe for complications such as bleeding and cardiac dysrhythmias

15. Name 4 assessment findings that would show R.J. is responding to the immediate actions.

CASE STUDY PROGRESS

R.J. is being transferred to the intensive care unit (ICU) for observation.

16. Using the SBAR framework, describe the report you will give the ICU nurse.

17. As the team prepares R.J.'s transfer, you go find R.J.'s wife to thank her for alerting you to the emergency so promptly and to tell her what has happened. Briefly, and in lay terms, how would you explain what happened to her husband?

18. As you both get up to leave, Mrs. J. suddenly turns pale and says she feels very dizzy. What should you do?

CASE STUDY OUTCOME

Once in the ICU, R.J. underwent placement of a central venous catheter and an emergency echocardiogram. After finding about 50 mL of additional fluid in the pericardial sac, the decision was made to take R.J. to the operating room. A thoracotomy was done with repair of a right atrium laceration. He made an uneventful recovery and was discharged home on postoperative day 5.

Case Study **21**

Name _____ Class/Group _____ Date _____

▶ Scenario

D.V. is a 34-year-old woman who had a ruptured appendix 8 days ago with subsequent peritonitis. Plans are in progress to discharge her to home care later this afternoon, with a left peripherally inserted central catheter (PICC) for IV antibiotic therapy. As you are doing your full assessment on D.V., you notice a large ecchymotic area over the right upper arm. You ask her whether she recalls any trauma to that area. She tells you, "You nurses have taken my blood pressure so many times it bruised."

1. Do you accept D.V.'s explanation? Why or why not?

2. In examining D.V. further, you find a fine, nonraised, dark red rash over her trunk (petechiae). What other questions would you ask D.V.?

CASE STUDY PROGRESS

D.V. had not noticed the petechiae before you pointed it out. She says the rash does not itch or cause pain and that she has never had one like it before. She denies any other bleeding.

3. What other information would you want to gather?

CASE STUDY PROGRESS

Her vital signs are within normal limits except for a temperature of 99.8° F (37.7° C). The abdominal wound is not discolored or draining; however, her abdomen is tender to light palpation. The rash is confined to the trunk. There is slight oozing of serosanguineous fluid around the PICC insertion site. She has no other signs of bleeding. You decide to call the provider with your findings.

4. Using SBAR, what information will you relay to the provider?

5. The provider orders blood to be drawn for coagulation studies and a CBC with differential. What tests would you expect to see performed in coagulation studies?

6. You draw D.V.'s blood and initiate her next ordered dose of IV antibiotic. She asks you, "What is going on?" How would you respond?

CASE STUDY PROGRESS

An hour later, just as you are about to go to into the room to discontinue the IV antibiotic infusion, D.V. turns on her light and asks you to come to the room "right now." She tells you that she went to the bathroom and urinated blood and shows you a tissue in which she has some bloody-appearing sputum. You perform a focused assessment and find that there is some bloody drainage from the blood draw site an hour earlier and more petechiae on her trunk. Her vital signs are unchanged.

Chart View

Laboratory Test Values	
PT	19 seconds
aPTT	96 seconds
INR	1.8
D-Dimer	4.8 mcg/mL (4.8 ng/mL)
Fibrinogen	56 mg/dL (0.56 g/L)
WBC	12,500/mm^3 (12.5 x 10^9/L)
Platelet count	46,000/mm^3 (46 x 10^9/L)

7. Interpret D.V.'s lab values.

CASE STUDY PROGRESS

The elevated WBC count is consistent with her diagnosis of peritonitis or other infection.

8. D.V. is diagnosed with disseminated intravascular coagulation (DIC). What is DIC?

9. What is the most likely cause of DIC in D.V.'s case?
   a. Acute liver failure
   b. Presence of an undetected pregnancy
   c. Development of toxic shock syndrome
   d. Presence of infection in the abdominal cavity

10. Are D.V.'s presenting signs and symptoms consistent with DIC? Explain.

11. What are the goals of care for D.V.?

12. What complications are associated with DIC?

CASE STUDY PROGRESS

You notify the provider of D.V.'s assessment and lab results. The provider writes for D.V. to be transferred immediately to the intensive care unit (ICU); however, no beds are available in the unit. The nursing supervisor informs you that it will be 2 to 3 hours before a bed will be available.

13. What medical interventions do you expect for D.V. and why?

14. List 3 nursing actions and the rationale for each that you need to implement until she is transferred.

 15. Describe 4 precautions you should begin to reduce the risk for further bleeding.

16. Which activities can you delegate to the UAP who is assisting you with D.V.'s care? Select all that apply.
   a. Recording intake and output every hour
   b. Evaluating foot sensation and peripheral pulses
   c. Assisting D.V. with repositioning every 2 hours
   d. Having D.V. sign a blood transfusion consent form
   e. Regulating IV fluid administration as prescribed the by provider

17. D.V. appears anxious about all that is going on. How you would offer her support?

CASE STUDY OUTCOME

Therapy for DIC is started with O₂, fluids, and IV heparin. She is transferred to the ICU in guarded condition. Her infection, however, quickly evolves into sepsis and she develops acute respiratory distress syndrome requiring ventilatory support. After 6 days, D.V.'s respiratory status improves, and she is extubated. She is discharged to home care with IV antibiotic therapy 19 days after her initial admission.

Case Study 22

Name _____ Class/Group _____ Date _____

▶ Scenario

A 57-year-old man named A.T. has been admitted to the telemetry unit for continuous cardiac monitoring. He has a past medical history of nonischemic cardiomyopathy, hypertension, chronic heart failure (HF) with an ejection fraction (EF) of 10%, implantable cardioverter-defibrillator (ICD) placement 1 month ago, alcohol abuse, and a past smoker (quit 3 years ago). He was admitted after reporting chest pain and his ICD firing 3 times at home, before admission. During his morning assessment, A.T. suddenly reports chest pain and feels like he was just kicked in the chest. There is no witnessed loss of consciousness.

1. The nurse suspects that what just occurred?

2. What is an ICD?

3. How does the ICD get power to work?

4. What cardiac rhythm would the nurse expect to see during the review of his continuous telemetry strip?

5. What conditions are indications for placement of an ICD?

The nurse receives a call from the telemetry monitor technician, who reports a 5-second episode of this dysrhythmia:

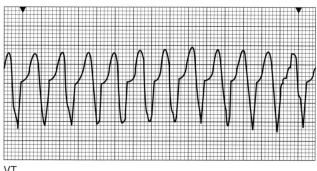

VT

(From Wesley K. Huszar's Basic Dysrhythmias. 4th ed. St. Louis, MO: Mosby; 2011.)

6. Identify this dysrhythmia

7. The nurse will assess and monitor for what other signs or symptoms?

The nurse calls the cardiologist to report the change in A.T.'s condition and receives orders for lab work.

8. What lab studies does the nurse expect to be ordered?

The nurse notes that the results from A.T.'s blood work are ready for review.

9. Considering A.T.'s condition, what lab results would require further management? Select all that apply.
   a. BTNP 435 pg/mL
   b. Calcium 9.4 mg/dL (2.35 mmol/L)
   c. Sodium 130 mEq/L (130 mmol/L)
   d. Glucose 107 mg/dL (5.9 mmol/L)
   e. Potassium 3.0 mEq/L (3.0 mmol/L)
   f. Hemoglobin 12.6 g/dL (126 g/L)
   g. Magnesium 1.3 mEq/L (0.5 mmol/L)

CASE STUDY PROGRESS

The nurse is asked to perform a medication reconciliation. The nurse makes a list of all of A.T.'s medications, which are listed in the following chart.

Chart View

Home Medications

Mexiletine hydrochloride 150 mg PO every 12 hours
Carvedilol 25 mg PO twice daily
Furosemide 80 mg PO twice daily at 8 a.m. and 2 p.m.
Lisinopril 10 mg PO once daily
Spironolactone 25 mg PO once daily
Isosorbide mononitrate 20 mg PO once daily
Aspirin EC 81 mg PO once daily
Rosuvastatin 20 mg PO every evening

10. For each drug listed, state its classification and specific use for A.T.

11. Which of A.T.'s medications would have a possible effect on his potassium level?

12. The hospitalist following A.T. ordered magnetic resonance imaging (MRI) because A.T. reported pain over his right middle quadrant. The patient escort has arrived to take him to the MRI room. Will you intervene? Explain your answer.

CASE STUDY PROGRESS

A.T. reports to the nurse that he feels overwhelmed at home managing his heart failure. He is saddened that he cannot play in his softball league but instead walks 1 mile every day in his neighborhood. He is proud that has quit smoking. He tells the nurse that he is "terrified" whenever his ICD "kicks him down." He also tells you that he doesn't really know what to do if his ICD goes off.

13. The nurse provides instructions about the ICD. Which statement by A.T. indicates a need for further instruction?
   a. "I will wear a medical alert bracelet at all times."
   b. "I will carry a list of my current medications with me."
   c. "If my ICD goes off, I need to call my doctor right away."
   d. "If my ICD goes off more than once, or if I feel sick, I will drive to the Emergency Room."

CASE STUDY OUTCOME

A.T. spends 3 days on the telemetry unit. His continuous telemetry monitoring now shows a normal sinus rhythm with a heart rate of 82. His BP is 116/72. A 2D Echo was performed that showed an EF of 25%. His ICD was interrogated without adverse reports. A CT scan of the abdomen showed no abnormalities. His most recent potassium level is 3.5 mEq/L (3.5 mmol/L). The cardiologist has agreed to discharge A.T. with a follow-up appointment 1 week from discharge. A.T. joins an ICD support group that meets monthly and enjoys talking with others who have the same concerns.

Case Study 23

Name_____ Class/Group_____ Date_____

▶ Scenario

You are a public health nurse working at a county immunization and tuberculosis (TB) clinic. B.A. is a 51-year-old woman who wants to obtain a food handler's license and is required to show proof of a negative tuberculosis skin test (TST) result before being hired. She came to your clinic 2 days ago for the first step of the TST. She has returned to have you evaluate her reaction.

1. What is TB and what microorganism causes it?

2. What is the route of transmission for TB?

3. The Centers for Disease Control and Prevention (CDC) recommends screening people at high risk for TB. List 5 populations at high risk for developing active disease.

4. Describe the 2 methods of TB screening.

5. How do you determine whether a TST result is positive or negative?

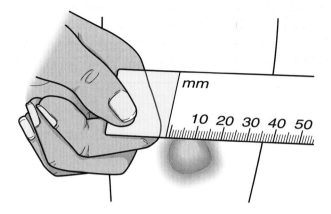

6. Interpret B.A.'s TST.

7. What other information do you need to obtain from B.A.?

8. You inform B.A. of the test result. She asks you what the result means. How will you respond?

CASE STUDY PROGRESS

B.A. is a natural-born American and has no risk factors for TB infection by the CDC guidelines. She has a 6-year history of type 2 diabetes mellitus that is well controlled with metformin (Glucophage). She admits that her mother had TB when she was a child but says she herself has never tested positive before. She is angry at the thought that she might have TB and says, "I feel just fine, and I don't think anything else is necessary."

9. What needs to be done to figure out whether B.A. has an active TB infection?

CASE STUDY PROGRESS

The provider orders a chest x-ray examination and informs B.A. that the image is clear, showing no signs of active TB infection. He tells her that she has class 2 TB, or a latent TB infection (LTBI), and that he will report her condition to the local public health department.

10. What is a LTBI?

11. What parameters are used to decide whether a person is treated for LTBI?

12. Is B.A. a candidate for LTBI treatment? State your rationale.

13. Outline the current CDC guidelines for the treatment of LTBI.

CASE STUDY PROGRESS

The provider decides to place B.A. on a 12-dose, once-weekly regimen of isoniazid and rifapentine as directly observed therapy (DOT).

14. How will you describe LTBI and DOT to B.A?

15. The medications used to treat LTBI have different side effects. Match the possible side effects to the tests used to assess for their presence:

_____A. Peripheral neuropathy   1. Audiogram
_____B. Hepatotoxicity   2. CBC
_____C. Fever and bleeding problems   3. BUN and creatinine
_____D. Nephrotoxicity   4. AST and ALT
_____E. Hyperuricemia   5. Monofilament testing
_____F. Optic neuritis   6. Red-green discrimination and visual acuity
_____G. Hearing neuritis   7. Uric acid

16. What other information does B.A. need to receive before leaving the clinic?

CASE STUDY OUTCOME

B.A. is hired under the condition that she complies with LTBI therapy and will immediately report any signs and symptoms of active disease to the clinic. She reports weekly for her medications and finishes her 12 weeks of therapy without experiencing any significant effects.

Case Study 24

Name_____ Class/Group_____ Date_____

▶ **Scenario**

It is 1130 and M.N., age 65, is being admitted to your surgical floor after having undergone an open cholecystectomy for acute cholecystitis. She has a nasogastric tube to continuous low wall suction, one peripheral IV line, and a large abdominal dressing. Her orders are as follows.

Chart View

Physician's Orders

Clear liquid diet; progress low-fat diet as tolerated

D_5 ½NS with 40 mEq KCl at 125 mL/hr

Turn, cough, and deep breathe q2hr

Incentive spirometer q2hr while awake

Oxygen per protocol to maintain Spo_2 at 95%

Dangle in a.m.

Morphine sulfate 10 mg IM q4hr prn for pain

Piperacillin/tazobactam (Zosyn) 3.375 grams IV q6hr

CXR in a.m.

1. Are these orders appropriate for M.N.? State your rationale.

2 Gas Exchange

CASE STUDY PROGRESS

At 1530, the UAP reports the following:

Chart View

Vital Signs

BP	148/82
Heart rate	118
Respiratory rate	24
Temperature	101° F (38.3° C)
SpO_2	92%

2. Based solely on her vital signs, what could be happening with M.N., and why?

3. You go to assess M.N. What do you need to include in your assessment at this time?

CASE STUDY PROGRESS

Your assessment of M.N. finds her with decreased breath sounds and crackles in the right base posteriorly. Her right middle and lower lobes percuss slightly dull. She splints her right side when attempting to take a deep breath. Her skin is pale, warm, and dry. She does not have a productive cough, chest pain, or any anxiety.

4. What complication do you suspect M.N. is experiencing? State your rationale.

5. Why is M.N. at risk for developing this complication?

6. What is your nursing priority at this time?

7. Describe 6 interventions you will perform over the next few hours based on this priority.

8. To promote optimal oxygenation with M.N., which actions could you delegate to the UAP? Select all that apply.
   a. Auscultating M.N.'s lung sounds
   b. Encouraging M.N. to splint the incision
   c. Assisting M.N. in getting up to the chair
   d. Reminding M.N. to cough and deep breathe
   e. Instructing M.N. on the use of incentive spirometry
   f. Taking M.N.'s temperature and reporting elevations

9. Identify 3 outcomes that you expect for M.N. as a result of your interventions.

CASE STUDY PROGRESS

At 1830, the UAP reports the following:

Chart View

Vital Signs

BP	136/72
Heart rate	104
Respiratory rate	24
Temperature	100.6° F (38.1° C)
Spo_2	93%

10. Has M.N.'s status improved or not? Defend your response.

11. You need to call the surgeon regarding M.N.'s status. Using SBAR, what would you report to the surgeon?

12. The surgeon orders a stat CXR. Afterward, the radiology department calls with a report, confirming that M.N. has atelectasis. Should this diagnosis change your plan of care for M.N.?

13. If M.N. had pneumonia, what changes might the surgeon have made to her plan of care?

14. M.N.'s sister questions you, saying, "I don't understand. She came in here with a bad gallbladder. What has happened to her lungs?" How would you respond?

CASE STUDY OUTCOME

M.N. stayed 2 extra days in the hospital, receiving IV antibiotics and continued care focusing on improving her respiratory status. Her atelectasis resolved, and she experienced no other complications from the cholecystectomy. She went home with her sister, and both thanked the staff for their care efforts by sending flowers.

Case Study 25

Name_____ Class/Group_____ Date_____

▶ Scenario

S.R. is a 59-year-old man who comes to the clinic because his wife complains "my snoring is difficult to live with."

1. As the clinic nurse, what routine information would you want to obtain from S.R.?

CASE STUDY PROGRESS

After interviewing S.R., you note the following: S.R. is under considerable stress. He owns his own business. The stress of overseeing his employees, meeting deadlines, and carrying out negotiations has led to poor sleep habits. He sleeps 3 to 4 hours per night. He keeps himself going by drinking 2 quarts (2 liters) of coffee and smoking three to four packs of cigarettes per day. He has gained 50 pounds (22.5 kg) over the 2 years, leading to a current weight of 250 pounds (114 kg). He tells you he has difficulty staying awake, wakes up with headaches on most mornings, and has midmorning somnolence. He says he is depressed and irritable most of the time and reports difficulty concentrating and learning new things. He has been involved in three auto accidents in the past year.

S.R.'s vital signs are 164/90, 92, 18, and SpO_2 90% on room air. His examination findings are normal, except for a few bruises over the right side of the rib cage. You inquire about the bruises, and S.R. reports that his wife jabs him with her elbow several times every night. In her own defense, the wife states, "Well, he stops breathing and I get worried, so I jab him to make him start breathing again. If I don't jab him, I find myself listening for his next breath and I can't go to sleep." You suspect sleep apnea.

2. Name the 2 main types of apnea and explain the pathology of each.

3. Based on your findings, which type of sleep apnea do you think S.R. has?

4. Name at least 5 signs or symptoms of this type of sleep apnea. Put a star next to those S.R. is experiencing.

5. How does the provider use diagnostic testing to diagnose sleep apnea?

CASE STUDY PROGRESS

The primary care provider examines S.R. and documents a long soft palate, recessed mandible, and medium-sized tonsils. S.R. undergoes an overnight home screening study, which shows 143 episodes of desaturation ranging from 68% to 76% with episodes of apnea. He is tentatively diagnosed with obstructive sleep apnea (OSA), and a full sleep study is ordered.

6. S.R. and his wife ask about a full sleep study. How would you explain a nocturnal polysomnogram to them?

7. S.R. and his wife ask why they need to be concerned about OSA. You tell them that treating OSA is necessary to prevent which common complications? Select all that apply.
   a. Stroke
   b. Hypotension
   c. Cardiac dysrhythmias
   d. Right-sided heart failure
   e. Early onset of chronic obstructive pulmonary disease (COPD)

8. The provider asks you to teach S.R. about lifestyle changes that he could make immediately to help with his situation. Describe 4 priority topics you would discuss with S.R.

CASE STUDY PROGRESS

The polysomnogram confirms S.R.'s diagnosis of OSA. At his 6-week follow-up visit, he reports he has lost 8 pounds (3.6 kg), but there has been little improvement in his symptoms. He says that he fell asleep while driving to work and wrecked his car. He wants to discuss further treatment options.

9. What are the treatment options for OSA? Describe 3.

CASE STUDY PROGRESS

S.R. and the provider decide to begin S.R. on continuous positive airway pressure (CPAP). The provider writes a prescription for CPAP.

2 Gas Exchange

 10. List 3 education topics you need to address with S.R. so he can safely self-manage CPAP therapy.

11. Which member of the interprofessional team will likely be involved in S.R.'s care and how?

12. S.R. calls 2 weeks later with complaints of dry nasal membranes, nosebleeds, and sores behind his ears. What instructions would you give S.R.?

13. Outline how you would document the phone call with S.R.

CASE STUDY OUTCOME

S.R. returns to the clinic 2 months after starting CPAP therapy. He reports that he is a "happier, healthier man." He says he now sleeps 7 hours a night, is not having to drink coffee just to get through the day, and his work performance has dramatically improved. S.R. tells you, "It is just remarkable, I never thought that sleep could be such a problem."

Case Study 26

Name_____   Class/Group_____   Date_____

▶ Scenario

G.C. is a 78-year-old widow who comes to the outpatient clinic saying that over the past 2 to 3 months she has felt increasingly tired, despite sleeping well at night. Over the past few years, she describes eating less and less meat because of her financial situation and has trouble preparing a meal "just for me." G.C. relates how she relies on her late husband's Social Security income for all her expenses. She struggles financially to buy medicines for the treatment of hypertension and arthritis. Her vital signs are 136/76, 16, 80. She denies any dyspnea or palpitations. The nurse practitioner orders blood work. G.C.'s chemistry panel findings are all within normal limits, and a stool fecal occult blood test result is negative. Her other results are shown in the chart.

Chart View

Laboratory Test Results

WBC	7600/mm^3 (7.6 x 10^9/L)
Hematocrit (Hct)	27.3%
Hemoglobin (Hgb)	8.3 mg/dL (83 g/L)
Platelets	151,000/mm^3 (151 x 10^9/L)

Red Blood Cell (RBC) Indices

Mean corpuscular volume (MCV)	65 fL (65 mm^3)
Mean corpuscular hemoglobin (MCH)	31.6 pg
MCH concentration (MCHC)	35.1%
Iron, total	30 mcg/dL (5 mcmol/L)
Iron-binding capacity	422 mcg/dL (75.5 mcmol/L)
Ferritin	8 mg/dL (18 pmol/L)
Vitamin B$_{12}$	414 pg/mL (305 pmol/L)
Folate	22 ng/mL (50 nmol/L)

1. Which lab values are normal, and which are abnormal?

2 Gas Exchange

2. Explain the significance of each abnormal result.

3. Based on these results and her history, what condition does G.C. have?

4. Who is at risk for this condition?

5. What other signs and symptoms of this condition do you assess for in G.C.?

6. Which question would *best* help you determine the impact of fatigue on her activities of daily living?
   a. "Are you upset about feeling more tired?"
   b. "Do you sleep more now than you used to?"
   c. "How far can you walk until you get short of breath?"
   d. "Have you been able to do what you would like to do?"

7. Discuss the treatment options for her condition.

8. When would parenteral iron therapy be indicated?

9. The nurse practitioner starts G.C. on ferrous sulfate 325 mg orally once per day. What teaching does G.C. need about this medication?

10. As you are evaluating your teaching, you determine that more instruction is needed if G.C. says:
    a. "My stools will likely turn a tarry, black color soon."
    b. "I can take the iron and my calcium supplements at the same time."
    c. "I will increase my fluid and fiber intake as long as I am on the iron."
    d. "Taking the tablets when I eat my meals will help my stomach not be upset."

11. Discuss some ideas that might help her with her meal planning.

12. You teach G.C. about foods she should include in her diet. You determine that she understands your teaching if she says she will increase her intake of which foods?
    a. Whole-wheat pastas and skim milk
    b. Lean cuts of poultry, pork, and fish
    c. Beans and dark green, leafy vegetables
    d. Cooked cereals, such as oats, and bananas

13. What community resources may benefit G.C.?

14. What parameters could you use to determine whether G.C.'s condition is improving?

15. Using a SOAP format, write a sample documentation entry for this encounter.

CASE STUDY OUTCOME

G.C. returns to the clinic in 3 months. She says she is feeling "a bit" less tired. Although her blood work shows some improvement, anemia is still present. G.C. and you discuss ways to promote better eating. She tells you she did not follow up on any of your suggestions about seeking community resources. She now agrees to speak with the social worker and explore available resources.

Case Study **27**

Name_____ Class/Group_____ Date_____

▶ **Scenario**

V.M. is a 29-year-old African American married man who has sickle cell disease (SCD) marked by frequent episodes of severe pain. His anemia has been managed with multiple transfusions. Six months ago, he started showing signs of chronic renal failure. His regular medications are acetaminophen, hydroxyurea (Hydrea), and folic acid. In the hematology clinic this morning, V.M.'s hemoglobin (Hgb) measured 6.7 g/dL (67 g/L). He received 2 units of packed red blood cells (PRBCs) over 3 hours and then went home. He developed dyspnea and shortness of breath about 1 hour later, and his wife called 911. The emergency medical system crew started O_2 at 8 L per nasal cannula and transported V.M. to the emergency department (ED).

1. What is SCD?

2. Evaluate each of the following statements about SCD. Enter "T" for true or "F" for false. Discuss why the false statements are incorrect.
   _____1. Only African Americans get SCD.
   _____2. There is currently no cure for SCD.
   _____3. Those with SCD should not receive childhood vaccinations.
   _____4. SCD cannot be diagnosed before an infant is 3 to 4 months old.
   _____5. An ophthalmologist should perform an eye examination every 1 to 2 years.
   _____6. Those with SCD should fly only on airplanes with pressurized cabins.

3. Which statement is true about the inheritance pattern of SCD?
   a. If V.M.'s wife has sickle cell trait, each child will either have SCD or be a carrier.
   b. If V.M.'s wife does not have sickle cell trait, each child has a 50% risk for having SCD.
   c. If V.M.'s wife has sickle cell trait, each child can either have SCD or be normal.
   d. If V.M. has children, each child will automatically have SCD regardless of his wife's status.

4. V.M.'s Hgb measured 6.7 g/dL (67 g/L). Why is anemia common in patients with SCD?

5. Why is it difficult to crossmatch blood to transfuse V.M.?

6. What role does hydroxyurea (Hydrea) play in managing V.M.'s SCD?

When V.M. arrives at the ED, you perform a quick assessment and note a grade III systolic murmur and crackles in V.M.'s bases bilaterally. Vital signs are BP 176/102, P 94, R 28, T 97.8° F (36.6° C), and Spo_2 78%. Peripheral pulses are equal and 3+. He is alert and oriented; he tells you he is nauseated. His abdomen is nontender, with hypoactive bowel sounds in ×4 quadrants. Acting according to the standing orders for your institution, you start an intravenous (IV) line, obtain arterial blood gas (ABG) values, and draw blood for complete blood count with differential and basal metabolic panel.

7. The ED resident asks him whether he is in pain and whether he needs pain medication. V.M. answers "no" to both questions. Why did the ED resident ask these questions?

8. V.M.'s ABGs on 8 L O_2 by simple face mask show Pao_2 74 mm Hg. Is V.M. being adequately oxygenated?

9. Are your assessment findings consistent with fluid overload or deficit? What findings led you to your conclusion?

10. Your institution uses electronic charting. Based on the assessment described, document your findings by providing a brief narrative note.

☐ Neurologic

☐ Respiratory

☐ Cardiovascular

☐ Gastrointestinal

☐ Psychosocial

Chart View

Laboratory Test Values

Sodium	137 mEq/L (137 mmol/L)
Potassium	4.9 mEq/L (4.9 mmol/L)
Chloride	110 mEq/L (110 mmol/L)
CO_2	16 mEq/L (16 mmol/L)
BUN	27 mg/dL (9.6 mmol/L)
Creatinine	2.7 mg/dL (239 mcmol/L)
WBC	4300/mm³ (4.3 x 10^9/L)
Hgb	7.8 g/dL (78 g/L)
Hct	20.9%
Platelets	208,000/mm³ (208 x 10^9/L)

11. Interpret V.M.'s lab results.

12. V.M. complains of being short of breath. Do you believe the low Hgb level is responsible for his complaints?

13. What action will you expect the ED resident to take next and why?

CASE STUDY PROGRESS

The ED resident prescribes furosemide (Lasix) 40 mg IV push now, methylprednisolone (Solu-Medrol) 75 mg IV push now, and ceftriaxone 1 g IV piggyback after the furosemide (Lasix).

14. Indicate the expected outcome for V.M. associated with each medication he is receiving.

15. The methylprednisolone 75 mg IV is supplied as a 125 mg/2 mL solution. Shade in the dose to be given on the syringe.

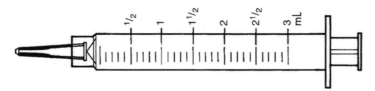

(From Gray Morris D. Calculate with Confidence. *5th ed. St. Louis, MO: Mosby; 2010.)*

16. Identify 3 outcomes that you expect for V.M. as a result of your interventions.

CASE STUDY PROGRESS

V.M. voids 1900 mL within 2 hours of giving the furosemide. As V.M.'s dyspnea is relieved, he shakes the ED resident's hand and thanks him for asking about the presence of pain and the need for pain medication. V.M. states, "One of my biggest fears is that I'll come in here in crisis and the doctor won't treat my pain aggressively enough. I don't want to be labeled as a drug seeker or an emergency room abuser."

17. Why would V.M. be concerned about obtaining adequate pain control in the ED?

18. What issues will you discuss with V.M. before discharge?

CASE STUDY OUTCOME

V.M. is discharged from the ED after being observed for 6 hours. He is instructed to follow up with his primary care provider about the episode and discuss with the hematology clinic staff longer transfusion times for any future transfusions.

Case Study 28

Name_____ Class/Group_____ Date_____

▶ Scenario

B.T., a 31-year-old man who lives in a small mountain town in Colorado, is highly allergic to dust and pollen and has a history of mild asthma. B.T.'s wife drove him to the emergency department when his wheezing was unresponsive to his fluticasone/salmeterol (Advair) inhaler, he was unable to lie down, and he began to use accessory muscles to breathe. B.T. is immediately started on 4 L O_2 by nasal cannula and IV D_5W at 75 mL/hr. A set of arterial blood gases (ABGs) is sent to the lab. B.T. appears anxious and says that he is short of breath.

Chart View

Vital Signs	
BP	152/84
Pulse rate	124
Respiratory rate	42
Temperature	100.4° F (38.4° C)

1. Are B.T.'s vital signs acceptable? Give your rationale.

2. What is the rationale for immediately starting B.T. on O_2?

3. Keeping in mind B.T.'s health history and presenting complaint, what are the critical areas you need to evaluate during your physical assessment?

Chart View

Arterial Blood Gases

pH	7.31
$Paco_2$	48 mm Hg
HCO_3	26 mEq/L
Pao_2	55 mm Hg

4. Interpret B.T.'s ABG results.

Chart View

Medication Orders

Albuterol 2.5 mg plus ipratropium 0.5 mg nebulizer treatment STAT, then q4hr
Methylprednisolone 100 mg IV now
Albuterol inhaler 2 puffs q4hr as needed

5. What is the rationale for the albuterol 2.5 mg plus ipratropium 0.5 mg nebulizer treatment STAT then q4hr?

6. Why is B.T. receiving methylprednisolone?

CASE STUDY PROGRESS

You assess B.T. and find that he has diminished lung sounds with inspiratory and expiratory wheezes in all lung fields with a nonproductive cough and accessory muscle use. His skin is pale, warm, and dry. The ECG shows sinus tachycardia without ectopy. He is alert and oriented ×4 spheres. He appears anxious and is sitting upright, leaning over the bedside table, and continuing to complain of shortness of breath.

7. What is your primary nursing goal right now?

8. Describe 6 actions you must implement based on this priority.

9. You will need to monitor B.T. closely for the next few hours. What is the most serious complication to anticipate?

10. Name 4 signs and symptoms of this complication you will assess for in B.T.

11. What are your responsibilities while administering aerosol therapy?

CASE STUDY PROGRESS

After several hours of rehydration and aerosol treatments, B.T.'s wheezing and dyspnea resolve, and he is able to expectorate his secretions. The provider discusses B.T.'s asthma management with him; B.T. says he has had several asthma attacks over the last few weeks. The provider discharges B.T. with prescriptions for fluticasone/salmeterol (Advair HFA 230/21) 1 inhalation every morning and evening, albuterol (Proair) metered-dose inhaler (MDI) 2 puffs q6hr as needed using a spacer, montelukast (Singulair) 10 mg/day each evening, and prednisone (5 mg tablets) 40 mg/day for 3 days, then taper by reducing the dose by 5 mg/day until discontinued. He gives him a prescription for a peak flow meter (PFM) and instructs B.T. to call the pulmonary clinic for follow-up with a pulmonary specialist.

12. How is montelukast (Singulair) different from other asthma medications?

13. Patients need to follow a specific sequence of administration when using multiple inhalers. Describe the instructions you will give B.T. about the correct sequence he should follow to safely use his inhalers.

14. Explain the drug class and expected outcomes associated with the drugs contained in fluticasone/salmeterol (Advair HFA).

15. B.T. states he had taken his Advair that morning, then again when he started to feel short of breath. He says, "It did not help," and wants to know why he has to stay on it. Is fluticasone/salmeterol (Advair) appropriate for use during an acute asthma attack? Explain.

16. Based on this information, what specific issue do you need to address in discharge teaching with B.T.?

17. You review with B.T the possible side effects he may experience, including hoarseness, dry mouth, fungal infection in the oral cavity, and coughing. What actions can you teach him to prevent or diminish the incidence of these effects? Select all that apply.
   a. Decrease his fluid intake.
   b. Use a spacer with the inhaler.
   c. Use the inhaler and Advair only as prescribed.
   d. Rinse his mouth with water immediately after taking the Advair.
   e. Clean the spacer in the dishwasher on "hot cycle with heated dry" daily.

18. What is the reason for the tapering doses of prednisone?

19. What is a PFM? Outline the instructions B.T. needs to perform the PFM maneuver.

20. B.T. asks why he has to use the PFM. Explain the purpose of the peak expiratory flow rate (PEFR) measurement, what an asthma action plan is, and the role the PEFR plays in an asthma action plan.

21. You set up an asthma action plan for B.T. What will you teach him to do if his PEFR value falls into the yellow or red zone?

22. You would recognize the need for additional teaching if B.T. makes which statements? Select all that apply and correct the incorrect answers.
    a. "I will keep a diary of all of my PEFR measures."
    b. "I will place a plastic cover on our mattress and my pillows."
    c. "I will use the albuterol inhaler 30 minutes before exercising."
    d. "My wife needs to know what to do in case I have a serious attack."
    e. "The bed linens need to be washed in cold water to reduce dust mites."
    f. "If the PEFR is in the yellow zone, I will use rescue drugs and go to the hospital."

23. B.T. states that he would like to read more about asthma on the Internet. List 3 credible websites to which you could direct him.

CASE STUDY OUTCOME

At the next follow-up visit, B.T.'s peak flow is 94% of the predicted. His symptoms have subsided, and he has not been experiencing any problems. He says he has been reading more about asthma and has a complete peak flow diary and asthma symptom journal on his smartphone.

Case Study **29**

Name_____ Class/Group_____ Date_____

▶ **Scenario**

L.S. is a 7-year-old who has been brought to the emergency department (ED) by his mother. She imme-diately tells you he has a history of ED visits for his asthma. He uses an inhaler when he wheezes, but it ran out a month ago. She is a single parent and has 2 other children at home with a babysitter. Your assessment finds L.S. alert, oriented, and extremely anxious. His color is pale, and his nail beds are dusky and cool to the touch; other findings are heart rate 136, respirations regular and even, rate 26, oral tem-perature T 37.3°C (99.1°F), Spo_2 89%, breath sounds decreased in lower lobes bilaterally and congested with inspiratory and expiratory wheezes, prolonged expirations, and a productive cough. As you ask L.S.'s mother questions, you note that L.S.'s respiratory rate is increasing; he is sitting on the side of the bed, leaning slightly forward, and having difficulty breathing. You are concerned that he is experiencing status asthmaticus.

1. You check the orders and need to decide which interventions are the priority at this time. Select all that apply and explain the rationale.
   a. Have L.S. lie flat.
   b. Have L.S. perform incentive spirometry.
   c. Administer oxygen via face mask to keep his Spo_2 above 90%.
   d. Administer albuterol (Proventil) and ipratropium bromide (Atrovent) via hand-held nebu-lizer (HHN) STAT.
   e. Reassess in 20 minutes, and if no improvement, administer salmeterol (Serevent Diskus) via dry-powder inhaler (DPI).
   f. Reassess in 20 minutes, and if no improvement, administer albuterol (Proventil) and ipra-tropium (Atrovent) via hand-held nebulizer again.
   g. Start IV normal saline (NS) at 15 mL/hr and administer methylprednisolone 2 mg/kg IV STAT × 1 dose.

2. Explain what the nurse will assess before, during, and after the nebulizer treatment with albuterol.

CASE STUDY PROGRESS

You give L.S. the albuterol and Atrovent twice. His O_2 saturation does not improve and remains at 88% with oxygen at 6 L/min via face mask. He says he "does not feel any better." He is retracting and his respiration rate remains 34. You have started his IV infusion and administered the methylprednisolone. L.S.'s mother is pacing and tells you she is very upset and worried. You overhead page the attending ED resident to assess, and you notify the patient-family advocate. The ED resident, Dr. S., arrives within 2 minutes to assess L.S. and to speak to L.S.'s mother. New orders are pending.

3. Chart your actions and the patient's response using the SBAR (*S*ituation, *B*ackground, *A*ssessment, and *R*ecommendation) format.

CASE STUDY PROGRESS

L.S. is admitted to the pediatric intensive care unit (PICU) for close monitoring. His condition improves, and 24 hours later he is transferred to the floor. Asthma teaching is ordered. You assess Ms. S.'s understanding of asthma and her understanding of the disorder.

4. Which statement by Ms. S. would indicate a need for further teaching? Explain your answer.
   a. "If he takes medications for a while, he will outgrow his asthma."
   b. "Part of his treatment should be avoiding things that irritate his lungs."
   c. "If I recognize early warning signs, he might be able to take medicine and not go to the ED."
   d. "He should go to the doctor regularly to make sure his asthma is being treated correctly."

5. You are educating L.S. and his mother on possible asthma triggers in their environment. They live in public housing in an apartment without air conditioning. Which statements indicate possible asthma triggers? Select all that apply.
   a. "We have a pet fish."
   b. "L. collects stuffed animals."
   c. "There are hardwood floors."
   d. "Our visitors smoke outside."
   e. "The building has copper pipes."
   f. "There are dark stains in our bathroom."
   g. "We had to get the housing authority to treat for bugs."
   h. "He coughs when we have cold nights after a warm day."

6. Discuss strategies to avoid the triggers you identified in the previous question.

CASE STUDY PROGRESS

The following day, L.S. gets the discharge orders shown in the chart.

Chart View

Discharge Orders

Discharge to home

Follow up with primary care provider in 3 days for evaluation

Albuterol (Proventil HFA) MDI: 2 puffs with spacer every 4 hours prn

Prednisolone (Prelone) 1 mg/kg PO every day for 5 days (L.S. weighs 23 kg.)

Fluticasone (Flovent HFA) MDI, 44 mcg/inhalation: 2 puffs with spacer twice a day

Montelukast (Singulair) 5 mg every evening PO

Provide peak flow meter and teaching

Regular diet

7. Ms. S. asks why she will use the spacer with the medicine L.S. inhales. Explain the purpose of using a spacer with the metered-dose inhaler (MDI).

8. Place the steps of using the MDI with the spacer in the correct order (1 = first step, 6 = last step)
   a. ____ Depress the top of the inhaler to release medication, and breathe in slowly for 3 to 5 seconds, holding the breath for 5 to 10 seconds at the end of inspiration.
   b. ____ Shake the inhaler well, 10 to 15 times, and attach to the spacer.
   c. ____ Wait 1 to 2 minutes between puffs if more than 1 puff of the quick-relief medication is ordered.
   d. ____ Remove and exhale slowly through the nose.
   e. ____ At the end of expiration, place mouthpiece into the mouth, forming an airtight seal.
   f. ____ Tilt the head back and exhale completely.

9. During your medication teaching session with Ms. S. and L.S., you ask Ms. S. to teach back what she has learned about taking 2 different inhalers. Ms. S. makes this statement: "So, if he has to take both inhalers at the same time, he should take the Flovent first, then the albuterol. Right?" Is this statement true or false? Explain your answer.

10. Ms. S. then asks, "How long should we wait between giving the two inhalers if they are both due at the same time? Can we just give them one after the other?" What is your response?

11. As you continue your medication teaching, you explain the difference between long-term controllers and quick relief medications. Place a *C* beside the controller medication(s) and an *R* beside the quick relief medication(s).
    _____a. Albuterol
    _____b. Prelone
    _____c. Flovent
    _____d. Singulair

12. After L.S. takes a dose of the inhaled corticosteroid Flovent, what is the most important action he should do next? Explain your answer.
    a. Hold his breath for 45 seconds.
    b. Rinse out his mouth with water.
    c. Repeat the dose in 5 minutes if he feels short of breath.
    d. Check his PFM reading for an improvement of function.

 13. Ms. S. comes back from the pharmacy with the Prelone and asks you to show her how much to give. Prelone is dispensed as 15 mg/5 mL. You give her a 10-mL oral dosage syringe. How much will she draw up for this dose? (Round to tenths.)

14. During the teaching session, you give L.S. a peak flow meter (PFM) and provide teaching for him and Ms. S. But L.S. looks puzzled and asks you, "Is this another medicine I have to take?" How would you explain the purpose of a peak flow meter to L.S.?

15. L.S. tells you that he loves to play basketball and football and asks you whether he can still do these activities. How will you respond?

16. Discuss the points to include in your discharge teaching regarding prevention of acute asthmatic episodes and symptom management.

17. List 3 Internet sites to which you can refer them for further information.

CASE STUDY OUTCOME

L.S. is discharged to home and has a follow-up appointment scheduled in 2 weeks. His mother has arranged for swimming lessons, and he plans to try out for his school's swim team.

Case Study 30

Name_____ Class/Group_____ Date_____

▶ **Scenario**

H.K.'s sister has brought her 71-year-old brother to the primary care clinic because he has had a fever for 2 days. She says he has shaking chills and a productive cough and he cannot lie down to sleep because "he can't stop coughing." After H.K. is examined, he is diagnosed with community-acquired pneumonia (CAP) and admitted to your floor at 1130. The resident is busy and asks you to complete your routine admission assessment and call her with your findings.

1. Name 4 priority areas to include in your assessment.

CASE STUDY PROGRESS

Your assessment findings are as follows: H.K.'s vital signs (VS) are 154/82, 105, 32, 103° F (39.4° C), SpO_2 84% on room air. You auscultate decreased breath sounds and coarse crackles in the left lower lobe anteriorly and posteriorly. His nail beds are dusky on fingers and toes. He has cough productive of rust-colored sputum and complains of pain in the left side of his chest when he coughs. He is a lifetime nonsmoker. His medical history includes coronary artery disease and myocardial infarction with a stent. He is currently on metoprolol, amlodipine, lisinopril, and furosemide; for his type 2 diabetes mellitus, he is taking metformin and glipizide. He has never gotten a pneumococcal or flu vaccination. He does report getting "hives" when he took "an antibiotic pill" a few years ago but does not remember the name of the antibiotic.

2. Which assessment findings are significant? Give your rationale.

Chart View

Admission Orders

Consistent carbohydrate diet
VS q2hr
IV of D_5 ½NS at 125 mL/hr
Ceftriaxone 1gram IV every 12 hours
Albuterol 2.5 mg/ipratropium 250 mcg nebulizer treatment STAT, then q4hr
Titrate O_2 to maintain Spo_2 over 90%
Obtain sputum for C&S
STAT blood cultures & sensitivity
Blood glucose ac and hs with sliding scale regular insulin per protocol #2
CBC with differential and basic metabolic panel
CXR now and in the morning
Continue home medications

3. You obtain orders from the resident. Outline a plan of what you need to do in the next 2 to 3 hours.

4. Is D_5 ½NS an appropriate IV fluid for H.K.? State your rationale.

5. What is the rationale for ordering O_2 to maintain Spo_2 over 90%?

6. What is a C&S test, and what role will blood and sputum cultures play in H.K.'s care?

7. What would you expect the CXR results to reveal?

8. You need to follow a specific protocol when obtaining peripheral blood cultures. Place in order the steps you will perform.
   _____1. Select venipuncture site. Cleanse and allow to dry.
   _____2. Inject 10 mL of blood into the aerobic bottle.
   _____3. Perform venipuncture and collect 20 mL of venous blood.
   _____4. Verify patient's identity and perform hand hygiene.
   _____5. Attach identification to specimens and send to lab within 30 minutes.
   _____6. Inject 10 mL of blood into the anaerobic bottle.

9. The pharmacy sends the ceftriaxone in 100 mL 0.9% NaCl with instructions to infuse over 40 minutes. At how many milliliters per hour will you regulate the IV infusion pump?

10. How will you ensure H.K.'s home medication list is accurate?

CASE STUDY PROGRESS

The next morning you are again assigned to care for H.K. Your assessment findings are as follows: VS 154/82, 92, 26, 100° F (37.8° C), SpO_2 94% on 2 L O_2 per nasal cannula. He appears to be in no apparent distress and denies any dyspnea. You auscultate decreased breath sounds and coarse crackles in the left lower lobe anteriorly. His skin is pale, warm, and dry. He has a cough productive of yellow-colored sputum and complains of pain in the left side of his chest when he coughs.

11. Is H.K. recovering as expected? Explain your rationale.

12. Based on your evaluation of H.K., write an outcome to achieve by the end of your shift, then list 6 priority interventions you will perform toward achieving this goal.

13. By the end of your shift, which assessment findings would *best* indicate that H.K. is responding to therapy?
    a. Cough productive of yellow sputum; lung sounds clear; SpO_2 96% on room air
    b. Complaints of dyspnea; respiratory rate of 26 on 2 L O_2; clear lung sounds
    c. Cough productive of white sputum; temperature 100.0° F (37.8° C); SpO_2 98% on 2 L O_2
    d. Coarse crackles in posterior lower lobes; respiratory rate 22; no complaints of chills

CASE STUDY PROGRESS

After continuing the plan of care for 2 more days, H.K. is recovering from his pneumonia and preparing for discharge.

14. You know that H.K. is at increased risk for contracting another CAP infection. Describe 4 strategies for preventing CAP infections you will include in H.K.'s discharge teaching plan.

15. H.K. confides in you, "You know, my wife died a year ago, and I live alone now. I've been thinking . . . this pneumonia stuff has been a little scary." How will you respond?

16. What are some community resources from which H.K. may benefit?

CASE STUDY OUTCOME

H.K. is discharged in the company of his sister. His plan is to stay with her for a few days. He thanks you for your care and taking the time to listen and talk with him. He says his sister and he talked, and they intend to join the local senior center after he is feeling better.

Case Study **31**

Name_____ Class/Group_____ Date_____

▶ Scenario

J.R., a 13-year-old with cystic fibrosis (CF), is being seen in the outpatient clinic for a biannual evaluation. J.R. lives at home with his parents and 7-year-old sister, C.R., who also has CF. J.R. reports that he "doesn't feel good," explaining that he has missed the last week of school, doesn't have any energy, is coughing more, and is having "a hard time breathing."

1. Discuss additional data that should be obtained from J.R. and his parents.

2. CF is a multisystem disorder. Describe the condition and its physiologic effect on the following systems: respiratory system, gastrointestinal system, reproductive system, skin, and electrolyte balance. Focus on factors that place J.R. at risk for developing respiratory infections.

CASE STUDY PROGRESS

J.R. is admitted to the hospital for a suspected respiratory tract infection and CF exacerbation. His mother helps get him settled into the room. Your assessment includes the following vital sign 115/76, 85, 28, oral T 38.8°C, and Spo_2 88% on room air. J.R. weighs 30 kg. His color is pale and skin is dry, with bluish-tinged nail beds and clubbing; capillary refill is 3 seconds. Respiratory effort is labored, with coarse productive cough and rhonchi noted throughout. He states his pain is 3 to 4 on a scale of 10, with coughing. His thorax has a barrel-chest appearance and appears thin with decreased muscle mass. His last void and bowel movement were this morning, with no problems. J.R. is anxious and answers questions in short phrases.

3. Your institution uses electronic charting. Based on the assessment just described, which of the following systems would you mark as abnormal as you document your findings? Mark abnormal findings with an "X" and provide a brief narrative note.

☐ Neurologic:

☐ Respiratory:

☐ Cardiovascular:

☐ Gastrointestinal:

☐ Genitourinary:

☐ Musculoskeletal:

☐ Skin:

☐ Psychosocial:

☐ Pain:

4. What are the common microorganisms that cause respiratory infections in children with CF?

Chart View

Medication Orders

Ceftazidime (Fortaz) 2 g IV q8hr
Gentamicin 100 mg IV q8hr
Vancomycin (Vancocin) 450 mg IV q8hr

5. You review the drugs that have been ordered to treat J.R.'s suspected infection. You are orienting a new nurse. Which statement would you question as you review the ordered medications with her?
   a. "I have assessed for possible allergies or hypersensitivities."
   b. "I will need to monitor serum levels for some of these medications."
   c. "I will verify dosage and medication compatibility with the pharmacy."
   d. "I will obtain a blood glucose level before administering the medications."

 6. Using a nursing drug reference, find the safe dosage ranges and calculate the dosage for the prescribed antibiotics. Are the prescribed doses within the safe ranges? Explain your answers and show all work.

7. You are reviewing the physician orders for respiratory care. State whether you would expect to perform each of the following interventions and give your rationale.
   a. Administer aerosolized albuterol (2.5 mg/3 mL)
   b. Administer chest physiotherapy (CPT) before administering the albuterol
   c. Monitor continuous pulse oximetry
   d. Administer aerosolized dornase alfa (Pulmozyme) after administration of bronchodilator
   e. Administer nebulized normal saline (NS)
   f. Administer tobramycin (TOBI) via jet nebulizer
   g. Limit fluid intake

8. Methods of providing CPT are changing. Traditionally, someone other than the patient had to administer the chest percussion or vibration to help loosen mucus secretions. Newer technology, such as high-frequency chest wall oscillation (the Vest) and the positive expiratory pressure (PEP) devices (the Flutter mucus clearance device) are available. Explain the benefits of these new devices.

9. J.R.'s weight is below the 5th percentile. He has been on a high-calorie, high-protein diet with unrestricted fat at home. J.R. reports that he hasn't been hungry and really hasn't been eating much. Describe the link between malnutrition and CF.

10. Which of the following actions can be delegated to the unlicensed assistive personnel (UAP)? Explain your answer.
    a. Charting daily weights and intake and output
    b. Increasing O_2 during an episode of desaturation
    c. Instructing the parents on correct administration of NS nebulizers
    d. Administering pancreatic enzymes from the home supply with each snack

11. Which strategy is appropriate to manage GI dysfunction that patients with CF often experience? Select all that apply.
    a. Restrict fat intake
    b. Encourage a high-protein diet
    c. Encourage snacks between meals
    d. Administer fat-soluble vitamins daily
    e. Hold proton pump inhibitor or H_2 blocker
    f. Breastfeeding is contraindicated in infants with CF
    g. Administer pancreatic enzymes with meals and snacks

12. What clinical sign assists in determining the effective dosage of pancreatic enzymes?

13. Which GI comorbidities might you see in a patient with CF? Select all that apply.
    a. Constipation
    b. Celiac disease
    c. Rectal prolapse
    d. Meconium ileus
    e. Chronic vomiting

J.R. will be spending 14 to 21 days in the hospital for treatment of his pulmonary infection.

14. List interventions that would foster development while J.R. is hospitalized.

15. J.R. asks you, "Will I be able to have children when I grow up?" While keeping his age in mind, which of these would be the best response? Explain your answer.
   a. "You should discuss this with your parents. I will let them know you asked."
   b. "Most males have a significant chance of being sterile, and you won't need to consider use of contraception."
   c. "CF does not affect the male reproductive system; however, it does affect the female reproductive tract."
   d. "Although nearly 95% of males are sterile, you should discuss this with your physician and family."

J.R.'s condition improves with antibiotic therapy, and he is being discharged to home.

16. As you provide your discharge teaching, discuss health promotion points to reinforce with J.R. and his parents.

J.R. is discharged to home, with a PEP device, and enjoys the fact that he is able to apply it himself.

Case Study 32

Name _____ Class/Group _____ Date _____

▶ Scenario

C.E., a 73-year-old married man and retired railroad engineer, visited his physician complaining, "Whenever I try to do anything, I get so out of breath I can't go on. I think I'm just getting older, but my wife told me I had to come see you about it." He has a history of hyperlipidemia and hypertension, which are managed with lisinopril, furosemide, atorvastatin, and metoprolol, and has a 30-pack-year smoking history. He had greenish-yellow sputum, an oral temperature of 100.4 ° F (38.4 ° C), and an Spo$_2$ of 83%. He was admitted to the local hospital with a new diagnosis of COPD exacerbation. After a 5-day stay during which the diagnosis of COPD was confirmed, he was discharged on continuous oxygen (O$_2$) therapy at a 2 L flow rate with new prescriptions for fluticasone/salmeterol (Advair Diskus) and albuterol (ProAir). You are the case manager at the home agency assigned to C.E.

1. What is the rationale for C.E.'s O$_2$ being at a 2 L flow rate?

2. What criteria need to be met for Medicare to pay for home O$_2$ therapy?

3. Which member of the interprofessional team would be involved in C.E.'s care and how?

4. How would you prepare for the initial home visit?

5. What would you address with C.E. and his wife at the first visit?

6. What manifestations of COPD would you expect C.E. to have? (Select all that apply.)
   a. Elevated temperature
   b. Complaints of fatigue
   c. Wheezing on auscultation
   d. Chronic, intermittent cough
   e. Prolonged expiratory phase
   f. Decreased anterior-posterior diameter

7. What patient problems would you to address as you develop C.E.'s plan of care?

8. What ongoing monitoring do you need to do at each visit with C.E.?

9. What are 2 specific questions you can ask C.E. to determine if he may be experiencing any complications?

CASE STUDY PROGRESS

Your first visit with C.E. and his wife is uneventful. You perform his baseline assessment, provide teaching, and establish a monitoring plan. The next time you visit, C.E. complains of sores behind his ears. He explains, "That long oxygen tubing seems to take on a life of its own. It twists around and gets caught under doors, chairs, everything. It darn near rips the ears off my head."

10. What can you tell him that could help?

11. You auscultate C.E.'s breath sounds and detect the odor of menthol rub. When you question C.E. about it, he tells you that he started to apply it in and around his nose to prevent his nose from becoming dry and sore. What specific teaching do you need to reinforce with C.E. and his wife?

 12. After you have finished, his wife seems upset and tells you that C.E. is still "smoking a couple of cigarettes" a day. How do you handle this situation?

CASE STUDY PROGRESS

At your next visit 2 weeks later, C.E. tells you that he has not smoked since your previous visit. He is upset, though, over an episode a few days ago. He says he walked to the kitchen for a snack and became short of breath. Per your instructions, C.E. removed the nasal cannula, tested the flow against his check, and felt no O_2 flowing from the catheter. He said he could not yell for help and was too short of breath to return to the living room to check his O_2 tank. He bent forward with his elbows on the countertop and struggled to breathe. He became more frightened with each passing second, and his breathing became increasingly more difficult. Several minutes later, C.E.'s wife found him and reconnected his O_2 tubing. C.E. sat at the table for 20 minutes before he could walk back to the living room.

13. Why did C.E. assume the peculiar position at the countertop?

14. C.E.'s wife states that since the incident, C.E. "doesn't want her out of his sight." She asks you to "talk some sense into him." She goes on to say that since then "All he does is sit in a chair all day. He won't even get up to get himself a glass of water. I've got a bad hip, and this is all very hard on me." What will you do to help C.E. and his wife cope with his condition?

15. What referrals could you consider at this time and why?

CASE STUDY PROGRESS

The next few visits are uneventful. C.E. has continued to not smoke and is doing better with managing episodes of dyspnea. At your next visit, you greet C.E., immediately note that he sounds congested, and comment that he sounds like he has a cold. He replies, "Oh, our great-grandchildren were over to visit several days ago and they all had snotty noses."

16. What is your immediate concern and why?

17. What assessment do you need to perform?

18. Which assessment finding would require your immediate intervention?
a. C.E.'s sputum is yellowish
b. The pulse oximeter reading is 93%
c. His oral temperature is 102.0° F (38.9° C)
d. He is dyspneic when walking to the bathroom.

19. What information would you want to review with C.E. and his wife about the signs and symptoms of infection and when to seek treatment?

20. What basic hygiene measures would you include in a teaching plan for C.E. and his wife to prevent his developing an infection? Select all that apply.

a. Avoid enclosed, public areas at all times.

b. Get pneumonia and flu vaccines every year.

c. Avoid people with cold and flu infections and screen visitors.

d. Practice good hand washing technique, and wash hands often.

e. Use the dishwasher to wash eating utensils, glasses, and plates.

f. Use antibacterial wipes daily to clean frequently touched surfaces.

21. C.E.'s wife says she would like to read more about COPD on the Internet. List 2 credible resources to which you could direct her.

CASE STUDY OUTCOME

You continue to visit C.E. and his wife and monitor his progress over the next several months. C.E. experiences an episode of pneumonia and experiences acute respiratory failure and sepsis, which leave him with residual neurologic deficits. He is discharged to a long-term care facility.

Case Study 33

Name_____   Class/Group_____   Date_____

▶ Scenario

D.Z., a 68-year-old man, is admitted at 1600 to a medical floor with an acute exacerbation of chronic obstructive pulmonary disease (COPD). His other medical history includes hypertension and type 2 diabetes. He has had pneumonia yearly for the past 3 years and has been a two-pack-a-day smoker for 38 years. His current medications include enalapril (Vasotec), hydrochlorothiazide, metformin (Glucophage), and fluticasone/salmeterol (Advair). He appears a cachectic man who is having difficulty breathing at rest. D.Z. seems irritable and anxious; he complains of sleeping poorly and states that lately he feels tired most of the time. He reports cough productive of thick yellow-green sputum. You auscultate decreased breath sounds, expiratory wheezes, and coarse crackles in both lower lobes anteriorly and posteriorly. His vital signs (VS) are 162/84, 124, 36, 102° F (38.9° C), and Spo_2 88%.

Chart View

Admission Orders

Diet as tolerated
Out of bed with one-person assistance
Oxygen (O_2) to maintain Spo_2 of 90%
IV of D_5W at 50 mL/hr
ECG monitoring
ABGs in a.m.
CBC with differential now
Basic metabolic panel now
Chest x-ray daily
Sputum culture
Albuterol 2.5 mg plus ipratropium 250 mcg nebulizer treatment STAT

1. Are D.Z.'s VS and Spo_2 acceptable? If not, explain why.

2. Describe a plan for implementing these orders.

3. What is the primary nursing goal at this time?

4. Based on this priority, name 3 independent nursing actions you would implement and why.

5. Identify 3 expected outcomes for D.Z. as a result of your interventions.

Chart View

Medication Administration Record

  Methylprednisolone (Solu-Medrol) 125 mg IV push every 8 hours
  Azithromycin (Zithromax) 500 mg IVPB q24hr
  Fluticasone/salmeterol (Advair) 100/50 mcg 2 puffs twice daily
  Heparin 4000 units subcutaneous every 12 hours
  Enalapril (Vasotec) 10 mg PO daily
  Albuterol 2.5 mg/ipratropium 250 mcg nebulizer treatment every 6 hours
  Metformin (Glucophage) 500 mg PO twice daily
  Nicotine patch 24 mg for 24 hours, daily

6. Indicate the expected outcome associated with each medication D.Z. is receiving.

7. Because D.Z. is on azithromycin, what interventions need to be included in his plan of care? Select all that apply.
   a. Place D.Z. on intake and output.
   b. Administer the medication over 30 minutes.
   c. Request a hearing test before initiating therapy.
   d. Monitor IV site for inflammation or extravasation.
   e. Assess liver function study results and bilirubin levels.
   f. Carefully dilute the medication in the proper amount of solution.

 8. D.Z is ordered heparin 4000 units subcutaneous q12hr. The following vial is available. How many milliliters will D.Z. receive? Shade in the dose on the syringe.

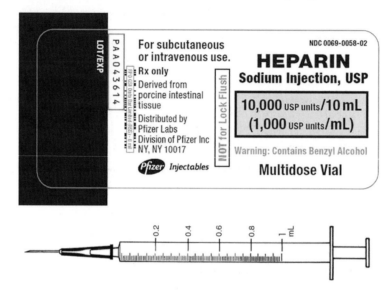

9. What common side effects of bronchodilator therapy do you need to assess for?

10. When you apply the nicotine patch, you take the opportunity to ask D.Z. if he would like information on smoking cessation. He tells you he is interested because he has to "stop while he is in here." How can you support his continuing cessation after discharge?

11. You deliver D.Z.'s dietary tray, and he comments on how hungry he is. As you leave the room, he is rapidly consuming the mashed potatoes. When you pick up the tray, you notice that he has not touched anything else. When you question him, he states, "I don't understand it. I can be so hungry, but when I start to eat, I have trouble breathing and I have to stop." Describe 4 interventions that might improve his caloric intake.

12. What other interprofessional team members could you involve in D.Z.'s care and how?

 13. After speaking with D.Z. about his diet and reviewing his medications, you are now concerned about his glycemic control. Hospital policy allows you to obtain as-needed blood glucose levels for patient with diabetes, so you direct the UAP to obtain D.Z.'s blood glucose level before the next meal. What is your responsibility in delegating this task to the UAP?

14. The UAP reports that D.Z.'s blood glucose level is 366 mg/dL. What action do you need to take and why?

CASE STUDY PROGRESS

The next morning, D.Z. is sitting in the bedside chair and appears to be experiencing less difficulty breathing. He states his cough remains productive of yellow-green sputum, although it is "easier to cough up" than it was the previous day. You auscultate decreased breath sounds and a few coarse crackles in both lower lobes posteriorly. His VS are 150/78, 94, 24, 99.7° F (37.6° C). His Spo_2 is 92% with O_2 on at L per nasal cannula.

Chart View

Arterial Blood Gases

pH	7.33
$Paco_2$	58 mm Hg
HCO_3	32 mEq/L (32 mmol/L)
Pao_2	65 mm Hg
Sao_2	92%

15. Interpret D.Z.'s ABG values.

16. Has D.Z.'s status improved or not? Defend your response.

17. What interventions would you include in your plan of care for D.Z. today?

CASE STUDY PROGRESS

D.Z.'s wife approaches you in the hallway and says, "I don't know what to do. My husband used to be so active before he retired 6 months ago. Since then he's lost 35 pounds (16 kg). He is going downhill so fast that it scares me. He wants me in the room with him all the time, but if I try to talk with him, he snarls and does things to irritate me. I have to keep working. We don't want to drain all of our savings, and I have to be able to support myself when he's gone. Sometimes I go to work just to get away from the house and his constant demands. He calls me several times a day asking me to come home, but I can't go home. I just don't know what to do."

18. How would you respond to her statement?

19. What topics do you need to address with D.Z. to reduce his risk for readmission?

CASE STUDY OUTCOME

D.Z. is discharged after 6 days with instructions to follow up with the primary care provider in 1 week. At the appointment, D.Z. reports he has been able to maintain his smoking cessation and is feeling less dyspnea. The provider continues the respiratory medication regimen and arranges for D.Z. to begin pulmonary rehabilitation therapy the next week.

Case Study 34

Name_____ Class/Group_____ Date_____

▶ Scenario

E.M., a 5-month-old girl, is brought to the emergency department (ED) with respiratory distress, hypoxia, and fever. Her parents state that she has had mild cold symptoms for a few days. She has breastfed poorly over the last few days, with a decreased number of wet diapers. You take her vital signs and complete an initial physical assessment and history.

Chart View

Vital Signs

Blood pressure	130/72
Respiratory rate	83
Heart rate	188
Temperature	38.6°C (101.5°F)
SpO_2	88% on room air
Weight	17.6 lbs (8 kg)

Initial Assessment

Neurologic	Alert, fussy; consoles briefly; anterior fontanel soft and slightly depressed
Cardiovascular	Tachycardia; capillary refill less than 3 seconds
Respiratory	Upper airway congestion; coarse cough; tachypnea, transient bilateral wheezing; coarse rhonchi and slightly decreased breath sounds at bases; mild intercostal retractions; mild nasal flaring
Gastrointestinal	Positive bowel sounds; last bowel movement yesterday
Genitourinary	Decreased urine output (per history); no urine output in last 4 hours
Skin	No rashes; slightly flushed
Other	Mucous membranes "sticky"; decreased tearing

Emergency Department Orders

Acetaminophen (Tylenol) 80 mg PO for fever × 1 dose
Start IV and administer normal saline (NS) bolus 20 mL/kg IV bolus over 30 minutes
Oxygen to keep saturation greater than 92%

1. Review the standing ED orders. Prioritize your interventions and give rationales.

2. Based on E.M.'s vital signs and assessment, what diagnostic tests would you anticipate?

3. Calculate how much normal saline E.M. will receive as a bolus.

CASE STUDY PROGRESS

E.M. begins coughing and has copious nasal secretions. You provide nasopharyngeal suctioning and obtain a large amount of thick secretions. Deep suctioning is used as infrequently as possible because it can be counterproductive, causing increased edema and secretions, and increased agitation of infant. She is allowed to recover and is reassessed. The respiratory rate and retractions have not changed significantly. Her breath sounds are less coarse but are diminished in the bases. The Spo_2 is now 92% to 93% on 1.5 L oxygen. After E.M. settles, her mother asks whether she can feed her because she has not eaten much for the past few days. You tell her that with a current respiratory rate higher than 65, she should not be fed.

4. What is the rationale for holding feedings?

5. When E.M.'s respiratory rate decreases, what teaching would you provide the parents concerning feeding?

Chart View

Medication Administration Record

Normal saline drops to nares q3hr with bulb suctioning
Acetaminophen (Tylenol) 80 mg PO q4hr prn for fever greater than 38.5°C (101.3°F)
Oxygen via nasal cannula (N/C) adjusted up to 2 L/min to maintain Spo_2 greater than 90%.
Amoxicillin (Amoxil) 45 mg/kg/day PO tid × 7 days

6. You are reviewing the medication administration record. Which order(s) would you question? Explain.

CASE STUDY PROGRESS

E.M.'s mother calls you to the room because her baby is "not right." You note E.M.'s respiratory rate is 23, and the intercostal retractions and nasal flaring have increased. She also has moderate subcostal retractions. The SpO_2 is 89% on 1.5 L/min of O_2. She is pale and listless and does not cry with stimulation. The oxygen is increased to 2 L/min with no change in status after 5 minutes.

7. Why is the respiratory rate significantly lower even though other signs of respiratory distress have increased?

CASE STUDY PROGRESS

You are concerned and call the rapid response team. You check her SpO_2 again with results of 88%. The senior resident orders a portable chest x-ray (CXR) examination and capillary blood gas (CBG). The CXR is consistent with bronchiolitis with atelectasis.

Chart View

Capillary Blood Gas

pH	7.31
$PaCO_2$	72 mm Hg
HCO_3	29 mEq/L (29 mmol/L)
PaO_2	57 mm Hg

8. Interpret E.M.'s CBG results.

CASE STUDY PROGRESS

E.M. is transferred to the pediatric intensive care unit (PICU) and placed on a heated high-flow nasal cannula, a noninvasive method that offers many of the same benefits as continuous positive airway pressure (CPAP), at 5 L/min. You know that patients with bronchiolitis generally have progressively increased symptoms from days 3 to 5. This is day 3 for E.M., and therefore she may stay in the PICU for several days until she starts improving and can be transferred to the general care floor. You explain this to the parents, who are very distressed.

9. What resources might you seek for E.M.'s parents during this unanticipated change in status?

10. You are considering measures to help E.M.'s parents deal with the anxiety and fear created by their infant's hospitalization and transfer to PICU. For each measure listed, explain why each answer is appropriate or not.
    a. The presence of the parents helps calm the infant.
    b. Parents need to put the needs of E.M. ahead of their own.
    c. Parental anxiety cannot be recognized by a 5-month-old infant.
    d. Provide detailed technical information about her care in the PICU to help the parents cope with the situation better.

CASE STUDY PROGRESS

After 2 days in the PICU, E.M. is transferred back to your unit. You note that she is taking increased oral fluids and requiring less suctioning. Her Spo_2 is 96% to 98% on room air. She is still having some mucus production and coughing. As you are preparing the parents for discharge, they want to know how they can prevent this in the future. They ask whether there is a "shot" E.M. can get to avoid getting this again.

11. How would you address their concerns?

12. E.M.'s parents ask you for instructions about the treatment of cold symptoms if E.M. develops them again. Which answer is correct? Explain your answer.
    a. "If a fever is present, you can treat the fever with baby aspirin."
    b. "Saline nose drops and bulb suctioning can be done before feedings."
    c. "Over-the-counter cough suppressants may be safely administered at night."
    d. "You do not need to worry if she is not drinking; intake should improve in a day or so."

13. What other specific teaching relating to fluid balance and normal signs and symptoms on discharge should be done before E.M. is discharged? E.M. now weighs 17 lbs (7.8 kg) and is drinking from a 6-oz bottle.

CASE STUDY OUTCOME

E.M. is discharged to home with her parents. The parents are instructed follow up with her pediatrician within the next few days and to call with any concerns.

Case Study 35

Name_____ Class/Group_____ Date_____

▶ Scenario

You are the trauma nurse working in the emergency department (ED) of a busy tertiary care facility. You receive a call from the paramedics that they are en route with the victim of gunshot wounds to the chest and abdomen. Perpetrators shot the 32-year-old man during a convenience store robbery. The victim was a customer; the clerk died at the scene. They started 2 16-gauge IV lines with lactated Ringer's solution and oxygen by nonrebreather mask at 15 L/min. The patient has a sucking chest wound on the left and a wound in the right upper quadrant of the abdomen. Vital signs in the field are 90/46, 140, and 42. The paramedics state they are having difficulty ventilating the patient, who is diaphoretic, very pale, and lethargic. The estimated time of arrival is 4 minutes.

1. To help determine the extent of the patient's injuries, the most important question the nurse needs to ask the paramedics is:
   a. "How long ago was the patient shot?"
   b. "Do you have the weapon that was used?"
   c. "What was the reason this incident occurred?"
   d. "Where are the assumed entry and exit wounds?"

2. Describe a sucking chest wound.

3. What are the classic assessment findings associated with a sucking chest wound?

4. Explain why the paramedics are having difficulty ventilating the patient.

5. List at least 6 things you will do to prepare for the patient's arrival.

6. Describe the priority roles of the nurse in a trauma situation.

7. Besides the lead provider, who usually responds to a trauma code and what are their roles?

8. What are your basic responsibilities regarding gathering forensic evidence?

CASE STUDY PROGRESS

On arrival, the patient, B.W., is cyanotic and in severe respiratory distress. His VS are 70/30, 160, and 42. When he is transferred to the trauma stretcher, you notice that there is an occlusive dressing over the open chest wound. It is taped down on all sides.

9. Is taping the occlusive dressing on all sides appropriate? Explain.

10. Which assessment findings would indicate B.W. may have a tension pneumothorax? Select all that apply.
a. Bilateral jugular vein distention
b. Tracheal deviation toward the affected side
c. Decreased breath sounds on the opposite side
d. Tracheal deviation toward the unaffected side
e. Decreased heart rate and decreased respirations

Chart View

Arterial Blood Gases (100% O_2)

pH	7.25
$Paco_2$	92 mm Hg
Pao_2	32 mm Hg
HCO_3	26 mEq/L (26 mmol/L)
Spo_2	53%

11. Interpret B.W.'s ABG results.

12. Based on B.W.'s vital signs and condition, what are the priority interventions?

CASE STUDY PROGRESS

The surgeon determines B.W. has a tension pneumothorax and performs a needle decompression followed by insertion of a size 32-Fr chest tube in the sixth intercostal space, midaxillary line. Treatments aimed toward stabilizing B.W.'s respiratory and volume statuses are started, and the anesthesiologist prepares to intubate B.W.

13. What are your responsibilities regarding endotracheal intubation?

14. How is endotracheal tube placement confirmed after intubation?

15. After B.W. is successfully intubated, describe the actions that you will perform as part of the secondary survey.

16. Would you expect his lung to reexpand immediately after the chest tube insertion and starting suction? Explain.

17. When evaluating the effectiveness of chest tube therapy, you would assess for:
   a. Increased drainage in the collection chamber
   b. Continuous bubbling in the water seal chamber
   c. A fall in the water seal chamber with inspiration
   d. Symmetrical breath sounds and chest expansion

18. You note the following ecchymotic area on B.W.'s abdomen along with distention and rigidity. What might this signify?

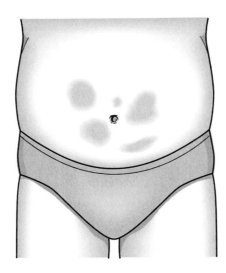

19. You report your findings to the physician, who orders a focused abdominal sonography for trauma (FAST). Why is this procedure appropriate for B.W.?

CASE STUDY PROGRESS

The FAST is positive. B.W. is sent for a CT of the abdomen, which shows a large liver laceration. The surgeon needs to take B.W. to the operating room (OR) for an exploratory laparotomy with repair of the liver laceration.

 20. Because B.W. is not able to give consent for surgery, how will consent be obtained?

21. When you return from transporting the patient to the OR, B.W.'s wife is in the ED, upset and frightened. The social worker has been called to another emergency. What information do you need to obtain from B.W.'s wife?

22. How would you support her?

CASE STUDY OUTCOME

Surgeons repaired B.W.'s wounds. He spent 3 days in the surgical intensive care unit, where he required continued fluid and respiratory support, and 14 days later he went home. After discharge, B.W. spent 3 months receiving physical therapy and counseling for victims of violent crime.

2 Gas Exchange

Case Study 36

Name_____   Class/Group_____   Date_____

▶ Scenario

A.B., a 68-year-old man, is admitted to your medical floor with a diagnosis of pleural effusion. He relates having shortness of breath; pain in his chest; weakness; and a dry, irritating cough. His vital signs (VS) are 142/82, 118, respirations 38 and labored and shallow, 102.1° F (38.9° C), and Spo$_2$ 85% on room air. Chest x-ray examination shows a large pleural effusion and pulmonary infiltrates in the right lower lobe consistent with pneumonia.

1. Given his diagnosis, are A.B.'s admission VS expected? Explain.

2. How does the underlying pathophysiology relate to A.B.'s presenting signs and symptoms?

CASE STUDY PROGRESS

The provider performs a thoracentesis and drains 1500 mL of fluid. A specimen for culture and sensitivity (C&S) is sent to the lab, and A.B. is started on ceftriaxone 500 mg IV every 12 hours.

3. What is a thoracentesis?

4. The order for the ceftriaxone reads to infuse the 100 mL 0.9% NaCl solution over 30 minutes. An IV pump will not be available for a few hours, so you decide to run the infusion by gravity. You have IV tubing that supplies 20 gtt/mL. At how many drops per minute will you regulate the infusion?

5. What interventions will you implement to help A.B.'s clear pulmonary secretions?

CASE STUDY PROGRESS

The pleural C&S results show a large amount of *Klebsiella* organism growth that is not sensitive to ceftriaxone.

 6. What action will you take next?

7. Because fluid continues to collect in the pleural space, the physician decides to insert a pleural chest tube under nonemergent conditions. What are your responsibilities as A.B.'s nurse regarding this procedure?

8. Part of your responsibilities after the chest tube has been inserted is to assess for fluctuation in the water-seal chamber and bubbling in the suction-control chamber. Label the areas on the chest drainage system that you would be monitoring.

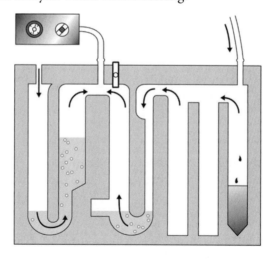

(Modified from Linton AL. Introduction to Medical-Surgical Nursing, *4th ed. St. Louis, MO: Saunders; 2007.)*

9. What interventions will you implement afterward to maintain A.B.'s chest tube system?

10. Evaluate each of the following statements about chest tube drainage systems. Enter *T* for true or *F* for false. State why false statements are incorrect.

_____1. The height of the water in the suction control mechanism limits the amount of suction transmitted to the pleural cavity.

_____2. A suction pressure of +20 cm H_2O is usually recommended for adults.

_____3. Bubbling in the water-seal chamber usually means that air is leaking from the lungs, the tubing, or the insertion site.

_____4. The rise and fall of the water level with the patient's respirations reflect normal pressure changes in the pleural cavity with respirations.

_____5. Water cannot evaporate from the system.

_____6. To declot the drainage tubing, put lotion on your hands, compress the tubing, and vigorously strip long segments of the tubing before releasing.

_____7. You lower the bed on top of the drainage system and break it. You immediately clamp the chest tube, leaving it clamped until you can reestablish the drainage system.

_____8. The collection chamber is full, so you need to connect a new drainage system. Briefly clamp the chest tube while you disconnect the old system and connect the new.

11. While A.B. has a chest drainage system, what instructions do you need to give to the UAP who is working with A.B.?

12. It is now the end of your shift and A.B.'s condition has stabilized. Using the SBAR framework, describe the bedside change-of-shift report you will give the oncoming nurse.

CASE STUDY PROGRESS

The next day you are again assigned to care for A.B. At the beginning of the shift, you assess A.B. and find that his condition is stable. His lung sounds remain diminished in the right lower lobe and his Spo_2 is 95% on oxygen at 2 L per nasal cannula. The chest drainage system is attached to suction at 20 mm Hg; there is still an air leak present. His morning chest x-ray examination showed some residual pleural effusion. Four hours into your shift, he pages you through the call system and tells you he feels "short of breath." You immediately go to his room. A.B. is sitting in the chair.

13. Describe the priority assessment you must perform at this time.

14. You find the chest tube has become disconnected from the drainage system and is now contaminated. What do you need to do?

15. After the chest drainage system has been reestablished, A.B.'s dyspnea resolves, and you need to document what happened. Write an example of a documentation entry describing this event.

CASE STUDY PROGRESS

The remainder of A.B.'s admission is uneventful. After 6 days of aggressive antibiotic and pulmonary therapy, the chest tube is removed and A.B. is ready for discharge.

16. What type of discharge instructions do you need to give to A.B.?

CASE STUDY OUTCOME

A week later, A.B. and his wife send a cookie tray to the floor, along with a note praising the staff for the quality care A.B. received. They also nominate you for one of your facility's nursing excellence awards, saying that you "provided amazing care" and were the type of nurse "everyone wants by their side."

Case Study 37

Name _____ Class/Group _____ Date _____

> ▶ **Scenario**

S.K., a 51-year-old roofer, was admitted to the hospital 3 days ago after falling 15 feet from a roof. He sustained bilateral fractured wrists and an open fracture of the left tibia and fibula. He was taken to surgery for open reduction and internal fixation (ORIF) of all his fractures. He is recovering on your orthopedic unit. You have orders to begin getting him out of bed and into the chair today. When you enter the room to get S.K. into the chair, you note he is agitated and dyspneic. He says to you, "My chest hurts really badly. I can't breathe." You auscultate S.K.'s breath sounds and find they are diminished in the left lower lobe. S.K. is diaphoretic and has circumoral cyanosis. His VS are 142/82, 118 and irregular, respirations 38 and labored and shallow, 99.8° F (37.7° C), and Spo_2 85% on O_2 at 2 L nasal cannula

1. Identify 5 possible reasons for S.K.'s symptoms.

2. List in order of priority 3 actions you should take next.

3. Using SBAR, what information will you give to the provider?

> **CASE STUDY PROGRESS**

The attending orders the following: STAT arterial blood gases (ABGs), chest x-ray (CXR) examination, 12-lead electrocardiogram, and a helical (spiral) computed tomography (CT) scan of the lungs.

Chart View

Arterial Blood Gases

pH	7.49
$Paco_2$	30.6 mm Hg
Pao_2	52 mm Hg
HCO_3	24.2 mmol/L
Sao_2	83%

4. Interpret S.K.'s ABG results.

5. Based on the ABGs and your assessment findings, what complication do you think S.K. is experiencing?

6. Why is S.K. at risk for developing this complication?

7. What are the typical manifestations of this complication? Underline those that S.K. has.

8. How is this complication best prevented from occurring?

9. The resident writes the following orders for S.K. Review each order. Mark with an *A* if the order is appropriate; mark with an *I* if the order is inappropriate. Correct all inappropriate orders and give rationales for your decisions.

_____ 1. Albuterol (Proventil) metered-dose inhaler, 2 puffs q6hr

_____ 2. Heparin 20,000 units IV now, then 25,000 units in 250 mL/D_5W to run at 18 units/kg per hour

_____ 3. Prothrombin time/international normalized ratio/partial thromboplastin time (PT/INR/PTT) q6hr; call house officer with results

_____ 4. Increase O_2 to 3 L by nasal cannula

_____ 5. Patient-controlled analgesia (PCA) pump with morphine sulfate: Loading dose 4 mg; dose 2 mg; lock-out time 15 minutes; maximum 4-h dose 30 mg

_____ 6. Streptokinase 250,000 international units IV over 30 minutes, then 100,000 international units/hr for 24 hr

_____ 7. Warfarin (Coumadin) 7.5 mg/day PO × 2 days

_____ 8. Complete blood count daily

 10. S.K. weighs 224 lb. Calculate the starting infusion rate in milliliters per hour for the heparin. (Round to the nearest tenth.)

11. S.K. asks why he is starting heparin. Your best response is:
a. "It will stop any blood clots from going to your lungs."
b. "The heparin will dissolve any other blood clots you have."
c. "Heparin will prevent any new blood clots from developing."
d. "The heparin will thin your blood so you will be able to breathe better."

CASE STUDY PROGRESS

All the orders are corrected. S.K.'s helical CT scan confirms the diagnosis of pulmonary embolism (PE) in the left lower lobe. Two hours later, repeat ABGs provide the values shown in the chart.

Chart View

Arterial Blood Gases

pH	7.46
$Paco_2$	33 mm Hg
Pao_2	82 mm Hg
HCO_3	24.1 mEq/L
Sao_2	90%

12. What do these ABGs indicate?

13. The attending orders furosemide 20 mg IV push now. What is the expected outcome associated with giving furosemide to S.K.?

14. What is your primary nursing goal at this time?

15. List 4 independent nursing interventions you would implement for S.K. that support this goal and the rationale for each.

 16. Because S.K. is receiving heparin therapy, he has the potential for bleeding. What interventions will be part of his plan of care to reduce this risk? Select all that apply.
a. Assess VS every 4 hours.
b. Use a central line to obtain blood specimens.
c. Apply direct pressure to any venipuncture site for 5 minutes.
d. Do not give any intramuscular medications unless absolutely necessary.
e. At least once a shift, check stool, urine, sputum, and vomitus for occult blood.

 17. To ensure S.K.'s safety, what instructions would you give to the UAP assisting with his care? Select all that apply.
a. Use an electric razor when shaving S.K.
b. Immediately report any signs of bleeding.
c. Inflate the BP cuff only as high as needed to obtain a reading.
d. Position S.K. with the head of his bed elevated, on his left side.
e. Use a sponge-toothed applicator when helping S.K. with oral care.

2 Gas Exchange

Chart View

Laboratory Test Values

PT	12.1 seconds
PTT	54 seconds
INR	1.4

Chart View

Weight-Based Heparin Protocol

1. Begin IV infusion of heparin at 18 units/kg per hour using 25,000 units heparin in 250 mL D_5 W. Obtain coagulation panel every 6 hours.
2. Adjust IV heparin based on activated partial thromboplastin time results:
   - ↓ 49 s, bolus with 80 units/kg and ↑ rate by 4 units/kg per hour
   - 50 to 59 s, bolus with 40 units/kg and ↑ rate by 2 units/kg per hour
   - 60 to 90 s, no change
   - ↑ 91 to 109 s, bolus with 80 units/kg and ↓ rate by 2 units/kg per hour
   - ↑ 110 s, stop infusion for 1 hour, then resume and ↓ rate by 3 units/kg per hour

18. Coagulation times are rechecked after S.K. has been on heparin therapy for 6 hours. What action do you need to take?

19. The heparin is supplied in a multiple-dose vial. How many milliliters will you administer? (Round to the hundredth.)

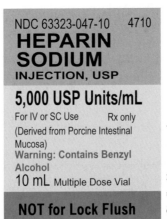

NDC 63323-047-10   4710

HEPARIN SODIUM
INJECTION, USP

5,000 USP Units/mL
For IV or SC Use   Rx only
(Derived from Porcine Intestinal Mucosa)
Warning: Contains Benzyl Alcohol
10 mL Multiple Dose Vial

NOT for Lock Flush

Sterile, Nonpyrogenic
Each mL contains: 5,000 USP Units
heparin sodium: 15 mg benzyl alcohol:
6 mg sodium chloride: Water for Injection
q.s. Hydrochloric acid and/or sodium
hydroxide may have been added for pH
adjustment.
Usual Dosage: See insert.
Use only if solution is clear and seal intact.
Store at 20° to 25°C (68° to 77°F) [see
USP Controlled Room Temperature].
This container closure is not made from
natural rubber latex.

APP Pharmaceuticals, LLC
Schaumburg, IL 60173

401796H

LOT/EXP

3 63323-047-10 8

CASE STUDY PROGRESS

S.K. is watched closely for the next several days for the onset of pulmonary edema. Anticoagulant therapy, O_2, pulse oximetry, daily CXR studies and ABG analysis, and pain management are continued.

20. On postoperative day 7, S.K. suddenly becomes very angry and throws the physical therapist out of his room. He yells, "I'm sick and tired of having everyone tell me what to do." How are you going to deal with this situation?

CASE STUDY OUTCOME

Ten days after the occurrence of the PE, S.K. was discharged to a long-term acute care facility for assistance with strengthening and ambulation.

Case Study 38

Name _____ Class/Group _____ Date _____

▶ Scenario

The intensive care unit (ICU) nurse calls to give you the following report: "D.S. is a 66-year-old man who is postop day 3 after a right lower lobe lobectomy. He had quit smoking 12 years ago and exercises regularly. He went to see his physician with complaints of increasing exertional dyspnea; CXR and imaging showed a mass in the right lung without any evidence of metastases. The pathology report came back today and confirming stage IB non–small cell lung cancer. The surgeon said there were clean margins. He has no neurologic deficits. His vital signs run 120/70, 110, about 30, with a fever around 100.2° F. His heart tones are clear, all peripheral pulses are palpable, and he is receiving IV D$_5$ ½ NS at 50 mL/hr in his PICC line. He has a right midaxillary chest tube; there is no air leak, and it is draining small amounts of serosanguineous fluid. He has pain at the insertion site, but the site looks good, and the dressing is dry and intact. He is on 4 L oxygen by nasal cannula. He has not had any pain medication today, nor has he slept since surgery. He'll be there in about 20 minutes."

1. What additional information would you ask the nurse to provide?

2. Smoking accounts for 60% of lung cancers. True or false?

3. D.S. presented with exertional dyspnea. What are other common manifestations of lung cancer?

4. Describe the type of surgery D.S. underwent and its role in lung cancer treatment.

5. What are the implications of D.S.'s cancer being a stage IB and the surgeon reporting clean margins?

6. What is the health care team's primary goal for D.S. at this time?

7. Outline interventions you will include in his plan of care to help achieve this goal and give a rationale for each.

CASE STUDY PROGRESS

D.S. is transported by wheelchair past the nurses' station to a room at the end of the hall. You enter his room for the first time to find him sitting on the edge of the bed with his left leg in bed and his right foot on the floor. As you introduce yourself, you note that he keeps rubbing his left hand over the right side of his chest. His respiratory rate is 30 with an SpO_2 of 90%. His respirations are slightly labored, and he appears dyspneic.

8. What issues or problems can you already identify?

9. Describe 3 things you need to do right now for D.S.

CASE STUDY PROGRESS

When asking D.S. about his reluctance to take pain medication, he replies, "I have a nephew who rolled his Jeep and busted himself up real bad. He got hooked on those drugs, and I don't want any part of them."

10. How would you respond to D.S.'s statement?

11. Which nonpharmacologic methods of pain relief may help D.S.? Select all that apply.
   a. Hypnosis
   b. Distraction
   c. Positioning
   d. Biofeedback
   e. Acupuncture

12. You administer morphine sulfate 4 mg IV and tell D.S. that you will return in 30 minutes; 15 minutes later, he turns on his call light. When you enter the room, D.S. says, "I think I'm going to throw up." What are the next 3 things you would do?

13. D.S. states, "I started to feel sick a couple minutes ago. It just kept getting worse until I knew I was going to throw up." What do you think caused the sudden onset of nausea?

14. Should you give D.S. another dose of morphine? What are your options?

15. You decide to call the surgeon to report the reaction. Using SBAR, what would you report?

16. The surgeon changes D.S.'s pain medication to fentanyl and orders ondansetron (Zofran) 4 mg IV every 6 hours as needed for nausea. You use a floor-stocked multidose vial to administer the first dose. How many milliliters will you give?

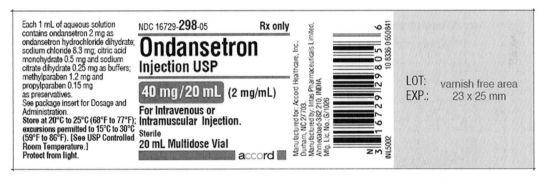

(From Macklin D, Chernecky C, Infortuna MH. Math for Clinical Practice. *2nd ed. St. Louis, MO: Mosby; 2011.)*

17. D.S. is having difficulty using his right arm. Given the type of surgery he underwent, is this expected and why?

18. D.S.'s pain and nausea are under control an hour later. The physical therapist arrives to perform passive exercises on D.S.'s right arm. The exercises are done to:
   a. Lower the risk for developing lymphedema
   b. Reduce spasticity of the shoulder and chest muscles
   c. Assist the patient in learning to reuse the affected arm
   d. Preserve muscle strength and reduce the effects of disuse

CASE STUDY PROGRESS

The next afternoon, the nurse giving you D.S.'s report says that he has been driving her crazy all morning. She tells you that he has been irritable and demanding. She says his assessment and VS are "okay" except for his Spo_2, which has been around 85%. The morning CXR showed infiltrates in the left lung.

19. What is your immediate concern?

CASE STUDY PROGRESS

You enter D.S.'s room to assess him and to tell him you are going to be his nurse again today. He is sitting on the side of the bed with his arms hunched up on the overbed table. You note that his head bobs up and his mouth opens, like a fish taking in water, every time he inhales. He says, "I just can't [breath] seem to [breath] get enough [breath] air."

20. Name 6 possible problems that D.S. could have that would account for his behavior.

21. What actions will you take next?

CASE STUDY PROGRESS

D.S.'s respiratory rate is 46, with an Spo_2 of 66%. You auscultate slight air movement over the large airways and no breath sounds distal to the third intercostal space. The chest drainage system is intact. His gown is in his lap, he is diaphoretic, you note intercostal retractions with inspiration, and all muscles of the upper torso are engaged in respiration.

22. What will you do next?

23. The rapid response team stabilizes D.S., and you go with him during transfer to the ICU. Why do you do this, and what information would you give to the ICU nurse?

2 Gas Exchange

CASE STUDY OUTCOME

After stabilizing D.S. in the ICU, the surgeon returns to your floor and is upset that he was not notified earlier about the change in D.S.'s condition. The next day you approach the nurse who gave you report, who is a new graduate, and explain how to better identify patients in early stages of respiratory difficulty. She thanks you for helping her learn from her mistake. D.S. experiences no further complications and completely recovers from the lobectomy after 2 months. He receives 6 months of external beam radiation therapy to the chest. His examination at 5 years shows no recurrence.

Case Study 39

Name_____ Class/Group_____ Date_____

▶ Scenario

P.R., a 66-year-old woman who has no history of respiratory disease, is being admitted to your intensive care unit (ICU) from the emergency department (ED) with a diagnosis of pneumonia and acute respiratory failure (ARF). The ED nurse tells you that P.R. was stuporous and cyanotic on her arrival to the ED. Her initial vital signs (VS) were 90/68, 134, 38, 101° F (38.3° C) an Spo_2 of 53%. She was endotracheally intubated orally, was placed on mechanical ventilation, and has equal breath sounds. Her ventilator settings are synchronized intermittent mandatory ventilation of 12/min, tidal volume (V_T) 700 mL, Fio_2 0.50, and positive end-expiratory pressure (PEEP) 5 cm H_2O. The nurse tells you P.R. had a chest x-ray (CXR) examination that confirmed the diagnosis of pneumonia before being intubated, but she needs an another CXR examination STAT.

1. Describe the pathophysiology of ARF.

2. How does the underlying pathophysiology relate to P.R.'s presenting signs and symptoms?

3. Describe each of P.R.'s ventilator settings and the rationale for each.

4. Why does P.R. need a second CXR examination?

Chart View

Arterial Blood Gases

pH	7.28
$Paco_2$	62 mm Hg
HCO_3	26 mEq/L
Pao_2	48 mm Hg
Spo_2	56%

5. The ABG results from the sample drawn in the ED before intubation are sent to you. Interpret P.R.'s ABG results.

CASE STUDY PROGRESS

The ICU attending assesses P.R. and after reviewing the ED orders, writes the following orders in addition to the mechanical ventilation protocol.

Chart View

Physician's Orders

Blood and sputum cultures STAT
ABGs via arterial line every 6 hours
NGT to intermittent, low suction
Insert indwelling urinary catheter
Enoxaparin (Lovenox) 40 mg subcutaneous q24hr at 1700
Apply anti-embolism and intermittent pneumatic compression stockings
Pantoprazole (Protonix) IV 40 mg daily
Lorazepam 1 mg IV every 4 hours
Ceftriaxone 1gram IV q8hr
D_5 ½ NS at 125 mL/hr

2 Gas Exchange

6. What is the rationale for each order?

7. What is your priority nursing goal at this time?

8. Describe the interventions you will perform over the next 2 hours based on this priority and the orders you need to implement.

9. P.R. is not heavily sedated and seems anxious about all that is going on. Describe how you can help her.

Arterial Blood Gases

pH	7.30
$Paco_2$	52 mm Hg
HCO_3	22 mEq/L
Pao_2	70 mm Hg
Spo_2	88%

10. ABGs are redrawn after P.R. has been on mechanical ventilation for 2 hours. What ventilator setting changes do you expect based on your interpretation? Select all that apply and explain your rationale.
    a. Decreasing the Fio_2 to 0.40
    b. Increasing the V_T to 850 mL
    c. Increasing the PEEP to 10 cm
    d. Increasing the rate on the ventilator to 16/min
    e. Changing to continuous mandatory ventilation

11. Evaluate each statement about caring for P.R. or a similar patient receiving mechanical ventilation with an endotracheal tube (ETT). Enter *T* for true or *F* for false. State why the false statements are incorrect.
    _____1. Give muscle-paralyzing agents to keep P.R. from "fighting the vent."
    _____2. Check ventilator settings at the beginning of each shift and then hourly.
    _____3. When suctioning the ETT, each pass should not exceed 15 seconds.
    _____4. Assign experienced UAP to take vital signs every 2 to 4 hours.
    _____5. Perform a respiratory assessment once per shift.
    _____6. Empty excess water that collects in the ventilation tubing back into the humidifier.
    _____7. Keep a resuscitation bag at the bedside.
    _____8. Monitor the cuff pressure of the ETT every 8 hours.
    _____9. Silence ventilator alarms when in the room to maintain a quiet environment.
    _____10. Change all ventilator tubings every 12 hours.

 12. What are 3 evidence-based practices you will need to implement to prevent ventilator-assisted pneumonia?

13. You hear the high-pressure alarm sounding on the mechanical ventilator and see that P.R.'s Sao$_2$ is 80%. What are potential causes of this problem?

14. You decide that P.R. needs to be suctioned. Place in order the steps for safely performing in-line or closed suctioning.

_____1. Hyperoxygenate the patient.

_____2. Use 5 to 10 mL of saline to rinse the catheter clear of secretions.

_____3. Insert catheter until you meet resistance or the patient coughs.

_____4. Assess patient's status and document procedure.

_____5. Put on clean gloves and face shield and attach suction.

_____6. Apply suction as you withdraw the catheter, not exceeding 10 seconds.

_____7. Reassess patient status and suction again as needed.

CASE STUDY PROGRESS

As P.R.'s primary nurse, you are responsible for her nursing care plan. Although the primary concern is her respiratory status, you are concerned about hydration, nutrition, oral hygiene, and skin integrity and decide to address each of these areas in P.R.'s plan of care.

15. Discuss 5 indicators you can use to assess her fluid status.

16. Write a nutrition-related outcome for P.R.

17. Describe 4 interventions that could assist in meeting P.R.'s nutrition goals.

18. You plan to assess P.R.'s skin every 4 hours. Name 4 other strategies that will help meet the expected outcome of maintaining skin integrity?

Over the next few days, P.R. progressively regains adequate respiratory functioning.

19. What factors would be considered in deciding when P.R. is ready to be weaned from mechanical ventilation?

20. What are your responsibilities during the weaning process?

21. Which assessment finding during the weaning process would indicate P.R. should be placed back on the ventilator?
a. Sao_2 of 94%
b. Heart rate 92
c. Temperature 99.3° F (37.4° C)
d. Respiratory rate 34

P.R. is easily weaned from the ventilator, and her respiratory function continued to improve. Unfortunately, she developed a urinary tract infection, experienced acute confusion for a few days, and had difficulty ambulating. She stayed 7 more days after being weaned before being discharged home.

Case Study **40**

Name _____ Class/Group _____ Date _____

▶ Scenario

G.S., a 56-year-old woman, was involved in a motor vehicle accident; a car drifted left of the center line and struck her head-on, pinning her behind the steering wheel. She was intubated immediately after extrication and flown to your trauma center. Her injuries were extensive: bilateral flail chest, right hemothorax and pneumothorax, fractured spleen, multiple small liver lacerations, open fractures of both legs, and a cardiac contusion. She was taken to the operating room for repair of her injuries. There she received 36 units of packed red blood cells, 20 units of platelets, 12 units of fresh frozen plasma, and 18 L of lactated Ringer's solution. G.S. was admitted to the ICU postoperatively, where she developed acute respiratory distress syndrome (ARDS).

1. What is ARDS?

2. What are the risk factors for developing ARDS? Which does G.S. have?

3. With her extensive injuries, how was ARDS diagnosed?

4. Describe the collaborative care patients generally receive in the ICU for ARDS.

CASE STUDY PROGRESS

After a 3-week stay in ICU, G.S. is being transferred to your unit. The ICU nurse gives you the following report: "She is awake, alert, and oriented to person and place. Both legs remain casted from hip to toe. She can wiggle her toes on both feet. Heart tones are clear, last vital signs were 138/90, 88, 26, 99.3° F (37.4° C); bilateral radial pulses 3 +. All the surgical incisions are healed. She has bilateral chest tubes to water suction with closed drainage, both dressings are dry and intact. She has a duodenal feeding tube, a Foley catheter to down drain, and a left double-lumen PICC line. Urine output is good; urine is clear yellow. Her morning labs are still pending."

5. What additional information do you need from the ICU nurse?

6. Describe the phase of ARDS G.S. is in.

7. What are the long-term complications of ARDS you need to monitor for in G.S.?

CASE STUDY PROGRESS

You complete your assessment of G.S. You note she is dyspneic and has fine crackles throughout all lung fields posteriorly and in both lower lobes anteriorly, and coarse crackles over the large airways. She has O_2 on at 2 L per nasal cannula and her Spo_2 is 94%.

8. What is the significance of the fine and coarse crackles?

9. The nurse from the previous shift charted the following statement: "Fine and coarse crackles that clear with vigorous coughing." Based on your knowledge of pathophysiology, determine the accuracy of this statement.

10. It is time to administer scheduled furosemide (Lasix) 60 mg intravenous push. What effect, if any, should furosemide have on G.S.'s breath sounds?

 11. What action do you need to take before giving the furosemide?

Chart View

Laboratory Results

Sodium	129 mmol/L
Potassium	3.0 mmol/L
Chloride	92 mmol/L
HCO_3	26 mEq/L
BUN	37 mg/dL
Creatinine	2 mg/dL
Glucose	128 mg/dL
Calcium	7.1 mg/dL

12. Which lab values concern you, and why?

 13. Given G.S.'s lab values, what action do you need to take and why?

CASE STUDY PROGRESS

The provider wants you to administer the furosemide and prescribes the following.

Chart View

Physician's Orders

STAT magnesium (Mg) level
Potassium chloride (KCl) 40 mEq IVPB
Calcium gluconate 2 g in 100 mL NS IVPB over 3 hours

14. Why did the provider order a magnesium level?

15. G.S. has 1 available port to use on the PICC line. Outline a plan for giving the potassium chloride and calcium gluconate.

 16. What interventions do you need to perform to safely administer IV potassium chloride? Select all that apply.
   a. Administer the infusion using an IV pump.
   b. Place G.S. on continuous electrocardiogram (ECG) monitoring.
   c. Assess the patency of the PICC line before initiating the infusion.
   d. Administer the potassium infusion over a period of at least 2 hours.
   e. Invert the potassium-containing IV bag several times before and during the infusion.

 17. You go to prepare G.S.'s furosemide dose and find only one 20-mg vial in the medication-dispensing system. The floor stock is empty. The pharmacist tells you that it will be at least an hour before he can send the drug to you. What are your options?

18. While you are giving the furosemide, G.S. says, "This is so weird. A couple times this morning, I felt like my heart flipped upside down in my chest, but now I feel like there's a bird flopping around in there." What are 2 actions you should take next?

2 Gas Exchange

19. G.S.'s pulse is 66 and irregular. Her blood pressure is 92/70 and respirations are 26. She admits to being "a little lightheaded" but denies having pain or nausea. Your co-worker connects G.S. to the code cart monitor for a "quick look." Interpret what you see.

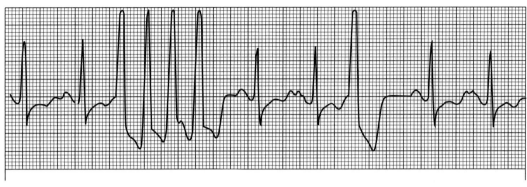

(From Aehlert B. ECGs Made Easy. *4th ed. St. Louis, MO: Mosby/JEMS; 2011.)*

20. Why is G.S. likely experiencing this dysrhythmia?

21. What will your next actions be?

Chart View

Arterial Blood Gases on 6 L O_2 by Nasal Cannula	
pH	7.30
Paco$_2$	59 mm Hg
Pao$_2$	82 mm Hg
HCO$_3$	36 mEq/L
Spo$_2$	91%

22. You increase her O_2 to 6 L, and the provider orders a STAT set of ABGs. How would you interpret G.S.'s ABGs?

23. What are your nursing priorities at this time?

24. Describe 5 interventions you will perform over the next few hours based on these priorities.

25. You notice that G.S. looks frightened and is lying stiff as a board. How would you respond to this situation?

CASE STUDY OUTCOME

G.S.'s pulmonary status does not improve after the furosemide, and she continues to have frequent ventricular dysrhythmias despite receiving the electrolytes. The provider transfers G.S. back to the ICU, where she is found to have a pulmonary embolus. Unfortunately, 1 week later she throws another embolus and all attempts at resuscitation fail.

Mobility

Case Study **41**

Name_____ Class/Group_____ Date_____

▶ **Scenario**

M.S., a 74-year-old woman, comes to your clinic for a complete physical examination. She has not been to a provider for 11 years because "I don't like doctors." Her only complaint today is "pain in my upper back." She describes the pain as sharp and knifelike. The pain began approximately 3 weeks ago when she was getting out of bed in the morning and hasn't changed at all. M.S. rates her pain as 6 on a 0- to 10-point pain scale and says the pain decreases to 3 or 4 after taking "a couple of ibuprofen." She denies recent falls or trauma.

M.S. admits she needs to quit smoking and start exercising but states, "I don't have the energy to exercise and, besides, I've always been thin." She has smoked one to two packs of cigarettes per day since she was 17 years old. Her last blood work was 11 years ago, and she cannot remember the results. She went through menopause at the age of 47 and has never taken hormone replacement therapy. The physical examination findings are unremarkable other than moderate tenderness to deep palpation over the spinous process at T7. There are no masses or tenderness to the tissue surrounding the tender spot. No visible masses, skin changes, or erythema are noted. Her neurologic findings are intact, and no muscle wasting is noted.

1. An x-ray examination of the thoracic spine reveals a collapsed vertebra at T7 and bone density changes in the spine. What could this result indicate?

2. The physician suspects osteoporosis. List 7 risk factors associated with osteoporosis.

3. Place a star or asterisk next to those risk factors specific to M.S.

M.S. has never had an osteoporosis screening. She confides that her mother and grandmother were diagnosed with osteoporosis when they were in their early 50s.

4. What diagnostic test is most commonly used to diagnose osteoporosis?

5. M.S.'s diagnostic test revealed a bone density T-score of −2.7. How will this be interpreted?

6. M.S. receives a prescription for alendronate (Fosamax) 70 mg/wk. Which instructions are appropriate as you provide patient teaching to M.S. about this drug? Select all that apply.
   a. "You can eat your breakfast along with this medication."
   b. "Take the medication with 8 ounces (236 mL) of water immediately on arising."
   c. "You can take this medication with your morning coffee or orange juice."
   d. "You need to sit or stand upright for at least 30 minutes after taking the medication."
   e. "If you experience any severe abdominal pain, vomiting, or jaw pain, notify your doctor immediately."

7. M.S. asks whether she needs to take a calcium supplement. How do you answer her?

M.S. asks you about foods that contain calcium. "I'd rather eat than take all these pills," she states. You review food sources of calcium with her.

8. Which foods are considered good sources of dietary calcium? Select all that apply.
   a. Banana
   b. Chicken salad
   c. 8 ounces (226 grams) of yogurt
   d. 1 cup (236 mL) of cooked spinach
   e. Baked potato with margarine

CASE STUDY PROGRESS

After reviewing her new prescription, you continue your teaching session about osteoporosis with M.S.

9. What nonpharmacologic interventions will you teach M.S. to prevent further bone loss?

10. M.S. begins to cry and says, "I cannot possibly stop smoking, change my diet, and exercise all at the same time." You encourage M.S. to start working on one problem at a time. How should it be decided which problem M.S. should attempt first?

CASE STUDY PROGRESS

One month later, M.S. comes in to the clinic and tells you that she stopped the Fosamax a week ago because it upset her stomach too much. The physician decides to start her on denosumab (Prolia), but asks M.S. to see her dentist first.

11. M.S. asks you why she needs to see a dentist before starting the new drug. Which problem may occur during therapy with denosumab?
   a. Gingivitis
   b. Tooth loss
   c. Tooth decay (cavities)
   d. Osteonecrosis of the jaw

12. How is denosumab given?

CASE STUDY OUTCOME

M.S. receives her first injection of denosumab 1 month later and has no significant adverse effects. At her 3-month check-up, she tells you that she finally stopped smoking and was excited to note a 5-pound (2.25 kg) weight loss.

Case Study 42

Name_____ Class/Group_____ Date_____

▶ Scenario

J.C. is a 41-year-old man who comes to the emergency department with acute low back pain. He states that he did some heavy lifting yesterday, went to bed with a mild backache, and awoke this morning with terrible back pain, which he rates as a 10 on a scale of 1 to 10. He admits to having had a similar episode of back pain years ago "after I lifted something heavy at work." J.C. has a medical history of peptic ulcer disease related to nonsteroidal antiinflammatory drug (NSAID) use. He is 6 feet tall (183 cm), weighs 265 pounds (120 kg), and has a prominent "potbelly."

1. What questions would be appropriate to ask J.C. in evaluating the extent of his back pain and injury?

2. What observable characteristic does J.C. have that makes him highly susceptible to low back injury?

3. J.C. took piroxicam (Feldene) 20 mg until he developed his duodenal ulcer. What is the relationship between the two? What signs and symptoms would you expect if an ulcer developed?

CASE STUDY PROGRESS

All serious medical conditions are ruled out, and J.C. is diagnosed with lumbar strain. The nurse practitioner (NP) orders a physical therapy consultation to develop a home stretching and back-strengthening exercise program and a dietary consultation for weight reduction. The NP gives J.C. prescriptions for cyclobenzaprine (Flexeril) 10 mg tid for 3 days only, and celecoxib (Celebrex) 100 mg/day for 3 months. He receives the following instructions: heat applications to the lower back for 20 to 30 minutes four times a day (using moist heat from heat packs or hot towels), no twisting or unnecessary bending, and no lifting more than 10 pounds (4.5 kg). J.C. is instructed to rest his back for 1 or 2 days, getting up only now and then to move around to relieve muscle spasms in his back and strengthen his back muscles. He is given a written excuse to stay off work for 7 days and, when he returns to work, specifying the limitation of lifting no more than 10 pounds (4.5 kg) for 3 months. He is instructed to contact his primary care provider if the pain gets worse.

3 Mobility

4. J.C. looks at the prescription for cyclobenzaprine and states, "I'm glad you didn't give me that Valium. They gave me Valium last time and that stuff knocked me out." How would you respond to J.C.?

5. Why do you think he was prescribed cyclobenzaprine instead of diazepam (Valium)?

6. J.C. states, "Well, I'm glad I'll still be able to take my sleeping pill." True or False? Explain.

CASE STUDY PROGRESS

J.C. asks, "What is Celebrex? I hope it won't do what that Feldene did to me years ago."

7. Why do you think it was prescribed for J.C., considering his gastrointestinal (GI) history?

8. It has been over 5 years since his last episode of GI bleeding. Are there any other conditions you need to assess for before J.C. begins to take the celecoxib? Explain.

9. Why would the NP prescribe an NSAID rather than acetaminophen for J.C.'s pain?

10. A physical therapist teaches J.C. maintenance exercises he can do on his own to promote back health. Describe 3 common exercises that would be included.

11. In addition to learning exercises, J.C. needs to learn proper body mechanics for lifting and performing day-to-day activities. Which statement by J.C. indicates a need for further instruction?
   a. "I will bend my knees when I lean forward."
   b. "When lifting heavy boxes, I will bend at the waist."
   c. "I will not lift anything above the level of my elbows."
   d. "I will avoid standing in one position for a long period of time."

12. J.C. tells you that when his back hurts, he has trouble getting comfortable when he goes to bed at night. What sleeping position would help him?
   a. Prone position
   b. Supine with legs out straight.
   c. Side-lying with knees and hips flexed.
   d. Position of the body during sleep does not affect back pain.

CASE STUDY OUTCOME

J.C. takes a week off from work to rest and uses warm compresses twice a day on his back. He returns to "light duty" at work for a period of 3 months.

3 Mobility

Case Study 43

Name_____ Class/Group_____ Date_____

▶ Scenario

D.M., a 25-year-old man, hops into the emergency department (ED) with complaints of right ankle pain. He states that he was playing basketball and stepped on another player's foot, inverting his ankle. You note swelling over the lateral malleolus down to the area of the fourth and fifth metatarsals, and pedal pulses are 3+ bilaterally. His vital signs (VS) are 124/76, 82, 18. He has no allergies and takes no medication. He states he has had no prior surgeries or medical problems.

1. In assessing D.M.'s injured ankle, what should you evaluate?

2. What will initial management of the ankle involve to prevent further swelling and injury?

3. You note significant swelling over the fourth and fifth metatarsals. How would you further evaluate this finding?

4. Which assessment finding would indicate that D.M. has a fracture instead of a sprain? Select all that apply.
   a. Bruising
   b. Slight swelling
   c. Inability to bear weight
   d. Increased pain with movement
   e. Deformity or abnormal position of the ankle

CASE STUDY PROGRESS

X-ray results are negative for fracture, and a second-degree sprain is diagnosed. The physician orders immobilization with an elastic bandage and an air stirrup brace, with instructions for crutches. The physician tells D.M. not to bear weight on his ankle for 2 days, then to use only partial weight bearing until the ankle heals.

5. Describe the technique for applying an elastic wrap. Give the rationale.

6. An hour after you apply the elastic wrap, D.M. states that his "toes are tingling" and his foot feels numb. What is the best action at this time?

7. When instructing D.M. to use crutches, D.M. states that he "likes it better" when the crutches rest under his arms while he walks with the crutches. Is this correct? Explain.

8. You instruct D.M. on using the three-point gait with the crutches. Which would be the correct first step for the three-point gait? Explain your answer.
a. Step first with the affected leg.
b. Step first with the unaffected leg.
c. Step first with both crutches and the affected leg.
d. Step first with the affected leg and the crutch opposite of the affected leg.

9. You are to instruct D.M. on application of cold, activity, and care of the ankle. What would be appropriate instructions in these areas?

10. D.M. is given a prescription for ibuprofen tablets, 400 mg, every 6 hours as needed for pain. Explain the purpose of this drug.

11. You provide instructions about the use of ibuprofen. Using the Teach-Back method, you ask D.M. to teach you what he has learned. Which statement by D.M. indicates a need for more teaching?

a. "I will take these pain pills with food or a snack."

b. "I will not take aspirin while taking this medicine."

c. "It would not hurt if I have a few beers while taking this."

d. "I will take no more than 2 pills every 6 hours if needed for pain."

CASE STUDY PROGRESS

Six days later, D.M. hobbles into the ED and boldly informs you that he "did it again, only this time it was touch football." He states that the pain pills worked so well, he thought it would be okay. You detect the odor of beer on his breath.

12. What are you going to do?

13. D.M.'s blood alcohol concentration (BAC) result is 0.06 mg%. Interpret this result. Does this level reflect legal intoxication?

14. Are there any concerns about his alcohol consumption and his prescription medicine? Explain.

15. You remove his sock and find a large hematoma forming on the lateral aspect of an already swollen ankle. The ankle shows the color of a bruise that is several days old. You inquire about D.M.'s pain perception. He states, "It doesn't feel too bad now, as long as I don't walk on it, but I sure saw stars when it popped." What is the significance of his statement?

CASE STUDY OUTCOME

D.M.'s ankle is fractured. His ankle is splinted for now with plans for a cast in a few days, after the initial swelling subsides. A referral to an orthopedic surgeon is obtained. You discuss his use of the pain medication and his drinking. He tells you that he did realize it could be harmful. He is now upset that it happened because he will not be playing any sports for some time.

Case Study 44

Name_____ Class/Group_____ Date_____

▶ Scenario

W.S., a 75-year-old man, was just admitted to an orthopedic surgery unit after undergoing right knee arthroplasty surgery. He is groggy but awake and states he is not in pain at this time. His right knee has a surgical dressing that is dry and intact. He has knee-high compression stockings on and is attached to sequential compression devices.

1. What is arthroplasty surgery of the knee?

2. What factors contribute to the decision to have knee arthroplasty surgery?

3. What immediate assessments will you perform?

Chart View

Post-Op Orders

Ice pack to operative site for 30 minutes every 4 hr
Cefazolin (Ancef) 1 gram IV q8hr × 2 doses
Acetaminophen (OFIRMEV) 1000 mg IV q6hr × 2, then acetaminophen 1000 mg PO q6hr
Ketorolac (Toradol) 15 mg IV q8hr × 3 doses, then start celecoxib (Celebrex) 100 mg PO q12hr
Morphine 4 mg IV q4hr prn for moderate to severe pain
Enoxaparin (Lovenox) 30 mg q12hr SubQ for 10 days
Advance diet as tolerated
Incentive spirometer
Knee-high compression stockings
SCDs
Begin PT/OT
Case Management referral

3 Mobility

4. Which interventions are part of pain management? Explain the purpose for each one.

5. What measures are ordered to prevent deep vein thrombosis (DVT)? Explain the function of each one.

6. Describe how you will assess for a DVT.

7. What are other possible postoperative complications of knee arthroplasty?

8. The UAP is assisting W.S. with positioning in the bed. Which position would you intervene to correct?
   a. The knee is hyperextended.
   b. The knee is in a neutral position.
   c. The knee is not rotated internally or externally.
   d. One pillow is placed under the lower calf and foot to encourage slight knee joint extension.

CASE STUDY PROGRESS

W.S. tells you that his friend had knee surgery that was "ruined" by an infection, and he is worried about that happening to him.

9. What signs and symptoms would alert the nurse to a possible infection?

 10. What is the most important intervention that can be done to prevent infection?

11. W.S. comments that the compression stockings are so difficult to put on, and asks you if they can be left on all the time. What would you teach W.S. about compression stockings? Select all that apply.
   a. "These stockings can be worn 24/7."
   b. "The stockings should be hand washed and air dried daily."
   c. "They should be applied before you get out of bed in the morning."
   d. "These stockings are used to strengthen the muscles in your lower legs."
   e. "We need to take them off daily to check the condition of the skin on your legs and feet."

12. Correct the incorrect statements in the previous question.

CASE STUDY PROGRESS

The next morning, the physical therapist works with W.S. on getting out of bed and walking with a walker. W.S. tolerates the session well but is glad to get back into the bed after all the activity.

13. After his first PT session, you notice a small amount of drainage on W.S.'s knee dressing. Which is the best action at this time?
   a. Remove the dressing
   b. Do nothing and continue to monitor
   c. Replace the dressing with a fresh dressing.
   d. Draw a circle around the drainage area, and date/time it with your initials

The next morning during your assessment, W.S. tells you that he wants to improve his walking, but he is afraid that the PT will "hurt too much."

14. When is the best time for W.S. to receive his pain medication? Explain your answer.

15. What types of exercises can W.S. perform in between PT sessions?

16. W.S. tells the physical therapist that he cannot wait to take long walks again when he gets home. Which answer by the physical therapist is correct?
   a. "Yes, that will be great exercise for you."
   b. "That should be fine after a month of therapy."
   c. "You will not be able to take long walks again now that you've had this surgery."
   d. "It takes time to reach your maximum strength and endurance, from 6 months to a year."

CASE STUDY OUTCOME

W.S. refused to go to a rehab facility and was discharged to his home with home health visits from a physical therapist and a nurse. He performed all the prescribed exercises, and his wife and daughter helped with his care. Within 3 months he was driving again and taking short walks in his neighborhood.

Case Study **45**

Name_____ Class/Group_____ Date_____

▶ Scenario

H.K. is a 26-year-old man who tried to light a cigarette while driving and lost control of his truck. The truck flipped and landed on the passenger side. H.K. was transported to the emergency department with a deformed, edematous right lower leg and a deep laceration wound approximately 2 inches (5 cm) long over the deformity. Blood continues to ooze from the wound.

1. What further assessment will you make of the leg injury and what precautions will you take in making this assessment?

2. What is the most appropriate method for controlling bleeding at this wound site?

3. What is the best way to immobilize the leg injury before surgery?

4. From the information given, it is clear that H.K. is a smoker. List at least 3 issues related to his smoking that can complicate his care and recovery. What interventions could be instituted to counter these complications?

CASE STUDY PROGRESS

H.K. is taken to surgery for open reduction and internal fixation (ORIF) of the tibia and fibula fractures. He returns with a full-leg fiberglass cast with windows over the areas of surgery.

5. Describe the assessment of a patient with a long leg cast involving trauma and surgery.

6. In assessing H.K.'s cast on the third day postoperatively, you notice a strong foul odor. Drainage on the cast is extending, and H.K. is complaining of pain more often and seems considerably more uncomfortable. Vital signs are 123/78, 102, 18, 102.2° F (39° C). What is your analysis of these findings, and what action is needed?

CASE STUDY PROGRESS

H.K. returns to surgery. The wound over H.K.'s fracture site has become necrotic with purulent drainage. The wound is debrided and cultured and a posterior splint is applied. H.K. returns to his room with orders for wet-to-moist dressing changes. The physician suspects osteomyelitis and orders nafcillin (Unipen) and ciprofloxacin (Cipro). Contact precautions are implemented.

7. Why are 2 antibiotics ordered?

8. H.K. asks you about the isolation precautions. "Does this mean I have something bad?" What is your best answer?
   a. "These are precautions that we use for every patient who has surgery."
   b. "These are precautions we are taking to help your infection get better."
   c. "This is an extremely serious infection; these precautions will keep the infection from getting worse."
   d. "These precautions prevent the spread of the infection to other patients and to health care personnel."

9. As you continue to assess H.K. over the following days, what evidence will you look for that antibiotics are effectively treating the infection?

10. Develop a teaching plan concerning the care of his cast.

11. After the teaching session, you use the Teach-Back method to assess H.K.'s learning. You ask H.K.: "We have reviewed a lot of information on how to care for your cast. To make sure that I explained it well to you, please tell me three things you will do." Which statements by H.K. indicates a good understanding of cast care? Select all that apply.
   a. "I will not get the cast wet."
   b. "I will keep plastic over the cast to protect it."
   c. "I will call my doctor if I notice a bad odor or see drainage."
   d. "I will keep my leg elevated above the level of my heart for the first 2 days."
   e. "I will use a long file if it gets itchy inside my cast to scratch my skin gently."

12. What nutritional needs does H.K. have and why?

CASE STUDY PROGRESS

To ensure pain management, H.K. is given hydromorphone (Dilaudid) 2 mg IV push every 4 hours prn pain. You prepare to give him the first dose.

13. Name this drug's therapeutic category.

14. What signs and symptoms would you see if he were to have a toxic or overdose reaction to the Dilaudid? Select all that apply.
   a. Nausea
   b. Pruritus
   c. Dilated pupils
   d. Respiratory depression
   e. Central nervous system (CNS) depression

15. What is the first thing you will need to do if you note a toxic or overdose reaction to the Dilaudid?

16. What is the antidote for toxic opioid reactions? How is it administered?

CASE STUDY PROGRESS

H.K. has no further complications with his leg wound and responds well to physical therapy. The discharge planner meets with him to discuss his posthospital care.

17. What issues would the discharge planner need to address with H.K.?

CASE STUDY OUTCOME

H.K. was discharged to his apartment, where he could stay with financial help from his parents. He continued on oral antibiotics for another month. Friends drove him to physical therapy on their way to classes at the university and took him back on their way home. He managed well and went back to work while still in his cast.

Case Study **46**

Name_____ Class/Group_____ Date_____

▶ Scenario

M.M., a 76-year-old retired schoolteacher, is postoperative day 2 after an open reduction and internal fix-ation (ORIF) for a fracture of his right femur. He has been on bed rest since surgery. At 0800, his vital signs (VS) are 132/84, 80 with regular rhythm, 18 unlabored, and 99° F (37.2° C), and Spo$_2$ 97% on room air. He is awake, alert, and oriented with no adventitious heart sounds. Breath sounds are clear but diminished in the bases bilaterally. Bowel sounds are present, and he is taking sips of clear liquids. He is receiving an intravenous (IV) infusion of D$_5$ ½ NS at 75 mL/hr in his left hand, and orders are to change it to a saline lock this morning if he is able to maintain adequate oral fluid intake. He has orders for oxygen (O$_2$) to maintain Spo$_2$ over 92%, but he has been refusing to wear the nasal cannula. Pain is controlled with morphine sul-fate 4 mg IV as needed every 4 hours, and he has ondansetron (Zofran) 4 mg IV every 4 hours as needed for nausea. He is receiving enoxaparin (Lovenox) 30 mg subcutaneously once daily, and taking docusate sodium (Colace) PO once daily.

At 1830 you answer M.M.'s call light and find him lying in bed breathing rapidly and rubbing the right side of his chest. He is complaining of right-sided chest pain and appears to be restless.

1. What will you do?

CASE STUDY PROGRESS

You check his VS, with these results: BP 98/60; P 120; R 24. You note he is restless and slightly confused. The pulse oximeter reads 86%, so you start him on 6 L O$_2$ by nasal cannula (NC). You identify faint crackles in the posterior bases bilaterally. The heart monitor on lead II shows nonspecific T wave changes.

2. Using *s*ituation, *b*ackground, *a*ssessment, *r*ecommendation (SBAR), what information, based on the findings, would you provide to the physician when you call?

3. The physician asks you to transfer M.M. to the ICU and orders blood coagulation studies, arterial blood gases (ABGs) on room air, continuous pulse oximetry, STAT chest x-ray (CXR), and STAT 12-lead ECG. What information will the physician gain from each of these?

4. Why would the physician order ABGs on room air as opposed to with supplemental O_2?

CASE STUDY PROGRESS

You evaluate the room air ABG results.

Chart View

Arterial Blood Gases	
pH	7.55
$Paco_2$	24 mm Hg
HCO_3	24 mEq/L (24 mmol/L)
Pao_2	56 mm Hg
Sao_2	86% (room air)

5. What is your interpretation of the ABGs, and what do you think the physician will order next, and why?

CASE STUDY PROGRESS

The CXR image shows a small right infiltrate. The physician suspects an embolism and orders a STAT spiral CT scan of the lungs. The interpretation of the results reads "strongly suggestive of a pulmonary embolus (PE)."

6. What are the most likely sources of the embolus?

7. For each characteristic in the following list, note whether it is a characteristic of a fat embolus *(F)*, a blood clot embolus *(BC)* in the lungs, or both *(B)*.
   a. Altered mental status
   b. Decreased Sao$_2$
   c. Petechiae
   d. Chest pain
   e. Crackles
   f. Increased respirations and pulse

CASE STUDY PROGRESS

The physician orders heparin using the Heparin Protocol listed below. M.M. weighs 76 kg.

Chart View

Heparin Protocol

Initial bolus: Give 80 units/kg.
Initial infusion: 18 units/kg/hr.
   Every 6 hours, check aPTT. Follow titration instructions:
   a. PTT less than 55 seconds
      Give bolus of 80 units/kg and increase infusion rate by 4 units/kg/hr
   b. 55 to 69 seconds
      Give 40 units/kg bolus and increase infusion rate by 2 units/kg/hr
   c. 70 to 105 seconds
      NO change in rate
   d. 106 to 140 seconds
      Decrease infusion rate by 2 units/kg/hr from previous rate
   e. Greater than 140 seconds
      i. Hold heparin infusion for 1 hour, then reduce infusion by 3 units/kg/hr
      ii. Notify MD

 8. How many units will M.M. receive for this bolus?

 9. What is the rate (milliliters per hour) for the initial infusion (round to the whole number)? The heparin solution is 25,000 units in 500 mL 0.45% NS.

10. After 6 hours, the lab calls you with a critical PTT result of 155 seconds. Per the protocol, what action will you take?

11. The physician is considering administering an antidote to the heparin. Which generic drug is considered an antidote to heparin therapy?
   a. Atropine
   b. Vitamin K
   c. Protamine sulfate
   d. Potassium chloride

CASE STUDY PROGRESS

The physician decides not to administer an antidote and orders the heparin to be held, with a second aPTT drawn in 2 hours. M.M. is monitored closely. After 2 hours, the aPTT is 95 seconds.

12. What is your evaluation of this aPTT level?

13. The physician resumes the heparin at a lower rate, and there are no further issues with the lab results. The next day, the physician's orders read, "Warfarin (Coumadin) 2.5 mg PO, PT/INR in a.m.; D/C heparin." Do you have any concerns about these orders? Explain your answer.

14. List 3 priority problems related to the care of M.M. in his current situation.

15. Several days later you hear M.M. asking his son to bring in a "decent razor" because he is tired of having beard stubble. How would you address this issue?

16. Before M.M. goes home, the physician switches the oral anticoagulant to rivaroxaban (Xarelto), after the heparin drip is discontinued. You inform him that he will be on this medication for several months to prevent another occurrence of VTE. Which statements will you include in the teaching? Select all that apply.

   a. "Take the Xarelto at the same time every day."
   b. "There are no dietary restrictions while on this drug."
   c. "Watch for bleeding from your gums, nose, and bowels."
   d. "You will need to have blood work done on a regular basis while on this drug."
   e. "It's a good idea to wear a medical alert bracelet or necklace while on this drug."

CASE STUDY PROGRESS

M.M.'s condition has improved, and he has had several physical therapy sessions. He is not permitted to bear weight on his affected leg, but the physical therapist has encouraged him to exercise.

17. What types of exercises are recommended after this type of surgery?

CASE STUDY OUTCOME

M.M. is discharged to a rehabilitation facility to help him to regain strength after his surgery and illness. He is thankful that the surgery is over and hopeful to get back to his retirement activities soon.

Case Study 47

Name_____ Class/Group_____ Date_____

▶ Scenario

J.F., a 67-year-old woman, was involved in an auto accident and flown by emergency helicopter to your facility. She sustained a ruptured spleen, fractured pelvis, and compound fractures of the left femur. On admission (5 days ago) she underwent a splenectomy. Her pelvis was stabilized with an external fixation device 3 days ago, and yesterday her left femur was stabilized using balanced suspension with skeletal traction. She has a Thomas splint with a Pearson attachment on her left leg. She has 20 pounds (9 kg) of skeletal traction and 5 pounds (2.25 kg) applied to the balanced suspension. Her left femur is elevated off the bed at approximately 45 degrees. The lower leg is parallel to the bed and lies in a sling that the nurse adjusts on the frame, and the foot hangs freely. This morning, J.F. was transferred to your orthopedic unit for specialized care. You are the nurse assigned to care for her on the night shift.

1. You enter J.F.'s room for the first time. What aspects of the traction will you inspect?

2. What are characteristics of skeletal traction? Select all that apply.
   a. Traction weights are usually 5 to 10 pounds (2.25 to 4.5 kg).
   b. Traction weights range from 5 to 45 pounds (2.25 to 20 kg).
   c. Used for short-term treatment, 48 to 72 hours.
   d. The primary goal is to align injured bones and joints.
   e. Tape, boots, or splints are attached directly to the skin.
   f. The primary goal is to reduce muscle spasms in the injured extremity.
   g. Traction is applied using pins or wires that are surgically inserted into the bone.

3. When inspecting the skeletal pin sites, you note that the skin is reddened for an inch (2.5 cm) around the pin on both the medial and lateral left leg. What does this finding indicate, and what action will you take?

CASE STUDY PROGRESS

You perform a neurovascular assessment and note the following findings: Left foot pale, temperature slightly cooler than right foot. Right foot color pink. Capillary refill less than 3 seconds on both sides. Edema +1 on left foot and lower leg; no edema on right leg. Dorsalis pedis palpable and equal on both feet. Sensation equal on both sides. Able to dorsiflex feet and rotate ankles freely. Rates pain in left femur as a 5 out of 10.

4. Your institution uses electronic charting. Based on the assessment just described, which of the following systems would you mark as abnormal as you document your neurovascular assessment? Mark abnormal findings with an "X" and provide a brief narrative note.

☐ Skin color:

☐ Skin temperature:

☐ Capillary refill:

☐ Edema:

☐ Peripheral pulses:

☐ Sensation:

☐ Motor function:

☐ Pain:

5. What other key points of the assessment will you document in the patient's record?

6. An hour later, you check on J.F. and find her body in the lower 75% of the bed and her left upper leg at an exaggerated angle (more than 45 degrees). The knot at the end of the bed is caught in the pulley, and the 20-pound (9 kg) weight is dangling just above the floor. What are you going to do?

7. When you lift J.F., you notice that her sheets are wet. You decide to change J.F.'s linen. How would you accomplish this task?

8. J.F. tells you that she feels like she needs to have a bowel movement, but it is too painful to sit on the bedpan. How would you respond?

9. J.F. expels a few small, hard, round pieces of stool. What could be done to promote normal elimination?

CASE STUDY PROGRESS

You ask J.F. whether she is ready for her bath, and she responds positively. You let her bathe the parts she can reach and engage her in a conversation as you attend to the rest of her body. While performing perineal care, you notice that the folds of skin around her perineal area are reddened and excoriated.

10. What is the likely cause of the problem and what needs to be done to encourage healing?

11. You ask J.F. what she is doing to exercise while she is confined to the bed. She looks surprised and states that she isn't doing anything. What activities can J.F. engage in while on bed rest?

12. You realize that maintaining skin integrity is a challenge in J.F.'s case. What measures will you take to prevent skin breakdown?

CASE STUDY PROGRESS

Although J.F. is recovering nicely, she is becoming increasingly withdrawn. You enter her room and find her crying. She tells you that she is all alone here, that she misses her family terribly. You know that her son is flying into town tomorrow but will only be able to stay a few days.

13. What can be done so that J.F. benefits from her family support system?

> ### CASE STUDY OUTCOME
>
> J.F. remains in the hospital for several weeks, then is discharged to a rehabilitation center. She talks to her grandchildren every other night via social media on her new electronic device. She is looking forward to an upcoming visit with them.

Case Study **48**

Name_____ Class/Group_____ Date_____

▶ **Scenario**

K.B. is a 16-year-old girl who fell while skiing. She briefly lost consciousness but is now alert and oriented. She was transported down the hill by the ski patrol after being stabilized and then was flown to the hospital. She has a fractured right femur and humerus. She will be admitted to your unit after an open reduction and internal fixation (ORIF) of the femur fracture and casting of her leg and arm.

1. You are taking the report from the postanesthesia care unit (PACU) nurse. K.B. is awake and taking ice chips. What information will you document on the admission form?

2. How will you use this information in planning your immediate assessment and care of K.B. on admission?

Chart View

Physician's Orders

Vital signs per routine for postop patient
Continuous pulse oximetry
Neurologic checks every 4 hours
Turn, cough, and deep breathe and incentive spirometer every 2 hours while awake
Heat pack and elevate right lower extremity and right upper extremity
Neurovascular checks every 1 hour
NPO
IV fluids NS at 100 mL/hr
Morphine sulfate 5 mg IV every 4 to 6 hours prn

3. For each order listed in the chart, state whether the order is appropriate or not and state why.

CASE STUDY PROGRESS

K.B. is settled into her room and begins to complain of pain (7/10) in her leg and arm. She weighs 65 kg. You note that the ordered dose of morphine sulfate was given 2 hours ago. Your drug reference states that the appropriate dose is 0.05 to 0.1 mg/kg every 2 to 4 hours.

 4. Is this dose safe and therapeutic for your patient?

 5. The morphine for injection comes in a concentration of 2 mg/mL. How much will you draw up and have a second RN double-check? Indicate the amount on the syringe.

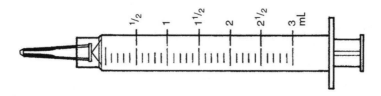

CASE STUDY PROGRESS

After K.B. has been on the unit for 6 hours, you identify the following changes in her assessment data: K.B. is difficult to arouse, but when awake she is able to identify who and where she is; PERRLA 1+ with slower reaction time than earlier; color pale, pink; skin cool and clammy; heart rate 126, respiratory rate 28, temperature (oral) 37.2 ° C (99° F); Spo$_2$ 90%. The findings of the neurovascular checks of the affected extremities are unchanged.

6. What will your immediate nursing interventions include?

7. K.B.'s Glasgow Coma Scale score begins to decline from 15 to 11. What are possible reasons for changes in her neurologic status?

8. What would you document about this incident?

CASE STUDY PROGRESS

K.B. is transferred to the pediatric intensive care unit (PICU) and treated for changes in her neurologic status. The next day her surgeon determines that her condition is stable and has her transferred back out to the pediatric unit. It is now 36 hours after surgery. K.B. suddenly begins to complain of extreme pain in her lower right leg. She had pain medication 2 hours ago and rates her pain as 10/10.

9. Which of these findings are early signs of compartment syndrome? Select all that apply.
   a. Edema
   b. Paresthesia
   c. Macular rash
   d. Increased pain
   e. Diminished pedal pulse
   f. Capillary refill less than 2 seconds

10. You page the orthopedic surgeon. Use SBAR (*s*ituation, *b*ackground, *a*ssessment, *r*ecommendation) to address patient status.

11. K.B.'s cast is split, and her foot pulses are restored. K.B. and her parents are extremely anxious. What education and support will be provided to K.B. and her parents?

CASE STUDY PROGRESS

K.B.'s status continues to improve. Physical and occupational therapists work with her on transfers and performing activities of daily living. She has many questions about how she will be able to go to school and resume her normal routine.

12. Recognizing K.B.'s developmental and cognitive stage, which of the following statements best supports your approach to discharge teaching?
   a. Adolescents are capable of thinking in concrete terms only.
   b. Family acceptance is more important than peer acceptance.
   c. Adolescents can anticipate future implications of current decisions.
   d. Adolescents are preoccupied with the immediate situation rather than future events.

 13. A new cast was applied several days later. Safety is an important issue for K.B. Describe what issues need to be addressed in discharge teaching in reference to safety?

14. The multidisciplinary team is made aware of K.B.'s progress in discharge rounds. Discuss how the following disciplines will be incorporated into her follow-up care after discharge: Discharge planning, PT, OT, dietitian, and hospital educator.

CASE STUDY OUTCOME

K.B. is discharged to home on postoperative day 5 with homebound schooling ordered, PT and OT ordered, and follow-up with orthopedics in 2 weeks.

Case Study 49

Name_____ Class/Group_____ Date_____

▶ Scenario

You are working in the emergency department when M.C., an 82-year-old widow, arrives by ambulance. Because M.C. had not answered her phone since noon yesterday, her daughter went to her home to check on her. She found M.C. lying on the kitchen floor, incontinent of urine and stool, and stating she had pain in her right hip. Her daughter reports a medical history of hypertension, angina, and osteoporosis. M.C. takes propranolol (Inderal), denosumab (Prolia), and hydrochlorothiazide, and uses a nitroglycerin patch. M.C.'s daughter reports that her mother is normally very alert and lives independently. On examination, you see an elderly woman, approximately 100 pounds (45 kg), holding her right thigh. You note shortening of the right leg with external rotation and a large amount of swelling at the proximal thigh and right hip. M.C. is oriented to person only and is confused about place and time, but she is able to say that her "leg hurts so bad." M.C.'s vital signs (VS) are 90/65, 120, 24, 97.5° F (36.4° C), Spo_2 89%. She is profoundly dehydrated. Preliminary diagnosis is a fracture of the right hip.

1. Considering her medical history and that she has been without her medications for at least 24 hours, explain her current VS.

2. Based on her history and your initial assessment, what 3 priority interventions would you expect to be initiated?

3. M.C.'s daughter states, "Mother is always so clear and alert. I have never seen her act so confused. What's wrong with her?" What are 3 possible causes for M.C.'s disorientation that should be considered and evaluated?

CASE STUDY PROGRESS

X-ray films confirm the diagnosis of intertrochanteric femoral fracture. Knowing that M.C. is going to be admitted, you draw admission labs and call for the orthopedic consultation.

4. What lab and diagnostic studies will be ordered to evaluate M.C.'s condition, and what critical information will each give you?

5. You insert an indwelling catheter and take careful note of the amount and appearance of M.C.'s urine. Why?

6. What are the 5 Ps that should guide the assessment of M.C.'s right leg before and after surgery?

7. In evaluating M.C.'s pulses, you find her posterior tibial pulse and dorsalis pedis pulse to be weaker on her right foot than on her left. What could be a possible cause of this finding?

8. You carefully monitor M.C.'s right extremity for compartment syndrome. Which are characteristics of compartment syndrome? Select all that apply.
   a. Pallor of the extremity
   b. Warmth of the extremity
   c. Petechiae over the extremity
   d. Numbness and tingling of the extremity
   e. Pain on passive stretch of the muscle traveling through the compartment

9. In planning further care for M.C., list 4 potential complications for which M.C. should be monitored and the reason for each.

10. M.C. keeps asking about "peaches." No one seems to be paying attention. You ask her what she means. She says Peaches is her little dog, and she's worried about who is taking care of it. How will you answer?

CASE STUDY PROGRESS

M.C. is placed in Buck's traction and sent to the orthopedic unit until an open reduction and internal fixation (ORIF) can be scheduled. Oxycodone-acetaminophen (Percocet 2.5/325) q4hr prn is ordered for severe pain and acetaminophen (Tylenol) 650 mg q4hr prn, for mild or moderate pain. She is placed on enoxaparin (Lovenox) 30 mg subQ bid. M.C.'s cardiovascular, pulmonary, and renal status is closely monitored.

11. As you assess the traction, you check the setup and M.C.'s comfort. Which are characteristics of Buck's traction? Select all that apply. Explain your answers.
   a. Weights need to be freely hanging at all times.
   b. The weights can be lifted manually as needed for comfort.
   c. Weights used for Buck's traction are limited to 5 to 10 pounds (2.25 to 4.5 kg).
   d. Pin site care is an essential part of nursing management for Buck's traction.
   e. A Velcro boot is used to immobilize the affected leg and connect to the weights.

12. What assessment is the priority when a patient is in Buck's traction?

13. Percocet can cause constipation. What will you do to prevent constipation?

 14. Between her admission at 1500 and the next day, she receives four doses of Percocet and one dose of acetaminophen (Tylenol). At 1300, she develops a fever of 101° F (38.3° C), and the physician writes an order to give acetaminophen (Tylenol), 650 mg PO every 4 hours for temperature over 100.5° F (38.1° C). Is there a concern with this order?

CASE STUDY OUTCOME

After an uneventful postoperative course, M.C. is transferred to a skilled-care facility for physical and occupational therapy rehabilitation.

3 Mobility

Case Study **50**

Name_____ Class/Group_____ Date_____

▶ **Scenario**

E.B., a 69-year-old man with type 1 diabetes mellitus (DM), is admitted to a large regional medical center complaining of severe pain in his right foot and lower leg. The right foot and lower leg are cool and without pulses (absent by Doppler). An arteriogram demonstrates severe atherosclerosis of the right popliteal artery with complete obstruction of blood flow. Despite attempts at percutaneous catheter-directed thrombolytic therapy with alteplase (tissue plasminogen activator [tPA]) over 48 hours and surgical thrombectomy, the foot and lower leg become necrotic. Finally, the decision is made to perform an above-the-knee amputation (AKA) on E.B.'s right leg. E.B. is recently widowed and has a son and daughter who live nearby. In preparation for E.B.'s surgery, the surgeons wish to spare as much viable tissue as possible. Hence, an order is written for E.B. to undergo 5 days of hyperbaric therapy for 20 minutes bid.

1. What is the purpose of hyperbaric therapy?

CASE STUDY PROGRESS

As you prepare E.B. for surgery, he is quiet and withdrawn. He follows instructions quietly and slowly without asking questions. His son and daughter are at his bedside, and they also are very quiet. Finally, E.B. tells his family, "I don't want to go like your mother did. She lingered on and had so much pain. I don't want them to bring me back."

2. You look at his chart and find no advance directives. What is your responsibility?

3. What is your assessment of E.B.'s behavior at this time?

4. What are some appropriate interventions and responses to E.B.'s anticipatory grief?

CASE STUDY PROGRESS

E.B. returns from surgery with the right residual limb dressed with gauze and an elastic wrap. The dressing is dry and intact, without drainage. He is drowsy and has the following vital signs: 142/80, 96, 14, 97.9° F (36.6° C), Spo$_2$ 92%. He is receiving a maintenance IV infusion of D$_5$ NS at 125 mL/hr in his right forearm.

5. The surgeon has written to keep E.B.'s residual limb elevated on pillows for 48 hours; after that, have him lie in a prone position for 30 minutes, 3 to 4 times a day. In teaching E.B. about his care, how will you explain the rationale for these orders?

6. In reviewing E.B.'s medical history, what factors do you notice that might affect the condition of his residual limb and ultimate rehabilitation potential?

CASE STUDY PROGRESS

You have just returned from a 2-day workshop on guidelines for the care of surgical patients with type 1 DM. You notice that E.B.'s daily fasting blood glucose has been running between 130 and 180 mg/dL. You recognize that patients with blood glucose values even slightly above normal levels experience impaired wound healing. However, you also recognize that the risks related to hypoglycemia, such as falls, might outweigh the risk for impaired healing from elevated glucose levels.

7. Identify 4 interventions that would facilitate timely healing of E.B.'s residual limb.

8. What should the postoperative assessment of E.B.'s residual limb dressing include?

9. You are reviewing the plan of care for E.B. Which care activities can be safely delegated to the UAP? Select all that apply.
   a. Checking E.B.'s vital signs
   b. Assessing E.B.'s IV insertion site
   c. Rewrapping the residual limb bandage
   d. Assisting E.B. with repositioning in the bed
   e. Asking E.B. to report his level of pain on a scale of 1 to 10

10. On the evening of the first postoperative day, E.B. becomes more alert and begins to complain of pain. He states, "My right leg is really hurting; how can it hurt so bad if it's gone?" What is your best response?
   a. "That is a side effect of the medication."
   b. "Are you able to rate that pain on a scale of 1 to 10?"
   c. "Don't worry, that sensation will go away in a few days."
   d. "You can't be feeling that because your leg was amputated."

11. What is causing E.B.'s pain?

12. A compression bandage was applied to E.B.'s residual limb after surgery. The next day, it is removed so that the surgical site can be assessed. Which actions by the nurse are correct? Select all that apply.
   a. Two elastic wrap bandages may be required.
   b. Use a figure-eight style of wrapping the residual limb.
   c. Remove and reapply the bandage several times daily.
   d. Apply the bandages very tightly to provide support and reduce edema.
   e. E.B. must wear the bandage at all times, even during physical therapy.

CASE STUDY PROGRESS

The case manager is contacted for discharge planning. E.B. will be discharged to an extended care facility for strength training. Once he receives his prosthesis, he will receive balance training. After that, he will be discharged to his daughter's home. A physical therapy and occupational therapy home evaluation are ordered. You have provided several sessions of teaching to E.B. and his daughter about care of the residual limb.

13. After your education sessions, you use the Teach-Back method to assess his understanding. Which statement by E.B. reflects a need for further instruction?
    a. "I will apply an alcohol-based lotion to my limb twice a day."
    b. "I will perform range-of-motion exercises to all my joints daily."
    c. "I will inspect my limb daily for signs of skin irritation and infection, such as redness, drainage, and odor."
    d. "I will wash my limb every night with warm water and a bacteriostatic soap and dry it gently, allowing it to air dry for 20 minutes."

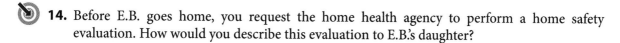 14. Before E.B. goes home, you request the home health agency to perform a home safety evaluation. How would you describe this evaluation to E.B.'s daughter?

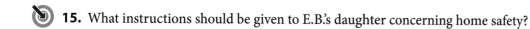 15. What instructions should be given to E.B.'s daughter concerning home safety?

16. What other discharge instructions should be given? Provide at least three.

CASE STUDY OUTCOME

E.B. makes a smooth transition from the hospital to the rehabilitation facility and then to the daughter's home. He was never able to adapt to independent living, so he eventually moved into his daughter's home.

Case Study **51**

Name_____ Class/Group_____ Date_____

▶ Scenario

T.M. is a 3-year-old boy with cerebral palsy (CP) who has been admitted to your unit. He is scheduled for surgery tomorrow morning for a femoral osteotomy and tendon lengthening to stabilize hip joints and to help reduce spasticity. You are orienting the parents to the unit and have a nursing student assisting you.

1. After getting the family settled, you return to the nurses' station and the nursing student asks you to explain what CP is and what might have caused it in this patient. How would you answer the student's question?

2. The nursing student asks what the family might have noticed that would indicate CP in T.M. when he was a baby. Which findings will you include in your discussion with the student? Select all that apply, and state your rationale.
   a. Leg scissoring
   b. Increased irritability
   c. Head lag at 5 months
   d. Use of pincer grasp at 9 months
   e. Ability to sit unassisted at 7 months
   f. Right hand preference at 12 months
   g. Positive Moro (startle) reflex at 2 months

CASE STUDY PROGRESS

You and the nursing student finish a health history with the family and determine that T.M. has impaired vision corrected with glasses, a speech impairment, a seizure disorder, and has had poor weight gain and feeding issues since birth. He has a skin-level feeding device (Mic-Key button) and receives supplemental tube feedings in addition to oral intake. He is not able to ambulate without braces and wears ankle-foot orthotics (AFOs). He receives physical, occupational, and speech therapy on an outpatient basis. T.M. is verbal and able to answer questions with simple phrases and responds to commands. He weighs 12 kg. The surgeon orders the following.

Chart View

Admission Orders

> Baclofen (Lioresal) 5 mg every 8 hours PO
> Diazepam (Valium) 2 mg twice a day PO
> Lamotrigine (Lamictal) 60 mg twice a day PO
> Diet as tolerated; NPO for solids and hold tube feedings at midnight; clear fluids until 4 a.m.
> Place IV on admission and begin D_5 ½NS at 10 mL/hr, increase rate to 45 mL/hr at midnight
> VS every 4 hours

3. Explain the rationale for each order.

4. Calculate T.M.'s maintenance fluid requirements. Do the IV fluids ordered meet this requirement? Show your work.

5. You ask T.M.'s mother about his history of seizures. She states that he has not had seizures since his medication doses were adjusted several months ago. With this knowledge, which admission orders would you question?

CASE STUDY PROGRESS

T.M. returns to your unit the next afternoon from the postanesthesia care unit (PACU). He is in a bilateral long leg hip spica cast, has an indwelling catheter, and has a family-controlled patient-controlled analgesia (PCA) device for pain control. You assess T.M. and chart the following findings.

Chart View

Postoperative Assessment

Neurologic	Awake and alert, verbalizes, and responds to commands. Periods of agitation and restlessness.
Respiratory	RR 25. Bilateral breath sounds, equal, clear, good air exchange. O_2 saturation 98% on room air.
Cardiovascular (CV)	IV line to right forearm infusing D_5 ½NS at 45 mL/hr. IV site is clean and dry, no signs of irritation or infiltration. HR 85. Temperature 36.8° C (98.2° F) (axillary).
Gastrointestinal (GI)	Positive bowel sounds; taking sips of juice PO; Mic-Key button to abdomen (left upper quadrant) clamped. Mic-Key site clean, no signs of breakdown.
Genitourinary (GU)	8 French Foley catheter intact and secured, draining yellow clear urine to collection bag. Diaper to spica cast opening.
Neuromuscular	Bilateral long leg hip spica casts with hip abductor bar intact. Toes warm to touch; able to move, unable to palpate pedal pulses due to cast. Cap refill less than 2 seconds.
Pain	T.M. occasionally whines and frowns but is comforted by parents. PCA is Y- connected to IV and infusing morphine at 0.01 mg/kg/hr continuous and 0.015 mg/kg per dose PCA with 15-minute lockout.
Psychosocial	Parents at bedside active in care.

6. What are your top 5 priorities while providing nursing care to T.M. postoperatively? Outline how you will you address each.

7. Score T.M. on the FLACC pain scale. Why is the FLACC scale an appropriate tool?

	Score		
Category	**0**	**1**	**2**
Face	No particular expression or smile	Occasional grimace or frown, withdrawn, disinterested	Frequent-to-constant quivering chin, clenched jaw
Legs	Normal position or relaxed	Uneasy, restless, tense	Kicking, or legs drawn up
Activity	Lying quietly, normal position, moves easily	Squirming, shifting back and forth, tense	Arched, rigid, or jerking
Cry	No cry (awake or asleep)	Moans or whimpers, occasional complaint	Crying steadily, screams or sobs, or frequent complaints
Consolability	Content, relaxed	Reassured by occasional touching, hugging, or being talked to, distractible	Difficult to console or comfort

Each of the five categories—(F) Face, (L) Legs, (A) Activity, (C) Cry, (C) Consolability—is scored from 0 to 2, which results in a total score between 0 and 10.

8. Which nonpharmacologic interventions would be age appropriate for T.M.? Select all that apply.
   a. Use guided imagery
   b. Read a favorite book
   c. Offer a favorite DVD or video
   d. Use bubbles to "blow the hurt away"
   e. Teach T.M. about pain and its relationship to the procedure
   f. Encourage "positive self-talk," such as, "I will feel better when the cast is off."

CASE STUDY PROGRESS

T.M.'s condition is stable throughout the day, and the surgeon writes the following orders:
   "Patient can PO ad lib. Resume home schedule of 520 mL PediaSure via G-tube from 10 p.m. to 6 a.m. Remove indwelling urinary catheter."

9. Place the steps for setting up a feeding with a Mic-Key button in the correct order.
   a. _____ Clean the skin-level device with alcohol
   b. _____ Wash hands and apply gloves
   c. _____ Place the correct amount of PediaSure in the feeding bag with overfill for priming
   d. _____ Insert extension set with secure lock, feeding and medication ports in to Mic-Key
   e. _____ Start the feeding
   f. _____ Attach the feeding bag to the pump and start "auto prime"
   g. _____ Attach feeding bag tubing to extension set feeding port

10. Calculate the hourly rate at which you will set the pump.

11. What nursing interventions and teaching will you include for T.M. and his family as you discontinue the indwelling urinary catheter?

CASE STUDY PROGRESS

T.M.'s condition continues to improve, and you provide discharge education. T.M.'s mother asks how she will care for his cast when he gets home. You discuss with her the care of a synthetic spica cast.

12. Which statements by T.M.'s mother would indicate that further education is needed? Select all that apply.
   a. "I need to keep his feet elevated when I get him home."
   b. "If he has an itch, it is okay to use a knitting needle to scratch under the cast."
   c. "Because T. uses pull-up diapers, I will need to use plastic tape to protect the cast opening."
   d. "It is okay if I give him a tub bath. Because it is a synthetic cast, I can dry it with a blow dryer."
   e. "I need to check the toes on his feet several times a day for the first week or so to see if they are warm and he is able to wiggle them."

13. What other information should you include in your discharge teaching?

14. The UAP, who is also a nursing student, offers to review the hospital "home medication" form with Mrs. M. True or False? This is an appropriate delegation of tasks. Explain your answer.

CASE STUDY OUTCOME

T.M.'s parents verbalize understanding of the discharge instructions. T.M. is discharged to home with a wheelchair and a home-health follow-up. He will return to the orthopedic surgeon in 2 weeks.

Case Study 52

Name_____ Class/Group_____ Date_____

▶ Scenario

You are working evenings on an orthopedic floor. One of your patients, J.O., is a 25-year-old Hispanic man who was a new admission on day shift. He was involved in a motor vehicle accident during a high-speed police chase on the previous night. His admitting diagnosis is status post (S/P) open reduction internal fixation (ORIF) of the right femur, multiple rib fractures, sternal bruises, and multiple abrasions. He speaks some English. He is under arrest for drug trafficking. He has one wrist shackled to the bed and a guard stationed inside his room. He says people are "coming to get him" because they think he is working with a rival group. Hospital security is aware of the situation.

Your initial assessment reveals stable vital signs (VS) of 116/78, 84, 16, 98.6° F (37° C). His only complaint is pain, for which he has a patient-controlled analgesia (PCA) pump. Lungs are clear to auscultation. His abdomen is soft and nontender. He is receiving IV D_5 LR through the proximal port of a left subclavian triple-lumen catheter at 75 mL/hr; the remaining two ports are locked. The right femur is connected to 10 pounds (4.5 kg) of skeletal traction. The dressing is dry and intact over the incision site.

1. What complications is J.O. at risk for because he has rib fractures and sternal bruising?

2. Outline the assessment you need to perform to detect these complications.

3. Which findings would you expect when performing his respiratory assessment?
   a. Continuous pain, with slow, shallow respirations
   b. Pain on inspiration, with deep, rapid respirations
   c. Pain on expiration, with slow, shallow respirations
   d. Pain on inspiration, with shallow, rapid respirations

4. J.O. has an antiembolism stocking ordered for his left leg. What is the rationale for putting a stocking only on this leg?

5. What other measures would be instituted as part of venous thromboembolism (VTE) prevention?

6. J.O. has an indwelling catheter inserted to drain his urine. What would you assess for in relation to the indwelling catheter?

7. J.O. has not had a cigarette since the accident and is irritable. Is J.O. a good candidate for nicotine replacement therapy? Give your rationale.

8. Because of the threat made on J.O.'s life and his vulnerable situation, what precautions should the nursing unit take to protect him?

CASE STUDY PROGRESS

The nurse in the emergency department phones to tell you that J.O.'s immunization status could not be determined when he arrived, but he did not receive a tetanus immunization. When you ask J.O. the date of his last tetanus shot, you find out that he was born and raised in Mexico and immigrated to the United States 5 years ago. He does not know whether he has ever had a tetanus shot. You inform the provider, and she orders diphtheria/tetanus toxoid 0.5 mL IM and tetanus immune globulin (HyperTET) 250 units deep IM.

9. Why is J.O. getting two injections?

10. When you give J.O. the tetanus injections, you find J.O. in the position shown in the illustration. Are any of these findings of concern to you? If so, how would you fix it?

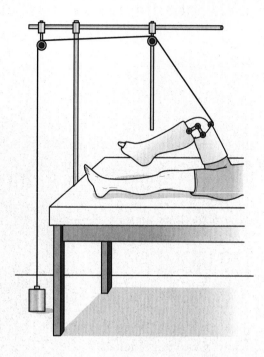

11. While assessing the leg distal to the fractured femur, you find his toes are slightly cool to the touch. Why does this concern you?

12. What assessment do you need to complete?

13. J.O.'s assessment is negative for any further signs and symptoms of an evolving complication. What do you think your best course of action is?

CASE STUDY PROGRESS

At 2100, J.O.'s guard summons you to his room. J.O. is pale, slightly confused, and reporting chest pain and dyspnea. Vital signs are 90/60, 120, 28, 100.0° F (37.8° C), and SpO_2 of 84%. His pulse is weak, and there are petechiae on his chest.

14. What do you expect is occurring and why?

15. Explain the pathophysiology of this complication and the reason J.O. is at risk for experiencing this complication.

16. List the priority actions you should take next and the reason for each.

Chart View

Arterial Blood Gases on 2 L Nasal Cannula

pH	7.32
$PaCO_2$	53 mm Hg
HCO_3	22 mEq/L (22 mmol/L)
PaO_2	84 mm Hg

17. Interpret J.O.'s ABG results.

CASE STUDY PROGRESS

The provider comes and examines J.O. She writes the following orders, then leaves, saying she will be back in 1 hour to check on J.O.

Chart View

Physician's Orders

Oxygen (O_2) to maintain SpO_2 of 90%
Increase IV D_5 LR to 125 mL/hr
ECG monitoring
Repeat ABGs in 1 hour
CBC with differential and serum lipase now
STAT chest x-ray (CXR)
Methylprednisolone (Solu-Medrol) 12 mg IV push now
Furosemide (Lasix) 60 mg IV push now
Digoxin 0.25 mg IV push now

18. Describe a plan for implementing these orders in order of priority.

Chart View

Arterial Blood Gases on 10 L Face Mask

pH	7.29
$PaCO_2$	56 mm Hg
HCO_3	22 mEq/L (22 mmol/L)
PaO_2	74 mm Hg

19. J.O. is placed on O_2 at 10 L via face mask. ABGs are redrawn after 1 hour. Interpret the results.

20. What intervention do you expect based on your interpretation of these values?

CASE STUDY PROGRESS

The provider returns to reexamine J.O. Because J.O.'s status is deteriorating despite receiving O_2 and the IV medications, the provider decides to transfer J.O. to the ICU for ventilator support.

21. You go with J.O. on the transfer to the ICU. Outline the report you would give the ICU nurse.

CASE STUDY OUTCOME

J.O. recovers for several weeks in the hospital before being transferred to jail to await trial. Shortly before his trial date, he is found stabbed to death in his cell. Although there is an investigation, the murder weapon is never found, and no one is ever charged in his death.

Case Study **53**

Name_____ Class/Group_____ Date_____

▶ Scenario

D.V., a 32-year-old man, is being admitted to the medical floor from the neurology clinic with symptoms of multiple sclerosis (MS). D.V. has experienced increasing urinary frequency and urgency over the past 2 months. D.V. recently had two brief episodes of eye "fuzziness" associated with diplopia and flashes of brightness. He has noticed ascending numbness and weakness of the right arm with the inability to hold objects over the past few days. Now he reports rapidly progressing weakness in his legs along with blurred, patchy vision.

1. MS is associated with scattered, patchy demyelination of the sheath around nerves in the brain and spinal cord. What does myelin do? What is demyelination?

2. MS is characterized by remissions and exacerbations. What happens to the myelin during each of these phases?

3. Is D.V. too young to get MS? What is the cause of MS?

4. Outline the subjective and objective assessment data associated with MS. Place a star next to those D.V. has.

5. The neurologist orders an MRI scan of the brain and spine. What role does this test play in diagnosing MS?

6. How will the neurologist determine whether D.V. has MS?

7. What are the overall goals of collaborative care for a patient with MS?

8. D.V. asks, "If this turns out to be MS, how will I be treated?" How would you respond?

9. D.V. is started on interferon beta-1a (Avonex) 30 mcg intramuscularly each week. What teaching do you need to provide regarding interferon therapy?

10. The neurologist also orders 500 mg methylprednisolone (Solu-Medrol) IV daily. What do you need to do to administer this medication safely? Select all that apply.
   a. Begin the infusion before 0900 each day
   b. Reconstitute with 8 mL of benzyl alcohol
   c. Use the solution within 60 minutes of reconstitution
   d. Administer a total dose of 8 mL of reconstituted solution
   e. Deliver the dose over 30 minutes using IV pulse administration

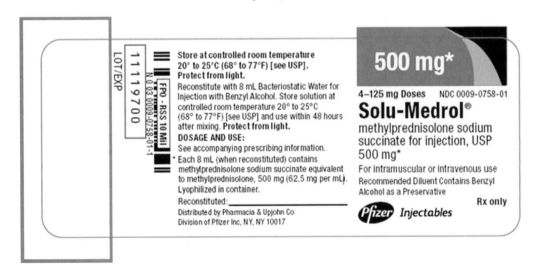

11. Because D.V. is experiencing urinary frequency and urgency, the neurologist orders oxybutynin. In addition to medication teaching, what will you teach him to do to assist in controlling urinary symptoms?

12. When planning D.V.'s care, what goal is the most appropriate goal for the clinical problem of activity intolerance related to muscle weakness?
    a. "D.V. is free of trauma related to muscle weakness."
    b. "D.V. will maintain muscle strength in his arms and legs."
    c. "D.V. can identify three factors that aggravate muscle weakness."
    d. "D.V. will participate in daily activities as desired without fatigue."

13. As part of your teaching plan, you want D.V. to be aware of situations or factors that are known to exacerbate symptoms. List 4.

CASE STUDY PROGRESS

After testing is complete, D.V. is diagnosed with MS. He confides in you that he has been depressed since his parents' divorce and the onset of these symptoms. He tells you that he knows his girlfriend has been unfaithful, but he is afraid of being alone. He is afraid if he tells her about his MS diagnosis, she will leave him.

14. What are you going to do with this information?

15. You are concerned with D.V.'s psychological status, particularly the negative feelings he expresses regarding himself and the concerns he has voiced. Write a nursing outcome addressing this issue and identify independent nursing actions you would implement.

16. In view of his personal history and current diagnosis, what 2 critical psychosocial issues require monitoring in his follow-up visits?

17. What community resources might D.V. find helpful?

CASE STUDY OUTCOME

D.V. takes advantage of his time with a psychiatric nurse specialist, joins a local MS support group, and tells his girlfriend to move out. He later marries a woman from the support group.

Case Study **54**

Name _____ Class/Group _____ Date _____

▶ Scenario

C.B. is a single, self-employed 54-year-old man. Three weeks ago, he saw his primary care provider because of symptoms of fatigue, myalgia, fever, and chills, which were accompanied by a hacking cough. He was diagnosed with viral influenza. Today he has weakness, numbness, and tingling of both lower extremities, which is progressing into his upper body. His brother brought him to the emergency department after recognizing the seriousness of his illness. The attending physician immediately suspects Guillain-Barré syndrome (GBS).

1. Describe the cause of GBS.

2. What factors in C.B.'s history support a diagnosis of GBS?

3. Describe the clinical manifestations of GBS.

4. How is GBS diagnosed, and what tests would you expect to be performed?

 5. What is your immediate concern for C.B. and why?

6. What assessment findings would tell you this is occurring?

7. Which set of arterial blood gases would be consistent with the presence of this complication?
   a. pH 7.50, P_{CO_2} 52 mm Hg
   b. pH 7.35, P_{CO_2} 40 mm Hg
   c. pH 7.25, P_{CO_2} 60 mm Hg
   d. pH 7.51, P_{CO_2} 31 mm Hg

8. Which assessment finding, if present, would require your immediate intervention?
   a. Diaphoresis
   b. Slurred speech
   c. Facial flushing
   d. Urinary retention

CASE STUDY PROGRESS

Shortly after arrival, C.B. becomes completely paralyzed and requires endotracheal intubation and mechanical ventilation. He is transferred to the neurologic ICU for further support.

9. What are the goals of medical management in GBS?

10. Describe the collaborative care patients generally receive in the ICU for GBS.

11. What are the overall goals of nursing care for C.B. at this time?

3 Mobility

12. The attending physician states C.B. will begin either IV immune globulin or plasmapheresis. What is plasmapheresis?

13. You are concerned about the possibility of disuse syndrome related to C.B.'s paralysis. Describe an outcome of nursing care for C.B., and 4 independent nursing interventions you would implement to meet that outcome.

14. How would performing passive ROM exercises benefit C.B. from a cardiovascular perspective?
   a. ROM will help prevent C.B. from developing contractures.
   b. Keeping his muscles active will assist in maintaining muscle tone.
   c. ROM is an effective way to help prevent VTE.
   d. The stretching motion accompanying ROM will decrease C.B.'s pain.

15. Name 5 interventions you would implement to meet the expected outcome of maintaining skin integrity.

16. What is foot drop? How can it be prevented?

17. How would C.B.'s nutritional needs be met?

18. What evaluative parameters would you use to determine whether C.B.'s nutritional needs were being met?

19. What interventions can you implement to help decrease C.B.'s fear and anxiety? Select all that apply.

    a. Speak calmly to him when providing care.

    b. Administer continuous intravenous sedation.

    c. Limit visitors only to immediate family members.

    d. Continually reassure him that his needs are being met.

    e. Use a communication system that allows C.B. to let his needs be known.

20. C.B.'s brother asks how long C.B. will be paralyzed. How should you respond?

CASE STUDY OUTCOME

After staying in the ICU for 8 days, C.B. is transferred to a special ventilator unit of an extended care facility because he shows no signs of improvement in respiratory muscle strength. After several weeks, he progressively regains neurologic function and is weaned from the ventilator. He is able to go home with his brother 5 months after the initial admission.

Digestion

4

Case Study 55

Name_____ Class/Group _____ Date _____

▶ Scenario

T.H., a 57-year-old stockbroker, has come to the gastroenterologist for treatment of recurrent mild to severe cramping in his abdomen and blood-streaked stool. You are the RN doing his initial workup. Your findings include a mildly obese man who demonstrates moderate guarding of his abdomen with both direct and rebound tenderness, especially in the left lower quadrant (LLQ). His vital signs are 168/98, 110, 24, 100.4° F (38° C); he is slightly diaphoretic. T.H. reports that he has periodic constipation. He has had previous episodes of abdominal cramping, but this time the pain is getting worse.

Past medical history reveals that T.H. has a "sedentary job with lots of emotional moments," he has smoked a pack of cigarettes a day for 30 years, and he had "two or three mixed drinks in the evening" until 2 months ago. He states, "I haven't had anything to drink in 2 months." He denies having regular exercise: "just no time." His diet consists mostly of "white bread, meat, potatoes, and ice cream with fruit and nuts over it." He denies having a history of cardiac or pulmonary problems and has no personal history of cancer, although his father and older brother died of colon cancer. He takes no medications and denies the use of any other drugs or herbal products.

1. Identify 4 general health risk problems that T.H. exhibits.

2. Identify a key factor in his family history that might have profound implications for his health and present state of mind.

3. Identify 3 key findings on his physical examination and indicate their significance.

CASE STUDY PROGRESS

The physician ordered a complete blood count (CBC), complete metabolic profile, and a CT scan of the abdomen with contrast. Based on the radiology and lab results, physical examination findings, and history, the physician diagnoses T.H. as having acute diverticulitis and discusses an outpatient treatment plan with him.

4. What is diverticulitis? What are the consequences of untreated diverticulitis?

5. While the patient is experiencing the severe crampy pain of acute diverticulitis, what interventions would you perform to help him feel more comfortable?

CASE STUDY PROGRESS

T.H. is being sent home with prescriptions for metronidazole (Flagyl) 500 mg PO q6hr and ciprofloxacin (Cipro) 500 mg PO q12hr.

6. For each medication, state the drug class and the purpose for T.H.

7. Given his history, what questions must you ask T.H. before he takes the initial dose of metronidazole? State your rationale.

8. Which are symptoms of a disulfiram-type reaction? Select all that apply.
   a. Headache
   b. Flushed skin
   c. Constipation
   d. Bradycardia
   e. Abdominal cramps
   f. Nausea and vomiting

9. When teaching T.H. about the metronidazole prescription, which instructions need to be included? Select all that apply.
   a. Take the medication with or after meals.
   b. This medication might cause a metallic taste.
   c. If his urine turns reddish brown, notify the doctor immediately.
   d. Avoid all alcohol-containing products while on this medication.
   e. Take the medication exactly as scheduled, without skipping doses.
   f. Some tingling or numbness might be felt in the hands, which is an expected effect.

 10. What specific information would you want to know before T.H. starts the antibiotics?

11. What are the signs and symptoms of an allergic reaction?

12. T.H. asks you if he can take a laxative for his occasional constipation. What is your answer?

13. T.H. asks you about his diet. "I'm confused. I was always told that I needed to be eating a high-fiber diet, which is difficult for me. But the doctor just told me that I need to be on a low-fiber diet for now, so now I'm confused. Which is it supposed to be?" How will you answer his question?

CASE STUDY PROGRESS

You discuss ways to manage while recovering. To help T.H. work through his dietary concerns, you obtain a referral to a registered dietitian.

14. What measures do you think the dietitian will discuss with T.H. to avoid recurrent diverticulitis once his acute symptoms have resolved? Name at least 5.

15. You discuss the need to avoid increased intraabdominal pressure. What are ways that he can avoid increasing intraabdominal pressure and why is this important?

CASE STUDY OUTCOME

T.H. returns for a checkup 14 days later; all signs and symptoms of diverticulitis are gone. He is working on his lifestyle changes, including smoking cessation, and reports he is walking 30 minutes every day.

Case Study **56**

Name_____ Class/Group_____ Date_____

▶ Scenario

J.V., a 56-year-old delivery truck driver, has been taken to the emergency department (ED) because he was experiencing chest pain. It started just after he had a quick lunch at a food truck. He told the paramedic that he often has chest pain but that it goes away when he "takes a swig of antacid," but this time the pain did not stop. On arrival he was given another dose of antacid and sublingual nitroglycerin, and the chest pain stopped. The first set of cardiac enzymes and basic metabolic profile (BMP) were drawn, and a 12-lead ECG was done. He weighs 275 pounds (125 kg), is 5 ft, 5 inches (165 cm) tall, and tells the nurse he has been overweight all his life. He said he's had the chest pains for about 2 years but did not go to get checked because they always went away when he took antacids and he was too busy with work to go to a doctor. He works late hours, "lives on coffee," and grabs fast food when he has time to eat. He smokes 1.5 to 2 packs of cigarettes a day, has a beer every evening once he is home, and usually finishes a 6 pack on the weekends. Vital signs: T 98.9° F (37.2° C), P 110, R 14, BP 148/98. The test results are listed below.

Chart View

Test Results

Test	Results	Test	Results
Sodium	142 mEq/L (142 mmol/L)	Creatinine	1.1 mg/dL (97 mcmol/L)
Potassium	4.1 mEq/L (4.1 mmol/L)	Calcium	5.1 mg/dL (1.28 mmol/L)
Chloride	102 mEq/L (102 mmol/L)	Hemoglobin	14.8 g/dL (148 g/L)
CO_2	28 mEq/L (28 mmol/L)	Hematocrit	48%
Glucose	168 mg/dL (9.3 mmol/L)	Cardiac troponin T	0.05 ng/mL (0.05 mcg/L)
BUN	12 mg/dL (4.3 mmol/L)	12-Lead ECG	Sinus tachycardia, rate 105

1. Review the test results and explain any abnormalities.

2. Six hours later, the second set of cardiac enzymes was normal. Do you think J.V. has had a myocardial infarction (MI)? Defend your answer.

CASE STUDY PROGRESS

After noting the ECG results and the normal second set of cardiac enzymes, the ED provider tells J.V. that the "chest pain" was more likely gastrointestinal (GI) in origin. J.V. was discharged from the ED with a referral to the hospital's GI clinic with a possible diagnosis of GERD. One week later, at the GI clinic, he is examined by the GI nurse practitioner (NP). The NP tells J.V. that she thinks he has GERD, but the diagnosis will be confirmed by an upper endoscopic examination. The upper endoscopy is scheduled for 0700 on Tuesday of the following week.

3. What is GERD, and what causes it?

4. List the signs and symptoms of GERD.

5. Which of these are potential risk factors for GERD? Select all that apply. Place an asterisk (*) by the ones that pertain to J.V.
   a. Obesity
   b. Alcohol use
   c. Caffeine use
   d. Cardiac history
   e. Cigarette smoking

6. J.V. has self-treated his pain with over-the-counter antacids for a few years. What concerns are there with this long-term self-treatment?

7. Describe the upper endoscopy procedure J.V. will undergo.

8. J.V. has several questions about the upper endoscopy. The nurse provides teaching about the procedure, required preparation, and what to expect afterward. Which statement by J.V. indicates a need for further teaching?
   a. "I will be wide awake during the procedure."
   b. "I will not eat or drink anything after midnight."
   c. "I will not take any antacid the morning of this test."
   d. "This test will help the doctor figure out why I have so much heartburn."

CASE STUDY PROGRESS

The upper endoscopy is performed successfully. The gastroenterologist tells J.V. and his daughter that the GERD diagnosis is confirmed, and that he has severe esophageal erosion but no visible ulcers. In addition, a gastric mucosal biopsy was sent for *Helicobacter pylori*. His postprocedure blood glucose level was 122 mg/dL.

9. What is *H. pylori*, and how is it treated?

10. *H. pylori* can be detected with other diagnostic testing. Which tests are potential diagnostic tests for *H. pylori*? Select all that apply.
    a. Urine test
    b. Stool culture
    c. Urea breath test
    d. Stool antigen test
    e. Serum or whole antibody tests

11. Which nursing actions are appropriate for delegation to the UAP after the procedure?
    a. Taking J.V.'s vital signs.
    b. Assessing J.V.'s level of consciousness.
    c. Reviewing J.V.'s point-of-care glucose results.
    d. Providing postop instructions to J.V. and his daughter.

CASE STUDY PROGRESS

J.V. was started on omeprazole (Prilosec) 20 mg every morning. The following week, J.V. has a follow-up appointment with the GI nurse practitioner. It turns out that the testing for *H. pylori* is negative, but he is told that his symptoms are caused by GERD and he will need to make some lifestyle changes in addition to taking the omeprazole for 6 months.

12. What is the mechanism of action of omeprazole?
    a. It neutralizes gastric acidity.
    b. It coats the stomach and provides relief of symptoms.
    c. It partially blocks histamine-2 receptors and reduces gastric acid secretion.
    d. It inhibits the proton pump, resulting in irreversible blocking of all gastric acid secretion.

13. The nurse has provided teaching regarding the omeprazole. Which statement by J.V. indicates a correct understanding of therapy with a proton pump inhibitor (PPI) such as omeprazole?
   a. "I will take it at night just before bedtime."
   b. "I will take the capsule with breakfast every day."
   c. "I will take it first thing in the morning, 30 to 60 minutes before breakfast."
   d. "I will open the capsule and chew the contents thoroughly to help it work better."

14. J.V. asks the nurse, "Why do I have to take this fancy medicine? The antacid made my heartburn go away. Isn't that enough?" How will you answer J.V.?

15. List at least 6 lifestyle modifications that J.V. can make to reduce the symptoms of GERD.

CASE STUDY OUTCOME

After 4 months, J.V. lost almost 40 pounds and is determined to lose at least 40 more. He stopped smoking "cold turkey" and has reduced his beer intake to once on the weekend. His daughter has helped him with his meal-planning, and he now brings his lunch and snacks with him instead of stopping for fast food. He is happy with his weight loss, how he is feeling, and the amount of money he has saved by not buying his lunches and the cigarettes.

Case Study 57

Name_____ Class/Group_____ Date_____

▶ **Scenario**

M.R. is a 56-year-old general contractor who is admitted to your telemetry unit directly from his internist's office with a diagnosis of chest pain. On report, you are informed that he has an intermittent 2-month history of chest tightness with substernal burning that radiates through to the mid-back off and on, in a stabbing fashion. Symptoms occur after a large meal, with heavy lifting at the construction site, and in the middle of the night when he awakens from sleep with coughing, shortness of breath, and a foul, bitter taste in his mouth. Recently he has developed nausea, without emesis, that is worse in the morning or after skipping meals. He reports having "heartburn" three or four times a day. When this happens, he takes a couple of Rolaids or Tums. He keeps a bottle at home, at the office, and in his truck. Vital signs (VS) at his physician's office were BP 130/80 lying and 120/72 standing, 100, 20, 98.6° F (37° C), Spo$_2$ 92% on room air. A 12-lead ECG showed normal sinus rhythm with a rare premature ventricular contraction (PVC).

1. Outline the common causes of chest pain.

2. What mnemonic can you use to help you better evaluate his pain?

3. What other history is important for you to obtain?

CASE STUDY PROGRESS

M.R. indicates that usually the chest pain is relieved by his antacids, but this time they had no effect. A "GI cocktail" consisting of Mylanta and viscous lidocaine given at his physician's office briefly helped decrease symptoms.

4. What tests can be done to determine the source of his problems?

CASE STUDY PROGRESS

M.R. has smoked one pack of cigarettes a day for the past 35 years, drinks 2 or 3 beers on most nights, and has noticed a 20-pound (9 kg) weight gain over the past 10 years. He feels "so tired and old now." M.R. has dark circles under his eyes and complains of constant daytime fatigue. His wife is even sleeping in another bedroom because he is snoring so loudly. He also reinjured his lower back a month ago at work, lifting a pile of boards, so his physician prescribed ibuprofen (Motrin) 400 mg twice a day for 4 weeks.

5. Which factors in M.R.'s life are likely contributing to his chest pain and nausea? Explain how.

CASE STUDY PROGRESS

M.R. explains that 6 months ago his physician prescribed ranitidine (Zantac) 150 mg PO at bedtime for heartburn, and that it helped a little, but that it never really "did the job," so he stopped taking it. Now he keeps a bottle of Tums or Rolaids in his truck and at his bedside "because I always seem to need them."

6. Why do you think the ranitidine did not help M.R.?

CASE STUDY PROGRESS

M.R.'s 12-lead ECG and the first set of cardiac enzymes were normal. The chest x-ray showed no abnormalities. Room air Spo$_2$ is 94% and breathing is unlabored. Other lab results are listed in the chart.

Chart View

Admission Laboratory Test Results

WBC	6000/mm^3 (6×10^9/L)
Hgb	15.0 g/dL (150 g/L)
Hct	47%
Platelets	220,000/mm^3 (220×10^9/L)
Na	140 mEq/L (140 mmol/L)
K	3.7 mEq/L (3.7 mmol/L)
BUN	18 mg/dL (6.4 mmol/L)
Creatinine	1.0 mg/dL (88 mcmol/L)
Lipase	20 units/L
Amylase	32 units/L
PT/INR	12.0 sec/1.0
Urea breath test	positive

---

7. What is the significance of the urea breath test result?

8. Are there any concerns with the other lab results?

CASE STUDY PROGRESS

Suddenly, M.R. begins to complain of nausea; as you hand him the emesis basin, he promptly vomits coffee-ground emesis with specks of bright red blood. VS remain stable.

9. What concerns do you have about the coffee-ground emesis?

10. How do you confirm that the emesis contains blood?

CASE STUDY PROGRESS

You ask the charge nurse to contact the gastrointestinal (GI) consulting physician to explain the recent events while you stay with M.R. The gastroenterologist gives several orders and states he will be there in 30 minutes. The orders are as follows.

Chart View

Physician's Orders

Nothing by mouth (NPO) status for emergent esophagogastroduodenoscopy (EGD)

Repeat CBC STAT

O_2 by nasal cannula; titrate O_2 to maintain Spo_2 over 94%

Type and crossmatch (T&C) 2 units packed red blood cells (PRBCs), and hold

Start a pantoprazole (Protonix) drip at 8 mg/hr, preceded by a 40-mg bolus IV over 2 minutes

Insert a Salem Sump nasogastric tube (NGT) and start a gastric lavage with 100 mL normal saline (NS)

Insert 2 large-bore IVs and start NS at 100 mL/hr

11. Place the previous orders in order of priority.

12. Explain the rationale for each of the preceding orders.

CASE STUDY PROGRESS

The gastroenterologist performs the EGD and finds erosive esophagitis Los Angeles (LA) class B, a moderately sized hiatal hernia, diffuse erosive gastritis, and an ulcer in the antrum of the stomach that is oozing blood. The duodenal bulb shows a normal endoscopic appearance. During the EGD, the bleeding is stopped with cautery. Biopsy specimens of the gastric mucosa are obtained, and his bleeding ulcer is attributed to the NSAIDs (i.e., ibuprofen). He is kept NPO until the next morning to allow sufficient hemostasis of the cauterized site. Clear liquids are allowed at breakfast. M.R. tolerates the liquid diet without any nausea and vomiting and is discharged to home the next day with the following instructions:

- Advance diet slowly, as tolerated, to mechanical soft.
- Take pantoprazole 40 mg PO q AM before breakfast
- Amoxicillin 1 gram PO twice daily for 2 weeks

- Clarithromycin extended-release 1 gram once daily for 2 weeks
- Sucralfate 1 gram 4 times a day (before meals and bedtime) for 3 months
- Make a follow-up appointment in 6 to 8 weeks with physician
- Stop all aspirin and over-the-counter or herbal pain relief medications, especially NSAIDs (ibuprofen, naproxen, and so on)
- Stop or limit alcohol intake and smoking

13. M.R. has prescriptions for 4 different drugs. You are providing teaching about the timing of the various drugs. Help M.R. map out a schedule for taking his new medications with regard to his meals. Explain your reasons for the times provided.

14. What is the purpose of the antibiotics?

15. After discussing lifestyle modifications for controlling acid reflux with M.R., which statement by M.R. indicates a further need for teaching?
a. "I will stop smoking."
b. "I will stop drinking alcohol."
c. "I will avoid eating 2 to 3 hours before my bedtime."
d. "I will wait 30 minutes before lying down or sitting in my recliner after meals."

CASE STUDY OUTCOME

M.R. goes home and vows to stop smoking, stop drinking alcohol, and take better care of himself. He calls his primary care physician to schedule a sleep study because of his snoring and cuts back his working hours. The biopsies were positive for *H. pylori* bacteria, and his symptoms disappeared after 2 weeks of antibiotic therapy. He will remain on the pantoprazole for another 3 months.

4 Digestion

Case Study 58

Name_____ Class/Group_____ Date_____

▶ Scenario

C.G. is admitted to your medical-surgical unit from the emergency department. He is 65 years old and presented with indigestion, loss of appetite (especially to meat), and a 30-lb (13.6 kg) weight loss over the last 6 months. He also reports that he has been having feelings of fullness that were only relieved by belching and vomiting. Other symptoms reported are abdominal pain, nausea, vomiting, and dysphagia. He has a history of smoking (20 pack-years), gastric ulcers, asthma, and pernicious anemia. He reports regular alcohol use of 3 to 4 beers each day. He reports, "I haven't had anything to drink in 2 weeks because of my stomach." He reports a family history of COPD, hypertension, Crohn's disease, and colon cancer. He denies any allergies or any previous hospitalizations.

1. Identify 4 health risk problems you have identified while reviewing C.G.'s admission information.

2. What are some possible medical diagnoses that will be considered, based on this initial assessment?

3. What diagnostic tests or exams would you anticipate being ordered? Select all that apply.
   a. Chest x-ray
   b. Hemoglobin A_{1C}
   c. Liver function tests
   d. Renal function tests
   e. Complete blood count
   f. Thyroid function tests
   g. CT scan of the abdomen
   h. Comprehensive metabolic panel
   i. Upper GI endoscopy and barium studies

CASE STUDY PROGRESS

After reviewing the test and pathology results, the physician has diagnosed C.G. with gastric cancer. Although he is upset by the news, C.G. states, "I am happy we caught it early and can cure it!"

4. How are the symptoms of gastric cancer related its disease progression?

Chart View

Laboratory Results

    Hgb 7.3 g/dL (73 g/L)

    Hct 27%

5. What is the significance of C.G.'s hemoglobin and hematocrit in relation to his diagnosis?

6. What condition in C.G.'s medical history could contribute to his anemia? Explain your rationale.

7. Which of these goals are appropriate pretreatment interventions for the patient with gastric cancer? Select all that apply.
   a. Treatment of anemia
   b. Eliminating infection
   c. Toleration of high-residue diet
   d. Replacement of blood volume
   e. Correction of nutritional deficits

CASE STUDY PROGRESS

After discussing his diagnosis, C.G. and his medical team have decided to perform surgical removal of the tumor. The treatment team spends several days improving his nutritional status by consulting nutrition services, encouraging several small meals per day and toleration of liquid supplements. He then undergoes a total gastrectomy and is admitted to the postsurgical unit. Postoperative care orders include nutrition consult, wound care consult, nasogastric tube (NGT) to low intermittent wall suction, and IV replacement of vitamins C, D, K, and B.

8. What is a total gastrectomy?

9. You note another postoperative order for cyanocobalamin, 100 mcg/day IM. What is this drug, and what is its purpose?

10. C.G. asks the nurse to explain why he needs to take all of the dietary supplements if the cancer is now gone. What teaching will you provide?

11. Explain the rationale for the NGT setting of "low intermittent suction" for this patient.

12. Postoperatively the patient has an NGT in place. The nursing student assigned to your patient comes to you and reports that the NGT has not drained any secretions in the last 2 hours. What response will you provide to the nursing student?

CASE STUDY PROGRESS

On postoperative day 3, C.G. is started on small amounts of clear liquids by mouth. He is tolerating the liquids without discomfort when suddenly, on postop day 7, C.G. begins to complain of severe abdominal pain and nausea. His VS are BP 96/68, P 117, R 24, T 102.1° F (38.9° C).

13. What condition do you anticipate based on C.G.'s symptoms?

14. What tests should the nurse expect to be ordered for evaluation of C.G.'s condition? Select all that apply.
    a. CT abdomen
    b. X-ray of the abdomen
    c. Upper GI endoscopy
    d. Upper GI series with gastrografin
    e. Complete blood count with differential

CASE STUDY PROGRESS

The UAP reports that the patient's VS are now BP 84/58, P 125, R 28, T 101.8° F (38.8° C), and Spo$_2$ 85%. The physician is notified, and you receive orders for oxygen, an IV fluid bolus, and broad-spectrum antibiotics. C.G. is transferred to the intensive care unit for management of a suspected anastomotic leak with development of a duodenal stump fistula.

15. Which of these conditions are an indication that the antibiotic treatment is unsuccessful in managing the leak and fistula? Select all that apply.
    a. Hemodynamic instability
    b. Decreased abdominal pain
    c. Hyperactive bowel sounds
    d. Increased body temperature
    e. Pain during abdominal palpation

16. For each intervention for an anastomotic leak with fistula that is listed, answer "Yes" if it is an appropriate intervention or "No" if it is not. For the "No" answers, explain the reason they are incorrect.
    a. Administration of IV fluids
    b. Clamping of the NGT tube
    c. Administration of IV antibiotics
    d. Acid suppression of the GI tract

17. The interventional radiologist is consulted to perform a percutaneous drainage procedure. What is the treatment goal of percutaneous drain placement?

CASE STUDY OUTCOME

C.G. was started on IV antibiotics, and a percutaneous drain was placed. His condition continued to deteriorate, and he was ultimately found to have acute abdomen and peritonitis with worsening sepsis. He was taken to the OR for laparoscopy with peritoneal washing. Postoperatively, he remained intubated and continued to receive IV antibiotic and fluid therapy. On postop day 2 after the laparoscopy, C.G. was found to be in septic shock and was started on IV vasopressors and IV fluids. His condition continued to deteriorate and progressed to cardiac arrest. After resuscitation efforts, C.G. succumbed to his condition secondary to severe septic shock from the anastomotic leak and peritonitis.

Case Study 59

Name_____ Class/Group_____ Date_____

▶ Scenario

You are on duty in the intermediate care unit and scheduled to take the next admission. The emergency department (ED) nurse calls to give you the following report: "This is Barb in the ED, and we have a 62-year-old man, K.L., with lower GI bleeding. He is a sandblaster with a 12-year history of silicosis. He is taking 40 mg of prednisone per day. During the night, he developed severe diarrhea. He was unable to get out of bed fast enough and had a large maroon-colored stool in the bed. His wife 'freaked' and called the paramedics. He is coming to you. His vital signs (VS) are stable—110/64, 110, 28, SpO_2 93%—and he's a little agitated. His temperature is 98.2° F (36.8° C). He has not had any stools since admission, but his rectal examination was guaiac positive and he is pale but not diaphoretic. We have him on 5 L O_2/NC. We started a 16-gauge IV with LR at 125 mL/hr. He has an 18-gauge Salem Sump to continuous low suction; that drainage is guaiac negative. We have done a CBC with differential, chem panel, coagulation times, a T&C for 4 units, ABGs, and a UA. He's all ready for you."

1. How do you prepare for the patient's arrival?

2. What are common causes of lower GI bleeding?

3. Given K.L.'s history, what do you think significantly contributed to the GI bleeding?

4. What other signs and symptoms would you ask him about?

5. Compare and contrast among melena, hematochezia, and occult blood in the stool.

CASE STUDY PROGRESS

K.L. arrives on your unit. As you help him transfer from the ED stretcher to the bed, K.L. becomes very dyspneic and expels 800 mL of maroon stool.

6. What immediate complication concerns you most?

7. What are the first 3 actions you should take?

CASE STUDY PROGRESS

K.L. reports that he is feeling nauseated. VS are 92/58, 116, 32, SpO_2 93%. The provider orders an IV fluid bolus of 500 mL 0.9% normal saline and 2 units packed red blood cells (PRBCs) STAT.

8. What other interventions do you need to do?

9. What assessment indicators would you monitor in K.L.?

10. In caring for K.L., which activities can be safely delegated to UAP? Select all that apply.
   a. Applying a pulse oximetry monitor
   b. Measuring his VS every 15 minutes
   c. Assessing K.L.'s peripheral circulation
   d. Monitoring K.L.'s hemoglobin and hematocrit levels
   e. Emptying the Foley catheter collection bag each hour
   f. Obtaining consent from K.L. for the blood transfusions

Chart View

Arterial Blood Gases

pH	7.47
$PaCO_2$	33 mm Hg
PaO_2	65 mm Hg
HCO_3	23 mEq/L (23 mmol/L)
SpO_2	91%

Complete Blood Count

WBCs	$4300/mm^3$ (4.3×10^9/L)
RBCs	4.0 million/mm^3 (4×10^{12}/L)
Hemoglobin (Hgb)	7.8 g/dL (78 g/L)
Hematocrit (Hct)	23%
Platelets	$208,000/mm^3$ (208×10^9/L)

11. K.L.'s ED lab results are sent to you. Interpret his ABGs. What do they tell you?

12. Discuss K.L.'s Hgb and Hct results.

13. You are preparing to administer the first of the 2 units of PRBCs. Evaluate each of the following statements about the safe administration of blood. Enter *T* for true or *F* for false. Tell why the false statements are incorrect.

_____ 1. Prime the correct tubing and filter with normal saline.
_____ 2. Verify K.L.'s identification with the secretary in the endoscopy suite
_____ 3. Obtain baseline vital signs before starting the transfusion
_____ 4. Begin the transfusion at a rate of 125 mL/hr
_____ 5. Take K.L.'s vital signs 30 minutes after starting the transfusion
_____ 6. Complete the transfusion within 6 hours of receiving the unit

CASE STUDY PROGRESS

The provider discusses K.L. with the gastroenterologist, who schedules K.L. for an immediate colonoscopy. You go with K.L. to the endoscopy suite and help the endoscopy nurse in giving him IV midazolam (Versed) and morphine sulfate during the procedure.

14. Why is K.L. receiving midazolam and morphine sulfate?

15. What is the priority nursing responsibility during the procedure?
   a. Reorienting K.L. as needed
   b. Monitoring K.L.'s IV fluid intake
   c. Assessing K.L.'s VS and oxygen saturation
   d. Documenting K.L.'s response to the procedures

4 Digestion

CASE STUDY PROGRESS

During the colonoscopy, K.L. begins passing large amounts of bright red blood. He becomes paler and more diaphoretic and begins to have an altered level of consciousness.

16. Name 3 immediate interventions you need to do.

CASE STUDY PROGRESS

The gastroenterologist finds the site of the bleeding and cauterizes the affected vessels. There is no further evidence of active bleeding. K.L. is transferred back to the unit and care continued with fluids and blood products to stabilize his condition. He received one dose of IV esomeprazole in endoscopy and is placed on twice-daily therapy.

17. Describe the ongoing assessment you need to obtain.

18. What assessment data would lead you to determine K.L.'s condition was stabilizing?

19. Which finding would warrant your immediate intervention?
   a. Palpable splenomegaly
   b. Hypoactive bowel sounds
   c. Complaints of abdominal cramping
   d. Orthostatic change in BP of 20

20. What is the expected outcome associated with giving esomeprazole?

21. Later, when he seems to be feeling better, K.L. tells you he is really embarrassed about the mess he made for you. How are you going to respond to him?

22. K.L. is being prepared for discharge. What do you need to address in your teaching with K.L.?

CASE STUDY OUTCOME

The gastroenterologist concludes that the GI hemorrhage was prednisone induced. Because the prednisone was being used to suppress the progression of silicosis, the provider will try to decrease his maintenance dose of prednisone while monitoring his respiratory status.

Case Study **60**

Name_____ Class/Group_____ Date_____

▶ Scenario

S.G. is a 6-month-old girl who is scheduled for sequential repair of her cleft lip (cheiloplasty) and palate (palatoplasty). She has recently been adopted from China and her medical history is unknown. S.G. is scheduled for her cleft lip repair, and Mrs. G. brings her to the same-day surgery unit the week before for her preoperative workup. As you do her workup, you recognize that care of the child with clefting uses a multidisciplinary approach.

1. Discuss the health problems for which these children are at risk and who on the craniofacial team would address each issue.

2. List at least 4 reasons why would it be important to include a social worker and/or psychologist to the craniofacial team following this infant?

3. S.G. weighs 6.5 kg. Plot this finding on the Centers for Disease Control and Prevention (CDC) growth chart (see http://www.cdc.gov/growthcharts/data/who/GrChrt_Girls_24LW_9210. pdf). Which statement best summarizes your findings?
   a. S.G.'s weight falls below the 5th percentile.
   b. S.G.'s weight is between the 10th and the 25th percentile.
   c. S.G.'s weight is between the 50th and the 75th percentile.
   d. S.G.'s weight is above the 95th percentile.

4. What information from her health history is important to obtain from her mother to plan her perioperative care? Select all that apply. Explain your rationale.
   a. Adoption status
   b. Immunization status
   c. Gross motor milestones
   d. Current method of feeding
   e. Parent's employment status
   f. Current known health status

5. Choose the lab tests that you expect to be obtained preoperatively. Discuss the rationale for your choices.
   a. CHEM-7
   b. Urinalysis
   c. Stool sample for fat content
   d. Arterial blood gases (ABGs)
   e. Complete blood count with differential

CASE STUDY PROGRESS

The lab test results and findings of S.G.'s preoperative workup are normal, and she is scheduled for her cheiloplasty.

6. What will you include in your preoperative teaching to S.G.'s parents?

7. Determine S.G.'s daily fluid maintenance requirements. How can her parents ensure this intake and determine adequate hydration status?

CASE STUDY PROGRESS

S.G. returns to the unit after her cheiloplasty. The surgeon notes on the chart that surgical glue was used to close the incision. You note standing postoperative orders to clean with normal saline and apply antibiotic ointment three times per day.

8. True or False? You would call the surgeon to question this order. Explain your answer.

 9. S.G. also has an order for acetaminophen 120 mg rectally or PO every 4 to 6 hours as needed for pain. Is the ordered dose safe and therapeutic?

10. Pain management is essential for healing. Which instructions should be given to the parents before S.G. is discharged? Select all that apply. Discuss your rationale for each.
   a. Administer pain medication with a teaspoon.
   b. You may add the pain medication to S.G.'s formula to help her take it more easily.
   c. Use distraction like a music box in the crib to act as an adjunct to pain medication.
   d. Give pain medication around the clock, every 4 to 6 hours for the first 24 to 48 hours after surgery.
   e. Provide diagrams to show parents how much pain medication to give with an oral medication syringe.

11. S.G.'s parents are advised that S.G. will return 6 months later for the palatoplasty. They are concerned about the delay between surgeries. What will your response be?

CASE STUDY PROGRESS

S.G. returns to your unit 6 months later for her cleft palate repair (palatoplasty).

12. Which nursing interventions are appropriate as you plan her care? Select all that apply. Discuss your rationale for each.
   a. Use elbow restraints as needed.
   b. Maintain strict intake and output.
   c. Administer pain medications as ordered.
   d. Oral suction with a plastic oral suction catheter as needed.
   e. Clear fluids; advance as tolerated. Patient may use a straw.
   f. Position patient side-lying or on abdomen postoperatively.

13. S.G. has a normal recovery and is being discharged. When giving her parents discharge instructions, what will you advise them concerning diet and signs and symptoms to report?

CASE STUDY OUTCOME

S.G. is discharged to home with instructions for follow-up with the surgeon and multidisciplinary team.

4 Digestion

Case Study **61**

Name_____ Class/Group_____ Date_____

▶ **Scenario**

As a nurse on a gastrointestinal (GI) unit, you receive a call from an affiliate outpatient clinic notifying you of a direct admission with an estimated time of arrival of 60 minutes. The clinic nurse gives you the following information: A.G. is an 82-year-old woman with a 3-day history of intermittent abdominal pain, abdominal bloating, and nausea and vomiting (N/V). A.G. moved from Italy to join her grandson and his family only 2 months ago, and she speaks very little English. All information was obtained through her grandson. Her medical history includes colectomy for colon cancer 6 years ago and ventral hernia repair 2 years ago. She has no history of coronary artery disease, diabetes mellitus, or pulmonary disease. She takes only ibuprofen (Motrin) occasionally for mild arthritis. Allergies include sulfa drugs and meperidine. A.G.'s tentative diagnosis is small bowel obstruction (SBO) secondary to adhesions. A.G. is being admitted to your floor for diagnostic workup. Her vital signs are stable, she is receiving an IV infusion of D_5 ½NS with 20 mEq KCl at 100 mL/hr, and 2 L oxygen by nasal cannula.

1. Based on the nurse's report, what signs of bowel obstruction does A.G. have?

2. Are there other signs and symptoms of a bowel obstruction that you should observe for while A.G. is in your care?

3. While A.G. is on the way, you secure the hospital's interpreter service on the telephone. A.G. arrives on your unit with her grandson. You admit A.G. to her room and introduce yourself as her nurse. As her grandson introduces her, she pats your hand. You know that you need to complete a physical examination and take a history. What will you do first?

4. Before you begin your examination, the grandson, an attorney, tells you that elderly Italian women are extremely modest and might not answer questions completely. He says he wants to stay in the room during the examination. How will you proceed?

5. What key questions must you ask this patient while you have the use of an interpreter?

6. For each characteristic listed, specify whether it is a characteristic of small bowel obstruction (SBO), large bowel obstruction (LBO), or both (B).

_____a. Persistent abdominal cramping

_____b. Colicky, cramping pain at frequent intervals

_____c. Upper or epigastric abdominal distention

_____d. Distention in the lower abdomen

_____e. Obstipation

_____f. Ribbon-like stools

_____g. Nausea and early, profuse vomiting, which may contain fecal material

_____h. Minimal or no vomiting

_____i. Severe fluid and electrolyte imbalances

7. What is obstipation?

8. During your examination, you note that she does not have muscle guarding or rebound tenderness on palpation. Is this important? Explain your answer.

9. A.G. vomits during your examination. Which indicates an obstruction that is more distal?
a. The emesis contains bile.
b. There is a minimal amount of emesis.
c. The emesis is foul-smelling and fecal.
d. The emesis is mostly mucus and clear liquid.

CASE STUDY PROGRESS

The physician orders the insertion of a Salem Sump nasogastric tube (NGT). You insert the NGT into A.G. and connect it to intermittent low wall suction.

10. How will you check for placement of the NGT?

11. List, in order, the structures through which the NGT must pass as it is inserted.

12. A.G.'s grandson asks you, "What is that blue thing at the end of the tube? Shouldn't it be connected to something?" How do you answer?

13. Which are appropriate nursing actions for a patient with an NGT? Select all that apply.
   a. Provide frequent oral care.
   b. Check the nares around the tube for signs of irritation.
   c. Apply a petroleum-based lubricant on the skin around the tube.
   d. Pull the tube tightly and pin to the patient's gown to prevent movement.
   e. Tape the tube to the nose so it does not pull on the nares or cause ulceration.
   f. Obtain an order for a topical antiseptic spray (i.e., Chloraseptic) if she has a sore throat.

14. You note that A.G.'s NGT has not drained in the last 3 hours. What can you do to facilitate drainage?

15. The NGT suddenly drains 575 mL; then drainage slows down to about 250 mL over 2 hours. Is this an expected amount?

16. You enter A.G.'s room to initiate your shift assessment. A.G.'s abdomen seems to be more distended than yesterday. How would you determine whether A.G.'s abdominal distention has changed?

CASE STUDY PROGRESS

After 24 hours, A.G.'s symptoms are unrelieved. She reports continued nausea, cramps, and sometimes strong abdominal pain; her hand grips are weaker; and she seems to be increasingly lethargic. You look up her latest lab values and compare them with the admission data.

Chart View

Laboratory Test Results

Test	Admission	Hospital Day 3
Sodium	136 mEq/L (136 mmol/L)	130 mEq/L (130 mmol/L)
Potassium	3.7 mEq/L (3.7 mmol/L)	2.5 mEq/L (2.5 mmol/L)
Chloride	108 mEq/L (108 mmol/L)	97 mEq/L (97 mmol/L)
Carbon dioxide	25 mEq/L (25 mmol/L)	31 mEq/L (31 mmol/L)
BUN	19 mg/dL (6.8 mmol/L)	38 mg/dL (13.6 mmol/L)
Creatinine	1 mg/dL (88.4 mcmol/L)	2.2 mg/dL (194.5 mcmol/L)
Glucose	126 mg/dL (7.0 mmol/L)	65 mg/dL (3.6 mmol/L)
Albumin	3.0 g/dL (30 g/L)	3.1 g/dL (31 g/L)
Protein	6.8 g/dL (68 g/L)	4.9 g/dL (49 g/L)

17. Which lab value is of most concern to you? Why? Are there others that are also of concern? Explain.

18. What measures do you anticipate to correct in each of the imbalances described in Question 17?

CASE STUDY OUTCOME

In view of A.G.'s continued deterioration, the surgeon meets with the patient and her family and they agree to surgery. The surgeon releases an 18-inch (46 cm) section of proximal ileum that had been constricted by adhesions. Several areas look ischemic, so these are excised, and an end-to-end anastomosis is done. A.G. tolerates the procedure well. Her recovery is slow but steady. A.G. goes home in the care of her grandson and his wife on the seventh postoperative day. Discharge plans include a home health nurse, home health aide, in-home physical therapy, and dietitian consultation. The grandson is included in the plans.

Case Study **62**

Name_____ Class/Group_____ Date_____

▶ **Scenario**

C.W., a 36-year-old woman, was admitted several days ago with a diagnosis of recurrent inflammatory bowel disease (IBD) and possible small bowel obstruction (SBO). C.W. is married, and her husband and 11-year-old son are supportive, but she has no extended family in the state. She has had IBD for 15 years and has been taking mesalamine (Asacol) for 15 years and prednisone 40 mg/day for the past 5 years. She is very thin; at 5 feet 2 inches (157 cm), she weighs 86 lbs (39 kg) and has lost 40 lbs (18 kg) over the past 10 years. She averages 5 to 10 loose stools per day. C.W.'s life has gradually become dominated by her disease, with anorexia, lactase deficiency, profound fatigue, frequent nausea and diarrhea, frequent hospitalizations for dehydration, and recurring, crippling abdominal pain that often strikes unexpectedly. The pain is incapacitating and relieved only by a small dose of diazepam (Valium), oral electrolyte solution (Pedialyte), and total bed rest. She confides in you that sexual activity is difficult: "It always causes diarrhea, nausea, and lots of pain. It's difficult for both of us." She is so weak she cannot stand without help. You indicate complete bed rest on the nursing care plan.

1. Identify 6 priority problems for C.W.

2. Considering C.W.'s weakness, chronic diarrhea, and lower-than-desired body weight, what nursing interventions need to be implemented to minimize skin breakdown? Name at least 6.

3. What is the mechanism of action of the mesalamine (Asacol) in relation to the IBD?
   a. It increases bulk and moisture content in the stool.
   b. It relaxes the smooth muscle of the intestines, thus reducing motility.
   c. It slows intestinal motility, prolonging transit time of intestinal contents.
   d. It blocks prostaglandin production, thus diminishing inflammation in the colon.

CASE STUDY PROGRESS

C.W.'s condition deteriorates. On the third day after admission she experiences intractable abdominal pain and unrelenting nausea and vomiting. C.W. is taken to the operating room because of probable SBO and is readmitted to your unit from the postanesthesia care unit. During surgery, 38 inches (96 cm) of her small bowel was found to be severely stenosed, with 2 areas of visible perforation. Much of the remaining bowel is severely inflamed and friable. A total of 5 feet (152 cm) of distal ileum and 2 feet (61 cm) of colon have been removed, and a temporary ileostomy was established. She has a Jackson-Pratt (JP) drain to bulb suction in her right lower quadrant (RLQ), and her wound was packed and left open. She has 2 peripheral IV lines, a Salem Sump nasogastric tube (NGT), and a Foley catheter. Her vital signs (VS) are 112/72, 86, 24, 100.8° F (38.2° C) (tympanic). You attach her NGT to low-continuous wall suction per the postoperative orders.

4. You begin a thorough postoperative assessment of C.W.'s abdomen. What does your assessment include? List the steps in the order in which the assessment should be completed.

5. A nursing student enters C.W.'s room and auscultates her abdomen. She looks at you and excitedly announces that she hears good bowel sounds. You take the opportunity to teach her the proper method of auscultating bowel sounds on a patient who has NGT to low-continuous wall suction. How would you correct her error?

6. Four hours later, you measure the drainage from the JP tube. Look at the following figure and state how much drainage you obtained.

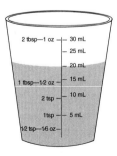

7. What else will you note about the drainage?

8. Describe the proper method for reestablishing suction on the JP drain after you have emptied the bulb container.

9. C.W. asks you, "I know why I have the pouch. Why do I have to have this other little tube?" How will you explain the purpose of the JP drain?

CASE STUDY PROGRESS

It is 4 days after C.W.'s surgery. During the routine dressing change, you note a small pool of yellow-green drainage in the deepest part of the wound. You obtain an order for a wound culture.

10. How will you obtain a culture specimen from C.W.'s wound?

11. What information do you need to send to the lab with the wound culture specimen?

12. You obtain a wound culture specimen, complete the dressing change, obtain a full set of VS, note a temperature of 100.4° F (38° C), and assess increased tenderness in C.W.'s abdomen. What orders do you anticipate receiving once you notify the surgeon of C.W.'s condition?

13. As you assess C.W.'s stoma and drainage, what would indicate that they are healthy? Select all that apply.
   a. The stoma will be level with the skin.
   b. The stoma will be in the shape of a donut.
   c. The drainage will be thick and dark brown.
   d. The skin around the stoma should be intact.
   e. The stoma will be a uniform medium cherry red.
   f. The stoma will be light pink, and an occasional dark spot might appear.

14. Will any aspect of C.W.'s history significantly affect the wound healing process? If so, how?

15. The surgeon tells you she will be there to examine C.W. As you tell C.W. that her doctor is coming to talk to her, C.W. says that she feels something wet running down her side. You find some leakage of intestinal drainage onto the skin. What should you do?

CASE STUDY PROGRESS

You change the ileostomy appliance before the surgeon arrives. C.W. is evaluated, and it is determined that she has developed peritonitis, and needs to return to surgery for exploratory laparotomy. The surgery revealed another area of perforated bowel and generalized peritonitis. Another 12 inches (30.5 cm) of ileum were resected. The peritoneal cavity was irrigated with normal saline (NS) and 3 drainage tubes were placed: a Jackson-Pratt (JP) drain to bulb suction, a rubber catheter to irrigate the wound bed with NS, and a sump drain to remove the irrigation fluid. The initial JP drain remains in place. A right subclavian triple-lumen catheter was also inserted.

16. A few hours later, C.W. is still experiencing pain from the peritonitis as well as from the surgical incision. Which position may help to make her more comfortable?
   a. Lying on her left side
   b. Lying on her right side
   c. Supine with legs extended
   d. Head of bed slightly elevated, with knees flexed

17. C.W. has been on NPO status since the surgery. The surgeon orders total parenteral nutrition (TPN) at a rate of 50 mL/hr. What is the purpose of these orders?

18. The pharmacy delivers C.W.'s first bag of TPN. You have an order to stop the maintenance IV infusion after starting the TPN. What is the purpose of this order?

19. During the night shift the TPN solution bag becomes nearly empty, and the night nurse discovers that the next bag of TPN has not been prepared. The hospital pharmacy does not prepare TPN during the night shift. What does the nurse need to do next?
a. Hang a bag of D_5W when the TPN is finished.
b. Hang a bag of $D_{10}W$ when the TPN is finished.
c. Convert the line to a saline lock until the TPN solution is ready.
d. Slow the TPN rate to 10 mL/hr until the next TPN bag can be prepared.

CASE STUDY PROGRESS

You discuss your concerns about C.W.'s nutritional status with C.W.'s surgeon. She agrees to request a consultation from a registered dietitian (RD). After gathering data and making several calculations, the RD makes recommendations to the surgeon. The TPN orders are adjusted, C.W. begins to gain weight slowly, and her wound shows signs of healing.

20. You discuss with the RD what specific digestive difficulties C.W. is likely to face. What problems might C.W. be prone to develop after having so much of her bowel removed?

21. The RD talks with C.W. about her dietary needs. You attend the session so you will be able to reinforce the information. What basic information is the RD likely to discuss with C.W.?

CASE STUDY OUTCOME

C.W. is successful in her battle with peritonitis. Gradually tubes are removed as she grows stronger with TPN and time. C.W. learns how to change her ostomy appliance and is discharged to home. She attends an enterostomal support group on a regular basis.

Case Study 63

Name_____ Class/Group_____ Date_____

▶ Scenario

Mr. and Mrs. B. arrive in the emergency department (ED) with their 6-week-old infant, S.B. As the triage nurse, you ask the couple why they have brought S.B. to the ED. Mrs. B. states, "My baby breastfed well for the first couple of weeks but has recently been throwing up all the time, sometimes a lot and really forcefully. He looks skinny and is hungry and fussy all the time." You determine that the couple is homeless and has been living out of their car for the past month. S.B. has had no primary care since discharge after delivery.

1. What additional information will you need to obtain from Mr. and Mrs. B.?

CASE STUDY PROGRESS

Your primary assessment of the infant reveals the following: S.B. is alert and fussy and consoles with a bottle of Pedialyte (per physician orders). His anterior fontanel is slightly depressed and posterior fontanel cannot be palpated. You auscultate regular breath sounds at a rate of 30 breaths/min. No adventitious sounds. Pulse oximetry is 98% on room air. Heart rate is 190 with regular rate and rhythm. Brachial and pedal pulses are +3 and equal. Abdomen is round and nontender to palpation. Positive bowel sounds. Diaper is dry. S.B. moves all extremities and there are no rashes noted. Rectal temperature is 37.2° C (98.9° F). There is a quarter-sized flat red area on occiput that "has been there since he was born" according to the mother. Slight "tenting" noted.

You transport S.B. to radiology, and he vomits a large amount of clear fluid. Patient returns to the room in his mother's arms, awake and alert. The mother appears anxious and states, "I don't know what's wrong with my baby! Why can't you people tell me anything?"

2. How do you respond to the mother?

3. Your institution uses electronic charting. Based on the assessment described, which of the following systems would you mark as abnormal as you document your findings? Mark abnormal findings with an "X," and provide a brief narrative note.

☐ Neurologic:

☐ Respiratory:

☐ Cardiovascular:

☐ Gastrointestinal:

☐ Genitourinary:

☐ Musculoskeletal:

☐ Skin:

☐ Psychosocial:

☐ Pain:

4. The emergency physician orders a complete blood count, complete metabolic profile, urinalysis, blood pH, and x-rays. The physician suspects dehydration and metabolic alkalosis secondary to hypertrophic pyloric stenosis. Which lab findings would you expect with metabolic alkalosis?
a. Na: 128 mEq/L (128 mmol/L), K: 2.6 mEq/L (2.6 mmol/L), Cl: 90 mEq/L (90 mmol/L), HCO_3: 30 mEq/L (30 mmol/L)
b. Na: 130 mEq/L (130 mmol/L), K: 5.7 mEq/L (5.7 mmol/L), Cl: 94 mEq/L (94 mmol/L), HCO_3: 22 mEq/L (22 mmol/L)
c. Na: 130 mEq/L (130 mmol/L), K: 3.9 mEq/L (3.9 mmol/L), Cl: 98 mEq/L (98 mmol/L), HCO_3: 17 mEq/L (17 mmol/L)
d. Na: 148 mEq/L (148 mmol/L), K: 4.1 mEq/L (4.1 mmol/L), Cl: 108 mEq/L (108 mmol/L), HCO_3: 13 mEq/L (13 mmol/L)

5. What is the underlying cause of S.B.'s diagnosis of metabolic alkalosis?

6. Which clinical manifestations might you find with metabolic alkalosis? Select all that apply.
   a. Tetany
   b. Hyperthermia
   c. Increased respiratory rate
   d. Increased risk for seizures
   e. Neuromuscular irritability

7. What additional assessment findings might reflect the consequences of frequent prolonged vomiting in the infant?

CASE STUDY PROGRESS

S.B. is diagnosed with hypertrophic pyloric stenosis, admitted to the pediatric unit, is NPO, and scheduled for surgery.

8. S.B.'s parents are concerned that their living situation contributed to S.B.'s diagnosis. How would you respond to their concerns?

9. Mr. and Mrs. B. have questions about the necessity of surgery and question what is going to be done next. What are your responsibilities as you respond to Mr. and Mrs. B.'s concerns?

Chart View

Preoperative Orders

Vital signs q4hr
Strict intake and output (I&O)
30 mL Pedialyte q3hr PO
Place IV and begin $D_5\frac{1}{3}NS$ at 50 mL/hr
Nasogastric (NG) tube placed to low continuous wall suction
Daily weights

10. Which preoperative orders would you question?

11. Which interventions can be delegated to unlicensed assistive personnel (UAP)? Select all that apply.
    a. Assessing for NG tube placement every shift
    b. Reminding parents to save diapers to be weighed
    c. Teaching parents the rationale for NG tube insertion
    d. Assisting parents in holding infant without removing NG tube
    e. Obtaining VS every 4 hours and reporting any abnormal findings to the RN

 12. You note that your patient was hypokalemic and the fluids you hung per orders do not include potassium. You contact the surgeon to clarify. You receive the following order: "Change IV to $D_5\frac{1}{3}NS$ with 20 mEq KCl at maintenance." You obtain the new fluids and hang per orders. True or False: This is an appropriate nursing action. Explain your answer.

CASE STUDY PROGRESS

S.B. returns to your unit after a pyloromyotomy. Mrs. B. is concerned about when she will be able to resume breastfeeding and what they need to do for their baby.

13. What postoperative teaching would you provide to them?

CASE STUDY OUTCOME

S.B. progresses well and is tolerating normal breastfeeding within 48 hours with minimal vomiting. He is discharged with follow-up in 2 weeks with the parents' new primary care provider. A social worker has helped Mr. and Mrs. B. obtain temporary housing and apply for available insurance and local resources.

Case Study 64

Name_____ Class/Group_____ Date_____

▶ Scenario

You are a nurse on an inpatient psychiatric unit. J.M., a 23-year-old woman, was admitted to the psychiatric unit last night after assessment and treatment at a local hospital emergency department for "blacking out at school." She has been given a preliminary diagnosis of anorexia nervosa. As you begin to assess her, you notice that she has very loose clothing, she is wrapped in a blanket, and her extremities are very thin. She tells you, "I don't know why I'm here. They're making a big deal about nothing." She appears to be extremely thin and pale, with dry and brittle hair, which is very thin and patchy, and she constantly complains about being cold. As you ask questions about weight and nutrition, she becomes defensive and vague, but she does admit to losing "some" weight after an appendectomy 2 years ago. She tells you that she used to be fat, but after her surgery she did not feel like eating and everybody started commenting on how good she was beginning to look, so she just quit eating for a while. She informs you that she is eating lots now, even though everyone keeps "bugging me about my weight and how much I eat." She eventually admits to a weight loss of "about 40 pounds (18 kg) and I'm still fat."

1. Using *Diagnostic and Statistical Manual of Mental Disorders,* Fifth Edition (DSM-V) criteria, how is the diagnosis of anorexia nervosa determined?

2. Identify 8 clinical signs or symptoms of anorexia nervosa. Place a star or asterisk next to those that J.M. has.

3. What other disorders might occur along with anorexia nervosa? Name at least 4.

4. How does bulimia nervosa differ from anorexia nervosa?

5. Name 5 behaviors that J.M. or any other patient with anorexia may engage in other than self-starvation.

6. What common family dynamics are associated with anorexia nervosa?

4 Digestion

You review her admission lab studies. An electrocardiogram (ECG) has also been ordered.

Chart View

Admission Laboratory Work

Sodium	135 mEq/L (135 mmol/L)
Potassium	3.4 mEq/L (3.4 mmol/L)
Chloride	99 mEq/L (99 mmol/L)
Magnesium	1.5 mEq/L (0.62 mmol/L)
Blood urea nitrogen	18 mg/dL (6.4 mmol/L)
Creatinine	1.0 mg/dL (88.4 mcmol/L)
Hemoglobin	11 g/dL (110 g/L)
Hematocrit	35%

7. Which lab results are of concern at this time? Explain your answers.

8. What clinical symptoms of anorexia nervosa, if present, should have the highest priority? Explain your answers.

J.M.'s ECG results show normal sinus rhythm with no ST segment or other changes. You meet with J.M. to formulate a plan of care.

9. Which of these are appropriate nutrition interventions for J.M.? Select all that apply.
   a. Do not prompt her to eat.
   b. Discuss food choices with her.
   c. Allow her to eat alone during mealtimes.
   d. Have normal conversations during meals.
   e. Allow her to select her menu on her own.
   f. Weigh her each morning after voiding, with her back to the scale.
   g. Restrict her from returning to her room or a restroom without staff supervision after meals.

10. List at least 6 psychologic aspects of the plan of care for J.M.

CASE STUDY PROGRESS

After 3 weeks, you are providing discharge teaching for J.M. You ask her whether she is ready to go home. J.M. states, "I'll be so glad to get out of this place. I'm so fat and ugly. I need to lose 10 pounds (4.5 kg). I bet I can do it in just a couple of days. Otherwise, I don't want to live anymore."

11. What will you discuss with the provider before any further discharge teaching or plans?

12. You report J.M.'s statements to the provider. What actions do you expect the provider to take?

13. What medications may help J.M. with resolution of both her anorexia nervosa and her depression?

14. Which statements by J.M. would indicate successful treatment? Select all that apply.
  a. "I just have to stay skinny to feel good."
  b. "When you say I look 'healthy' I feel fat."
  c. "Lately I've been feeling a little better about things."
  d. "I am looking forward to going out with my friends again."
  e. "It's up to me to take care of my body by eating enough food."

CASE STUDY OUTCOME

After 2 weeks, J.M. has gained 5 lbs (2.25 kg) and seems to be more willing to eat. She still expresses fears of "getting fat," but she states that she is ready to go home and back to school. The provider arranges for J.M. to participate in an outpatient partial hospitalization program that specializes in eating disorders. J.M. expresses interest in meeting others with the same problems.

Case Study **65**

Name_____ Class/Group_____ Date_____

▶ Scenario

You are working on the postoperative surgical unit and admitted S.B., a 42-year-old woman with a history of morbid obesity, hypertension, sleep apnea, and diabetes mellitus. She underwent a laparoscopic Roux-en-Y procedure. For the past year, she had tried to lose weight with diet and exercise, but the progress was minimal. Her preoperative weight was 298 pounds (135 kg), and she is 5 feet, 5 inches (165 cm) tall.

1. What is BMI? Calculate S.B.'s BMI and specify the degree of obesity her BMI reflects.

2. What is the Roux-en-Y procedure? What are the intended outcomes of this surgery?

3. Using arrows, specify the direction of food passage and the direction of digestive juices after Roux-en-Y gastric bypass surgery.

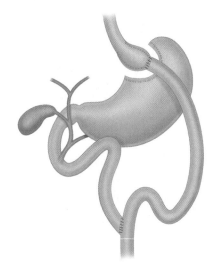

4. In preparing the room for S.B.'s admission, what equipment would you ensure is in place to eliminate embarrassment and promote patient safety? Explain your rationale.

CASE STUDY PROGRESS

S.B. is admitted to the bariatric unit and positioned in a bariatric bed. Postoperative orders include placing the nasogastric (NG) tube on low continuous suction. S.B.'s family asks, "How can she eat if this tube is in her nose?"

5. What education will you need to offer the patient and family about the need for the NG tube and delivery of nutrition?

6. How much volume is the gastric pouch able to hold after a Roux-en-Y surgery?
   a. 10 to 15 mL
   b. 15 to 30 mL
   c. 30 to 50 mL
   d. 50 to 100 mL

Chart View

Post-Op Orders

  1000 mL normal saline with thiamine 100 mg, folic acid 1 mg, and multivitamins 10 mL, once daily to infuse at 125 mL/hr
  Famotidine (Pepcid) 20 mg IVP twice daily
  Head of bed at 30 degrees
  Ambulate every 4 hours
  Out of bed to chair twice daily
  Incentive spirometry

7. What is the purpose of the IV infusion?

Digestion

8. What type of medication is famotidine, and what is its purpose?

9. What is the purpose for raising the head of the bed 30 degrees?

CASE STUDY PROGRESS

On postoperative day 2, S.B. is refusing to get out bed to ambulate or to transfer to the bedside recliner. She is requesting to lie in bed with the head of bed flat.

10. List at least 4 interventions you should encourage for the immobile patient with risk for postsurgical complications.

11. What are the risks associated with immobility and bed rest after surgery?

12. What education should you give to S.B. about the importance of using the incentive spirometer (IS)?

13. You are giving S.B. instructions on how to use the IS. Which statements are correct about the proper use of the IS? Select all that apply.
   a. "Incentive spirometry should be done every hour."
   b. "If able, sit in the chair or as far up in bed as possible to use the IS."
   c. "Place the mouthpiece in your mouth, but there should not be an airtight seal."
   d. "After each set of deep breaths using the IS, cough to make sure your lungs are clear."
   e. "Breathe in slowly and as deeply as possible, until you see the piston reach the goal amount for volume."
   f. "After breathing in, hold the breath and the piston in place for 3 to 5 seconds and then release the breath."

CASE STUDY PROGRESS

On postoperative day 3, S.B. has been out of bed to the chair once and has ambulated in the hall twice. She has been using the IS based on your instructions and has been able to meet her volume goal. Suddenly, S.B. reports that she is not able to achieve the IS goals and is having increased abdominal pain. The UAP takes vital signs and reports them as follows: BP 100/76, P 113, R 12, T 101.4° F (38.6° C).

14. What is the nurse's priority assessment?

15. What information would the nurse document while assessing the surgical incision?

16. Based on the patient's vital signs, what does the nurse suspect?

17. The surgical incision showed no drainage or other abnormal findings. Which tests would the nurse expect to be ordered? Select all that apply, and explain your answers.
   a. Lactic acid
   b. Chest x-ray
   c. Urine culture
   d. Blood cultures
   e. Abdominal CT scan
   f. Liver function panel
   g. CBC with differential

CASE STUDY PROGRESS

The lab results all come back within defined limits for the patients, but the cultures are pending. S.B. has been able to achieve adequate pain control and has been more mobile. Her temperature is down to 98.7° F (37.1° C). The NG tube was removed, and she is now taking a full liquid diet and advancing as tolerated. You overhear the patient state, "I have probably lost 15 pounds (6.8 kg) already because of the surgery. I can eat whatever I want now."

18. How would you address this comment? What education should you offer the patient about gastric bypass and weight loss?

19. Once S.B. begins eating regularly, what complication should the nurse anticipate and assess for?

20. Which nutrient deficiencies are common with this type of surgery? Select all that apply.
   a. Iron
   b. Calcium
   c. Vitamin C
   d. Magnesium
   e. Cobalamin (B12)

CASE STUDY OUTCOME

The dietitian follows up with S.B. and discusses healthy eating practices and smart food choices. They develop a plan and goals for managing and maintaining S.B's weight loss. S.B. was discharged home with home health care, home physical therapy, and nutritional services. After 8 months, S.B. successfully lost 88 lbs (40 kg) after gastric bypass surgery and is an active member of a local bariatric surgery support group.

Case Study 66

Name_____ Class/Group_____ Date_____

▶ Scenario

You are a nurse working on a surgical unit and take the following report from the registered nurse in the emergency department. "We are sending you a patient with rule out small bowel obstruction and/or food blockage. Dr. N., the gastrointestinal specialist, is on his way in to see the patient. D.S. is a 68-year-old obese man who has had a sudden onset of severe abdominal cramping, distention, and nausea and vomiting; he denies passing of flatus or stool within the past 12 hours. Past medical history includes heart failure, hypertension, colon cancer, and ulcerative colitis. He underwent a total colectomy 6 years ago and had an enterocutaneous fistula 4 years ago. Lab samples have been drawn, and the results will be sent to your floor. We started an IV and placed a Salem Sump nasogastric tube (NGT). His vital signs are 143/76, 82, respirations 26 and slightly labored, and 101.1° F (38.4° C). He is on his way up."

1. Given that D.S. previously had a total colectomy, would he have a colostomy or an ileostomy? Explain your answer.

2. What would you expect to see if D.S.'s ostomy has normal function?

CASE STUDY PROGRESS

After D.S. is settled into his room, the NGT and IV line are functioning well, and he receives pain medication, you begin your admission assessment. His abdomen is extremely large, firm to touch, with multiple scars and an ileostomy pouching system in his right lower quadrant (RLQ).

3. Describe 3 common complications of an ileostomy.

4. D.S.'s past medical history of fistula, combined with the probability of blockage or obstruction, places him at an increased risk for which problems?

5. As you assess the stoma, you look for signs that it is healthy. Which assessment findings are characteristics of a healthy stoma? Select all that apply.
   a. The stoma is dry.
   b. The stoma is moist.
   c. The stoma is pale pink in color.
   d. The stoma is flat against the skin.
   e. The stoma is cherry red to dark pink in color.

6. What stoma changes would you report immediately to the physician? Name at least 4.

7. Why are transparent ostomy pouches recommended for postoperative patients or for patients who are hospitalized?

8. True or False: The stoma will present visual clues of D.S.'s bowel blockage or obstruction. Explain your answer.

CASE STUDY PROGRESS

D.S. continues to complain of abdominal pain and cramping and becomes increasingly restless. You notice that the abdomen behind and around his stoma and pouch appears larger when compared with the other side of his abdomen.

9. How would you assess for a possible peristomal hernia?

10. Why is a peristomal hernia a problem?

CASE STUDY PROGRESS

You note the ostomy pouch has liquid brown effluent along the lateral edge of the wafer. You check to see that the pouch is properly attached to the wafer and discover that stool is indeed leaking from under the barrier. D.S. apologizes for not bringing any supplies with him, stating, "My ostomy nurse told me to always carry extra supplies for times like this." Right now, D.S. cannot remember what size he needs. You note he is wearing a two-piece system with a plastic ring-flange that attaches to the pouch with a matching ring.

11. How will you determine the correct pouching size and system?

CASE STUDY PROGRESS

You finish your general head-to-toe assessment and order the appropriate pouching products for D.S. You take clean towels, washcloths, and underpads into his room, along with a hamper for soiled linens. You gather scissors, Skin-Prep, and adhesive remover to assist with the pouching change.

12. As you return to his room, you review the steps for changing an ostomy pouch. What are the steps you will need to follow?

CASE STUDY PROGRESS

You have gathered all needed supplies, and D.S. is as comfortable as possible. You begin the pouching change. Using the adhesive remover, with the push-pull method, you gently remove the wafer. As you lift the wafer, you note that the peristomal skin has severe erythema directly encircling the stoma. There is denudation (partial-thickness breakdown) at the medial stoma-skin edge.

13. How should the skin around the stoma look?

14. In general, there are 4 different causes of erythema or skin breakdown. Identify 2.

15. After you discover the reddened skin, how will you proceed with the ostomy care?

16. As you clean the site, D.S. tells you, "You need to scrub that with strong soap! It's dirty!" How do you reply to D.S.?

17. As you plan care for D.S. for the shift, which activities may be performed by UAP? Select all that apply.
   a. Empty ostomy bag.
   b. Provide skin care around the ostomy.
   c. Assess and document stoma appearance.
   d. Measure liquid contents from ostomy bag.
   e. Teach ostomy care and skin care to the patient and caregiver.

CASE STUDY PROGRESS

The next day, D.S.'s vital signs return to normal and his abdomen is less distended. The ileostomy is steadily draining greenish-brown liquid stool. The NGT is removed, and D.S. is started on sips of clear liquids. When you go to check his ileostomy pouch, D.S. tells you, "I know I've had this a long time, but I still can't stand to look at this thing. My wife usually helps me with it, and I hate that."

18. What will you suggest for D.S. at this time?

CASE STUDY OUTCOME

D.S. is discharged from the hospital and has no further complications. He and his wife now attend the local ostomy support group.

Urinary Elimination

Case Study 67

Name _____ Class/Group _____ Date _____

▶ **Scenario**

You are working in an extended care facility when M.Z.'s daughter brings her mother in for a week's stay while she goes on a planned vacation. M.Z. is an 89-year-old widow with a 4-day history of nonlocalized abdominal discomfort, incontinence, new-onset mental confusion, and loose stools. Her most current vital signs are 118/60, 88, 18, 98.4° F (37.4° C). The medical director ordered a postvoid catheterization, which yielded 100 mL of cloudy urine that had a strong odor, and several lab tests on admission. Urine culture and sensitivity (C&S) results are pending; the other results are shown in the chart.

Chart View

Laboratory Test Results

Complete metabolic panel (CMP): Within normal limits except for the following results:

BUN	25 mg/dL (8.9 mmol/L)
Sodium	131 mEq/L (131 mmol/L)
Potassium	3.2 mEq/L (3.2 mmol/L)
White blood cell count	11,000/mm^3 (11 x 10^9/L)

Urinalysis

Appearance	Cloudy
Odor	Foul
pH	8.9
Protein	Negative
Nitrites	Positive
Crystals	Negative
WBCs	6 per low-power field
RBCs	3

1. What condition do the lab reports point toward?

2. Which assessment findings are typical of an older adult with the condition in Question 1?
   a. Fever
   b. Hematuria
   c. Bladder spasms
   d. Nonlocalized abdominal discomfort

3. Considering her history and lab results, what other condition is a possibility?

4. The medical director makes rounds and writes orders to start an IV of D_5 NS at 75 mL/hr. Because M.Z. is unable to take oral medications, the medical director orders ciprofloxacin (Cipro) 400 mg q12hr IV piggyback (IVPB). Are the type of fluid and rate appropriate for M.Z.'s age and condition? Explain.

5. While the IVPB ciprofloxacin is being administered, which adverse effects might occur? Select all that apply.
   a. Nausea
   b. Headache
   c. Drowsiness
   d. Hypotension
   e. Restlessness
   f. Tendon rupture

6. You enter the room to start the IV infusion and find that the UAP had taken M.Z. to the bathroom for a bowel movement. M.Z. asks you to help her, and, as you open the door, you observe her wiping herself from back to front. What do you need to do at this time?

7. Later that day, M.Z. has difficulty voiding, and palpation of the bladder reveals distention. A bedside bladder scanner indicates at least 250 mL of urine in the bladder. A Foley catheter is ordered and inserted. Because M.Z. has been having diarrhea, what special instructions should you give the UAP assigned to give basic care to M.Z.?

CASE STUDY PROGRESS

The next day, you are the nurse assigned to M.Z.'s care. You notice that the UAP emptying the gravity drain is not wearing personal protection devices. You observe that the drainage port of the drainage bag was contaminated during the process because the UAP allowed it to touch the floor.

8. What issues need to be considered in protecting M.Z.'s safety? Describe your actions in working with the UAP.

9. As you assess M.Z., you notice that her catheter tubing is not secured. Why does the tubing need to be secured? Where is the correct place for the catheter tubing?

CASE STUDY PROGRESS

On the third day after M.Z.'s admission, the urinary C&S results are as follows: *E. coli,* more than 100,000 colonies, sensitive to ciprofloxacin, trimethoprim-sulfamethoxazole, and nitrofurantoin.

10. What changes, if any, will be made to the antibiotic therapy?

11. The UAP reports that M.Z.'s 8-hour intake is 520 mL and the output is 140 mL. Identify 2 possible reasons that could account for the difference and explain how you would assess each.

CASE STUDY PROGRESS

Further monitoring of M.Z.'s urine output reflects adequate output amounts. After a week, M.Z. has completed her antibiotic therapy. Her mental status has cleared, the Foley catheter has been discontinued, and she is voiding without difficulty. She is ready for discharge.

12. What instructions should you discuss with the daughter?

13. She needs to notify the primary care physician if her mother develops which problems? Name at least 6.

CASE STUDY OUTCOME

The diarrhea subsides, and M.Z.'s urine is more clear and normal in appearance. She goes back to her daughter's home after a week and is more alert.

Case Study **68**

Name_____ Class/Group_____ Date_____

▶ Scenario

You are working in the emergency department (ED) when M.B., a 72-year-old man, comes in and states he is unable to void. His initial vital signs (VS) are 168/92, 88, 20, 98.2° F (36.8° C).

1. Are M.B.'s VS appropriate for a man of his age? If not, offer a rationale for the abnormal readings.

2. Given M.B.'s statement, what would you expect to find during your initial assessment?

CASE STUDY PROGRESS

While you are taking M.B.'s history, he tells you he is generally in good health and leads an active life. His current medications include finasteride (Proscar) 5 mg/day and vitamin supplements. He reports that he has been unable to void for 12 hours and is very uncomfortable. He asks you to help him.

3. Which of these statements best describes the therapeutic effect of the finasteride?
   a. It reduces urinary flow.
   b. It strengthens the detrusor muscle.
   c. It reduces the size of the prostate gland.
   d. It causes relaxation of the urinary sphincter.

4. What do you need to know about the history of his use of the finasteride?

 5. If you are going to administer the finasteride, what precautions are necessary?

6. What are your priorities for this patient?

7. After examining M.B., the ED physician asks you to insert an indwelling urethral Foley catheter. What will you include in M.B.'s teaching before placing the Foley?

8. You have just finished providing peri-care and are preparing to insert the Foley catheter. Put in order the steps to follow when inserting a Foley catheter, with 1 being the first step:

_____ a. Apply sterile gloves.

_____ b. Anchor the catheter to the patient's inner thigh.

_____ c. Ensure that the drainage bag is secured to the bed, below the level of the bladder.

_____ d. Position and drape the patient.

_____ e. Cleanse the urethral meatus, following the proper procedure for a male patient.

_____ f. Open lubricant container, antiseptic container. Most catheter manufacturers no longer recommend testing the balloon.

_____ g. Inflate the balloon fully with the amount of fluid recommended for the catheter.

_____ h. Gently insert the catheter 7 to 9 inches (17 to 22.5 cm) or until urine flows into the catheter tubing, then insert catheter at least 1 inch further.

_____ i. Perform hand hygiene.

_____ j. Lubricate catheter.

_____ k. Open the catheterization kit and place the underpad, if present, under the patient.

9. After two unsuccessful attempts to advance the catheter into the bladder, you stop. What is your next intervention? Why? What could be causing this problem?

10. The ED physician successfully inserts the indwelling catheter with the use of the type of catheter illustrated in the accompanying figure. What type of catheter is this, what is its advantage in this situation, and how is it inserted?

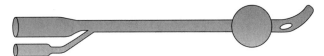

11. As the physician begins to inflate the catheter balloon, M.B. winces in pain and states, "*Ouch, you're hurting me!*" What happened, and what will the physician do?

12. You watch the urine drain into the bag and note that the amount is approaching 500 mL. What do you do at this time?

13. After the catheter is in place, the ED physician writes orders to discharge M.B. with instructions to see his primary care provider (PCP) on the following day. It is your responsibility to give discharge instructions. Outline your care plan.

14. The next day, M.B. is seen by his PCP, who changes M.B.'s medication to alfuzosin (Uroxatral). The catheter will be discontinued 2 days later. What teaching is essential regarding this new medication?
    a. Alfuzosin needs to be taken in the morning.
    b. M.B. needs to take each dose on an empty stomach.
    c. This medication might cause fainting when he first starts taking it.
    d. M.B. can stop taking the alfuzosin once the urinary symptoms subside.

15. You provide teaching on managing episodes of urinary retention. You use the Teach-Back technique and ask M.B. to teach back the concept he has learned. Which statement by M.B. indicates a need for further teaching?
   a. "A warm shower may help me urinate."
   b. "I will drink small amounts of water throughout the day."
   c. "I will limit alcoholic drinks to 1 per day if I have any."
   d. "I will drink large amounts of water at mealtimes to help me urinate."

CASE STUDY OUTCOME

M.B. is discharged but continues to have difficulty emptying his bladder. He is referred to a urologist who eventually recommends surgery for an enlarged prostate gland.

Case Study 69

Name_____   Class/Group_____   Date_____

▶ Scenario

N.H., an 89-year-old widow, recently experienced a left-sided cerebrovascular accident (CVA). She has right-sided weakness and expressive aphasia with minimal swallowing difficulty. N.H. has a medical history of a minor left-sided CVA 2 1/2 years ago, chronic atrial flutter, and hypertension. She has lived with her daughter's family in a rural town since her previous stroke. Since admission to an acute care facility 5 days ago, N.H. has gained some strength, has become oriented to person and place, and is anxious to begin her rehabilitation program. She is transferred for rehabilitation to your skilled nursing facility with the orders shown in the chart.

Chart View

Admission Orders

Hydrochlorothiazide 25 mg/day PO
Digoxin 0.125 mg/day PO
Warfarin (Coumadin) 5 mg/day PO
Acetaminophen 325 mg q6hr PO prn for pain
Zolpidem (Ambien) 5 mg PO at bedtime prn for sleep
Diet: Mechanical soft, low sodium with ground meat
Foley catheter to gravity drainage, and then begin bladder training
Referrals for speech therapy, occupational therapy, and physical therapy to evaluate and treat
    swallowing, communication, and functional abilities

1. What lab orders would you anticipate as a result of this specific list of orders? With each response, describe your rationale.

CASE STUDY PROGRESS

A week later, at the interdisciplinary care conference, you report that bladder training is progressing and recommend removing the catheter if N.H.'s mobility and communication abilities have progressed sufficiently. The group and N.H. agree that she is ready for the Foley catheter to be removed.

2. Identify 3 problems that N.H. is at risk for developing after catheter removal and describe specific interventions for each problem.

CASE STUDY PROGRESS

Two days after the Foley catheter is removed, you observe that N.H.'s urine is cloudy and concentrated and has a strong odor, even though the volumes voided have been adequate.

3. What are your immediate actions?

CASE STUDY PROGRESS

N.H. is started on sulfamethoxazole 800 mg/trimethoprim 160 mg (Bactrim DS) 1 tab PO bid × 10 days for a urinary tract infection (UTI). However, 2 days later, N.H. is in the bathroom and she is very upset. She has just voided; there is blood on the toilet, and the water is bright red with blood. You help the UAP clean N.H. and help her into bed.

4. Describe your assessment steps.

5. Identify at least 2 potential causes for N.H.'s hematuria.

6. Using SBAR, what information would you provide to the physician when you call?

CASE STUDY PROGRESS

N.H.'s physician changes her antibiotic to oral ciprofloxacin (Cipro) and holds the warfarin for 2 days. Two days later, N.H.'s UTI is responding to antibiotics and she has had no further bleeding in the urine. You want to prepare her and her daughter for eventual discharge.

7. You have provided teaching about preventing a recurrent UTI to N.H. and her daughter. You use the Teach-Back technique to confirm understanding. Which statement by N.H.'s daughter indicates an adequate understanding of the information provided?
   a. "She needs to limit how much water she drinks each day."
   b. "When Mom uses the toilet she needs to wipe from back to front."
   c. "She needs to try to urinate every 2 to 3 hours and not delay it if she needs to go."
   d. "If she thinks she might be getting an infection, I will mention it at her next appointment."

8. You discuss with N.H.'s daughter how certain foods and drinks may irritate the bladder and should be avoided. These foods include which of the following? Select all that apply.
   a. Bananas
   b. Chocolate
   c. Spicy foods
   d. Citrus juices
   e. Caffeinated beverages

9. You talk with N.H.'s daughter about her understanding of caregiving responsibilities for her mother. What kind of questions do you ask to assess whether she is capable of taking care of her mother since her mother's health has declined? List at least four.

CASE STUDY OUTCOME

N.H.'s right-sided weakness and expressive aphasia do not resolve. Her daughter takes N.H. home and, with the help of her sister, nieces, and a home health aide, they have adjusted well to living together.

Case Study **70**

Name_____ Class/Group_____ Date_____

▶ Scenario

S.M. is a 68-year-old man who is being seen at your clinic for routine health maintenance and health promotion. He reports that he has been feeling well and has no specific complaints, except for some trouble "emptying my bladder." Vital signs at this visit are 148/88, 82, 16, 96.9° F (36.1° C). He had a complete blood count and complete metabolic panel completed 1 week before his visit, and the results are listed in the chart.

Chart View

Laboratory Test Results

Sodium	140 mEq/L (140 mmol/L)
Potassium	4.2 mEq/L (4.2 mmol/L)
Chloride	100 mEq/L (100 mmol/L)
Bicarbonate	26 mEq/L (26 mmol/L)
BUN	19 mg/dL (6.8 mmol/L)
Creatinine	0.8 mg/dL (72 mcmol/L)
Glucose	94 mg/dL (5.2 mmol/L)
RBC	5.2 million/mm³ (5.2×10^{12}/L)
WBC	7400/mm³ (7.4×10^9/L)
Hgb	15.2 g/dL (152 g/L)
Hct	46%
Platelets	348,000/mm³ (348×10^9/L)
Prostate-specific antigen (PSA)	4.23 ng/mL (4.23 mcg/L)
Urinalysis	Within normal limits

1. What can you tell S.M. about his lab work?

2. What is the significance of the PSA result?

3. What other specific examination will S.M. need to have along with the PSA test?

CASE STUDY PROGRESS

While obtaining your nursing history, you record no family history of cancer or other genitourinary problems. S.M. reports frequency, urgency, and nocturia × 4; he has a weak stream and has to sit to void. These symptoms have been progressive over the past 6 months. He reports he was diagnosed with a "large prostate" a number of years ago. Last month, he began taking saw palmetto capsules but had to stop taking them because "they made me sick."

4. Why did S.M. try taking the saw palmetto, and why do you think he stopped taking it?

5. S.M. is curious why his enlarged prostate would affect his urination. He is concerned that he has prostate cancer. What would you teach him?

CASE STUDY PROGRESS

The primary care provider (PCP) performs a digital rectal examination (DRE) and asks for a post-void residual (PVR) urine test.

6. Which findings from the DRE indicate BPH? Select all that apply.
   a. Prostate is firm.
   b. Prostate feels nodular.
   c. Prostate feels spongy.
   d. Prostate feels smooth.
   e. Prostate is symmetrically enlarged.

7. You use a bedside bladder scanner and document that S.M. voided 60 mL and his PVR is 120 mL. You report the PVR to the PCP. What is the significance of his PVR?

8. Which of these are considered risk factors for BPH? Select all that apply.
   a. Aging
   b. Obesity
   c. Smoking
   d. High cholesterol levels
   e. Lack of physical activity
   f. History of urinary tract infections

9. Commonly used medications for BPH are 5-alpha-reductase inhibitors, such as finasteride (Proscar), and alpha-blocking drugs, such as tamsulosin (Flomax). How do these drugs differ?

10. The PCP orders tamsulosin (Flomax) 0.4 mg/day PO. You enter S.M.'s room to teach him about this medication. What side effects will you tell S.M. about? Select all that apply.
    a. Diarrhea
    b. Dizziness
    c. Headache
    d. Heartburn
    e. Dry mouth
    f. Orthostatic hypotension

11. S.M. asks, "Will this condition affect my relationship with my wife?" What should you tell him?

12. What would you expect S.M. to report if the medication was successful?

CASE STUDY PROGRESS

S.M. returns in 6 months to report that his symptoms are worse than ever. He has tried several different medications, but medication management failed, and he is told that surgical intervention is necessary.

13. What surgical options are available to S.M.? Describe at least 3.

CASE STUDY OUTCOME

S.M. chose an outpatient procedure. He did well postoperatively and was discharged to home.

Case Study **71**

Name_____ Class/Group_____ Date_____

▶ Scenario

G.W., a 34-year-old African American man, presents with increasing right knee swelling. He states that the swelling has gotten worse over the past 2 weeks and on presentation is now having difficulty ambulating. He reports taking over-the-counter ibuprofen 200 mg tablets at least 4 to 8 tablets per day for nearly 1 year for persistent back and knee pain. He has not seen his primary care physician (PCP) in nearly 2 years. G.W. also complains of weakness, fatigue, decreased urine output, and joint pain and stiffness. He also tells you that when he does urinate, it looks "rusty." His vital signs are as follows: BP 210/100, P 86, R 24, T 98.7° F (37.1° C).

1. What are the health risks associated with taking ibuprofen for an extended period?

2. What specific questions would you ask G.W. based on his reported symptoms?

CASE STUDY PROGRESS

G.W. tells you that a few years ago he was diagnosed with high blood pressure, but he did not like the medication's side effects, so he stopped taking it. He said that he was told that he had "kidney problems" but never kept the appointments to check his kidneys. After further assessment, the nurse finds that the abdomen appears firm, round, and distended with edema. He has +2 edema on his ankles and shins bilaterally. He reports decreased urine output; on admission urine is dark and rust-colored. G.W. is alert and oriented to person, place, time and situation. He is lethargic but easily arousable and coherent. His blood work shows a BUN of 35 mg/dL (12.5 mmol/L), serum creatinine of 4.7 mg/dL (415 mcmol/L), albumin 1.2 g/dL (12 g/L), and H&H 7.1 g/dL (71 g/L) & 23.5%. The results of his urinalysis are listed here:

Chart View

Urinalysis

Appearance	**Clear**
Color:	Rust
Odor:	Aromatic
pH	6.2
Protein	14 mg/dL
Glucose	Negative
White blood cells	5
WBC casts	Many
Red blood cells	10
RBC casts	Many

---

3. The physician suspects glomerulonephritis. Which assessment findings and lab results support this diagnosis?

4. What risk factors, if any, does G.W. have for developing glomerulonephritis?

5. Differentiate acute and chronic glomerulonephritis. Which one does G.W. have? Defend your answer.

6. What diagnostic tests are used to confirm the diagnosis of glomerulonephritis?

7. G.W. asks you, "What is glomerulonephritis? Do I have a kidney infection?" Which answer is correct?
   a. "No, you have had an allergic reaction to the ibuprofen."
   b. "Yes, glomerulonephritis is a chronic infection of the kidneys."
   c. "Yes, you had a bladder infection that led to a kidney infection."
   d. "No, glomerulonephritis is an inflammation of a section of the kidneys."

CASE STUDY PROGRESS

The nephrologist is consulted and the results of a renal biopsy confirm the diagnosis of chronic glomerulonephritis. G.W. received a furosemide (Lasix) drip, and had a total urine output of 450 mL in the next 24 hours. G.W.'s BP has improved but remains elevated at 198/102. The nephrologist ordered lisinopril 5 mg PO once daily, IV methylprednisolone (Solu-Medrol) and cyclophosphamide 2 mg/kg PO daily.

8. How does lisinopril work to reduce blood pressure?
   a. Increases the heart rate.
   b. Increases preload and afterload.
   c. Causes systemic vasoconstriction.
   d. Prevents the conversion of angiotensin I to angiotensin II.

9. What nursing considerations are important when giving lisinopril?

10. What are the expected outcomes of furosemide (Lasix) therapy? Select all that apply.
   a. Diuresis of excess fluid
   b. Reduced blood pressure
   c. Decreased BUN and creatinine levels
   d. Increased systemic vascular resistance
   e. Increased water, sodium, and potassium excretion

11. What do you need to monitor while G.W. is on a furosemide (Lasix) infusion?

12. Which findings would indicate potential adverse effects of a furosemide (Lasix) infusion? Select all that apply.
   a. Tinnitus
   b. Dizziness
   c. Weakness
   d. Dry mouth
   e. Increased blood pressure

13. Cyclophosphamide comes in 50 mg tablets. G.W. weighs 110 pounds (50 kg). How many 50 mg tablets will he receive for each daily dose of cyclophosphamide?

14. Discuss at least 3 nursing interventions that are important while the patient is on cyclophosphamide therapy.

CASE STUDY PROGRESS

Orders for G.W. include fluid restriction and a "renal diet." The dietitian visits G.W. to discuss the changes to his diet.

15. Which of these reflect a renal diet? Select all that apply.
   a. High protein diet
   b. Reduced salt intake
   c. Increased potassium intake
   d. Reduced phosphorus intake
   e. Taking calcium supplements

16. Discuss the rationale behind the fluid restriction and renal diet.

CASE STUDY OUTCOME

After 3 days, G.W.'s creatinine and BUN remained elevated with continued hypertension, edema, and decreased urine output. He was started on hemodialysis for management of renal function and the Solu-Medrol was changed to PO prednisone. He remained in the hospital for 3 weeks before being transferred to a rehabilitation facility.

Case Study **72**

Name_____ Class/Group_____ Date_____

▶ Scenario

K.B. is a 32-year-old woman being admitted to the medical floor for fatigue and dehydration. While taking her history, you discover that she has diabetes mellitus (DM) and has been insulin dependent since the age of 8. She has undergone hemodialysis (HD) for the past 2 years because of end-stage renal disease (ESRD). Your initial assessment of K.B. reveals a pale, thin, slightly drowsy woman. Her skin is warm and dry to the touch with poor skin turgor, and her mucous membranes are dry. Her vital signs are 140/88, 116, 18, 99.9° F (37.7° C). She tells you she has been nauseated for 2 days so she has not been eating or drinking. She reports severe diarrhea. The following blood chemistry results are back.

Chart View

Laboratory Test Results	
Sodium	145 mEq/L (145 mmol/L)
Potassium	6.0 mEq/L (6.0 mmol/L)
Chloride	93 mEq/L (93 mmol/L)
Bicarbonate	27 mEq/L (27 mmol/L)
BUN	48 mg/dL (17.1 mmol/L)
Creatinine	5.0 mg/dL (442 mcmol/L)
Glucose	238 mg/dL (13.2 mmol/L)

1. What aspects of your assessment support her admitting diagnosis of dehydration?

2. Explain any lab results that might be of concern.

3. Identify 2 possible causes for K.B.'s low-grade fever.

CASE STUDY PROGRESS

The rest of K.B.'s physical assessment is within normal limits. You note that she has an arteriovenous (AV) fistula in her left arm.

4. What is an AV fistula? Why does K.B. have one?

5. What steps do you take to assess K.B.'s AV fistula, and what physical findings are expected? Explain.

6. As you continue the assessment, you notice that the UAP comes in to take K.B.'s BP. The UAP places the BP cuff on K.B.'s left arm. What, if anything, do you do?

CASE STUDY PROGRESS

K.B.'s admission CBC yields the following results:

Chart View

Laboratory Test Results

WBC	7600/mm³ (7.6 x 10⁹/L)
RBC	3.2 million/mm³ (3.2 x 10¹²/L)
Hgb	8.1 g/dL (81 g/L)
Hct	24.3%
Platelets	333,000/mm³ (330 x 10⁹/L)

7. Are these values normal? If not, what are the abnormalities?

8. K.B.'s physician notes that she is anemic, which most likely is the cause of her increasing fatigue. Why is K.B. anemic?

CASE STUDY PROGRESS

K.B. is sent for an HD treatment. Over the next 24 hours, K.B.'s nausea subsides, and she is able to eat normally. While you are helping her with her morning care, she confides in you that she does not understand her diet. "I just get blood drawn every week and meet with the dialysis dietitian every month—I just eat what she tells me to eat. It's so hard!"

9. Because K.B. is on HD and has DM, who would be the best resource to help her with her nutrition questions?

10. What are her special nutritional needs? Name at least 4 specific components of the diet recommended for K.B.

11. Which of these statements about fluid intake for dialysis patients is correct? Select all that apply.
a. There are no fluid restrictions for dialysis patients.
b. Dialysis patients need to restrict fluid intake to water only.
c. Fluids are restricted to 600 mL plus the amount equal to the previous day's urine output.
d. A fluid is anything that is liquid at room temperature, such as coffee, popsicles, and ice cream.
e. Hypertension may occur if large amounts of fluid are retained between dialysis treatments.

12. Patients in renal failure have the potential to develop comorbid conditions. Identify 5 potential problems, determine how you would assess the problem, then delineate nursing interventions and patient education strategies for each.

CASE STUDY PROGRESS

The following day, K.B. is discharged feeling much better and with a good understanding of her dietary restrictions. Her iron stores have been evaluated and found to be low. Her physician has instructed her to resume her preadmission medications, with the addition of ferrous fumarate oral suspension 100 mg PO bid between meals with water, if tolerated (or with meals if GI distress occurs) and epoetin (Epogen) to be given 3 times a week intravenously with dialysis. She is also given a prescription for Nephrocaps vitamin supplements to be taken daily.

13. Explain the purpose of the new medications for K.B.

14. You spend some time with K.B. to explain the new medications. Using the Teach-Back technique, you ask K.B. to explain what she has learned. Which statement by K.B. reflects need for further teaching?
   a. "The liquid iron will cause my bowel movements to turn black or dark green."
   b. "I should dilute the liquid iron and drink it with a straw so that it won't stain my teeth."
   c. "I won't need to take the iron supplements as long as I get the Epogen during dialysis."
   d. "Hopefully I will feel less tired all the time when these medicines start building up my red blood cells."

15. K.B. asks, "Why do I need a prescription for vitamins? I can just take something on sale at the drugstore, right?" How do you respond?

16. The ferrous fumarate suspension comes in a bottle that is labeled 100 mg/5 mL. Indicate on the measuring cup how much medication will be used for each dose.

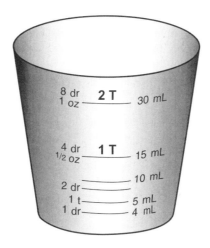

17. K.B. asks you, "I can just use a teaspoon to measure this medicine when I'm at home, right?" What is your response?

18. In monitoring K.B.'s response to the epoetin, what adverse effects would you expect? Select all that apply.
   a. Diarrhea
   b. Headache
   c. Arthralgia
   d. Drowsiness
   e. Tachycardia
   f. Hypertension

19. Which vital sign will you monitor carefully while K.B. is on epoetin therapy? Explain your answer.

20. During the following weeks, which lab result is most important to monitor while K.B. is on the epoetin? Explain.

CASE STUDY OUTCOME

K.B. is discharged to home and goes to the local dialysis center 3 times a week. She also keeps appointments with the registered dietitian and reports that she is feeling much better.

Case Study **73**

Name_____ Class/Group_____ Date_____

▶ Scenario

You are a registered nurse in the emergency department (ED). It is a hot summer day and S.R., a 25-year-old woman, comes to the ED with severe left flank and abdominal pain and nausea with vomiting. S.R. looks very tired, her skin is warm, and she is perspiring. She paces about the room doubled over and is clutching her abdomen. S.R. tells you the pain started early this morning and has been pretty steady for the past 6 hours. She gives a history of working outside as a landscaper and takes little time for water breaks. Her past medical history includes three kidney stone attacks, all occurring during late summer. Her abdomen is soft and without tenderness, but her left flank is extremely tender to touch. You place S.R. in one of the examination rooms and take the following vital signs: 188/98, 90, 20, 99° F (37.2° C). A voided urinalysis shows RBCs of 50 to 100 on voided specimen and WBCs of zero.

1. What could be the cause of the blood in her urine? How could you rule out some of these causes?

2. The physician orders an intravenous pyelogram (IVP). What questions do you need to ask S.R. before the test is conducted? What blood test results do you need to check before she has an IVP?

3. S.R. states she had an allergic reaction during her last IVP and was instructed, "Don't let anyone give you dye for any testing." The physician cancels the IVP. What alternative test will be conducted?

CASE STUDY PROGRESS

The noncontrast CT scan shows a left 2-mm ureteral vesicle junction stone.

4. What are the most common types of stones? Select all that apply.
   a. Cystine
   b. Struvite
   c. Uric acid
   d. Calcium oxalate
   e. Calcium phosphate

5. What is the most likely cause of S.R.'s stone?

6. What is a possible complication if S.R.'s stone is not removed?
   a. Trabeculation
   b. Hydronephrosis
   c. Nephrosclerosis
   d. Nephrotic syndrome

7. Identify 2 methods of treating a patient with a ureteral vesicle junction stone.

CASE STUDY PROGRESS

S.R. was discharged with instructions to strain all urine and return if she experienced pain unrelieved by the pain medication or increased nausea and vomiting.

8. What specific instructions will you give S.R. about straining her urine, fluid intake, medications, and activity?

CASE STUDY PROGRESS

S.R. returns to the ED in 6 hours with pain unrelieved by the pain medication and increased blood in her urine. She is being held in the ED until she can be transported to surgery.

9. What is the immediate plan of care for S.R.?

CASE STUDY PROGRESS

A 2-mm calculus was removed by basket extraction. Pathologic examination reported the stone to be calcium oxalate.

10. If S.R. continues to form calcium oxalate stones, what recommendations would the physician make for S.R.?

11. Because S.R.'s stone has been reported as calcium oxalate, she is referred to a registered dietitian for guidance on a diet that will prevent further development of stones. Which statements are true regarding recommendations for S.R.'s diet? Select all that apply.
   a. Decrease fat intake.
   b. Decrease sodium intake.
   c. Drink at least 3 to 4 liters of water each day.
   d. Avoid eating organ meats, bacon, citrus fruits, and red wine.
   e. Avoid chocolate, spinach, tomatoes, dried fruits, beans, sardines, and nuts.

12. After an education session, you use the Teach-Back technique to assess S.R.'s understanding of her new dietary guidelines. Which statement by S.R. indicates a need for further teaching?
   a. "I will avoid coffee, cocoa, and chocolate."
   b. "I will not add salt to my food when cooking."
   c. "I will drink at least 3 liters of water each day."
   d. "I will increase my intake of milk and cheese daily."

CASE STUDY OUTCOME

S.R. recovers from this most recent episode and continues to follow the protocol for fluid intake and dietary measures. One year later, she has yet to report a recurrence of stones.

Case Study 74

Name _____ Class/Group _____ Date _____

▶ Scenario

You are working on a telemetry unit and have just received a transfer from the ICU. The 70-year-old male patient, T.A., is postoperative day 2 after three-vessel coronary bypass graft surgery. He has a history of hypertension, hyperlipidemia, and type 2 diabetes mellitus requiring insulin for the past 6 months to control glucose levels. The ICU nurse tells you that there were complications during surgery and he received 3 units of blood to treat hypotension. Since surgery, T.A. has experienced intermittent atrial fibrillation that is under control with amiodarone and metoprolol. The nurse voices concern his urine output seems to be decreasing.

1. Four hours after his admission to your floor, you note that T.A. has had a total urine output of 75 mL of dark amber urine. Why are you concerned?

2. You check the urinary catheter and tubing for obstructions and find none. What other assessments do you need to gather?

CASE STUDY PROGRESS

You notify the surgeon of the decreased urine output. The surgeon orders a stat electrolyte panel and asks you to call with the results.

Chart View

Laboratory Test Results

Potassium	5.8 mEq/L (5.8 mmol/L)
Sodium	132 mEq/L (132 mmol/L)
Glucose	224 mEq/L (12.4 mmol/L)
BUN	86 mg/dL (30.7 mmol/L)
Creatinine	4.4 mg/dL (389 mcmol/L)

3. Interpret T.A.'s lab results.

 4. What actions do you need to take because of the serum potassium level?

CASE STUDY PROGRESS

Chart View

Medication Administration Record

> Dopamine IV infusion at 2 mcg/kg/min
> Furosemide 80 mg IV push daily
> Sodium polystyrene sulfonate (Kayexalate) 1 gram PO twice daily
> Sevelamer hydrochloride (Renagel) 800 mg PO with meals

5. The surgeon writes new orders. Identify the expected outcome associated with each medication he will be receiving.

 6. T.A. weighs 164 lbs. The pharmacy-supplied IV bag reads "dopamine 400 mg/250 mL." Calculate the hourly rate for the dopamine infusion. Round to the tenth.

CASE STUDY PROGRESS

The surgeon determines that T.A. is in the oliguric phase of acute kidney injury (AKI). T.A. is sent to radiology for placement of a dialysis catheter.

7. What is the likely reason T.A. developed AKI?

8. The RIFLE criteria delineate the three stages of AKI based on:
   a. Glomerular filtration rate (GFR)
   b. Serum creatinine and urine output
   c. Urine osmolality and specific gravity
   d. Blood pressure and BUN/creatinine ratio

9. You decide to assess T.A. for indications of AKI. What do these include?

10. What are your priority nursing problems right now?

11. The dialysis catheter is inserted into T.A.'s left subclavian vein. You are preparing to give the IV furosemide and find that his only other IV access, a peripheral line, is the site of the dopamine infusion. What are your options?

12. T.A. asks if he is going to be on dialysis for the rest of his life. How would you respond?

13. T.A. is placed on a fluid restriction and a renal diet. T.A. asks how much he is going to be able to drink. What is your reply?

14. Briefly describe a renal diet.

15. What referral may be needed and why?

16. What are some interventions you can use to help T.A. be more comfortable while on a fluid restriction?

17. As you plan your care of T.A. for the rest of the shift, identify which aspects of his care you can delegate to the UAP. Select all that apply.
   a. Measure vital signs every 2 hours
   b. Assist him with oral hygiene as needed
   c. Obtain T.A.'s glucose level before dinner
   d. Monitor T.A.'s lung sounds every 4 hours
   e. Obtain and record an accurate daily weight
   f. Evaluate T.A.'s I/O trends for the past 48 hours

18. You note that T.A.'s postoperative blood glucose levels range from 62 to 387 mg/dL (3.4 to 21.6 mmol/L). He comments, "That's funny, you're giving me almost twice the amount of insulin that I give myself at home. I don't understand why it's not working." How should you respond?

 19. In addition to ongoing assessment, describe nursing interventions to place in T.A.'s plan of care that are part of patient safety initiatives aimed at minimizing his risk for a VTE developing.

CASE STUDY PROGRESS

The next morning, T.A. is scheduled for his first dialysis treatment at 0800.

20. What type of assessment data do you need to gather before his dialysis treatment?

21. Doses of IV amiodarone, metoprolol, and furosemide are scheduled for 0800. What should you do?
   a. Give all three medications 1 hour before dialysis
   b. Hold all three medications and notify the surgeon
   c. Give the amiodarone and hold the metoprolol and furosemide
   d. Hold all three medications and give them immediately upon return

22. T.A. is off the unit 4 hours for therapy. When he returns, what assessments do you need to make?

23. Shortly after his return, T.A. tells you he has a headache and severe nausea. He is restless and slightly confused, and his BP is 180/102. What is the significance of these findings?

24. You page the surgeon. What will you do while waiting for a return call?

CASE STUDY OUTCOME

T.A. recovers from the episode of disequilibrium syndrome. During the rest of his hospitalization, he continues to have trouble maintaining fluid and electrolyte balance between his dialysis treatments. He spends two weeks in a rehabilitation center before being discharged on dialysis and with home health. He eventually regains kidney function.

Case Study 75

Name_____ Class/Group_____ Date_____

▶ Scenario

W.V. is a 51-year-old man who lives with his wife and two teenage sons. W.V. developed chronic kidney disease 15 years ago after using a drug for migraine headaches that was later shown to cause severe nephrotoxicity. W.V. underwent hemodialysis for 5 years before receiving a cadaveric transplant, or a cadaver kidney. He recovered without complications, and his serum lab values returned to normal. He started immunosuppression therapy with prednisone and tacrolimus before his discharge to home.

1. Why are kidney transplants done?

2. What histocompatibility studies are usually done before a transplant? Why are they important?

3. By what criteria was W.V. considered a suitable candidate for a kidney transplant?

4. True or False? During transplant surgery, the old kidney is surgically removed and the new one is sewn in its place. Defend your response.

5. Why is W.V. receiving prednisone and tacrolimus?

6. Name 4 ways in which W.V. might have difficulty adjusting after an organ transplant.

7. If W.V.'s kidney is producing enough urine and he is feeling well, why is ongoing lab monitoring necessary?

8. Why should W.V. be concerned about infection?

9. Which statement would show W.V. needs further teaching regarding posttransplant care and immunosuppressant therapy?
   a. "I should wash my hands often."
   b. "I will need to have regular lab testing."
   c. "I will call the doctor if I urinate less frequently."
   d. "It will be nice to go to all of my grandkids' activities now."

CASE STUDY PROGRESS

Today, W.V. reports to his provider for a 12-week follow-up. W.V. has gained 5 pounds since his last appointment 2 weeks ago.

Chart View

Vital Signs

Blood pressure (BP)	148/82
Pulse rate	88
Respiratory rate	24
Temperature	99.2° F (37.3° C)

Laboratory Test Results

Sodium	148 mmol/L (148 mmol/L)
Potassium	4.0 mmol/L (4.0 mmol/L)
Glucose	198 mg/dL (11.0 mmol/L)
Calcium	10.1 mg/dL (2.5 mmol/L)
Creatinine	2.2 mg/dL (194 mcmol/L)
Blood urea nitrogen (BUN)	42 mg/dL (15.0 mmol/L)

10. What is the possible significance of W.V.'s BP?

11. Interpret W.V.'s lab results.

CASE STUDY PROGRESS

The provider suspects W.V. is experiencing acute rejection and orders a renal biopsy, which confirms a diagnosis of acute rejection.

12. What other signs and symptoms may be present with acute rejection?

13. Explain the pathophysiology of acute rejection.

14. What are the collaborative care options to save the kidney when rejection is present?

15. The provider decides to add mycophenolate (CellCept) 1 gram orally twice daily to W.V.'s immunosuppressive regimen. How does mycophenolate help protect W.V.'s kidney?

16. What do you need to teach W.V. about mycophenolate therapy?

17. Glipizide is prescribed for W.V.'s hyperglycemia. W.V. asks if this means he is now a diabetic. How would you answer him?

18. W.V. asks you if this means he is going to lose the kidney and go back on dialysis. How would you respond?

19. How can you best support W.V. and his family during this time?

CASE STUDY OUTCOME

W.V. does not experience any further episodes of acute rejection and within 6 months is able to be on lower doses of immunosuppressive therapy. With the lower level of immunosuppression, his elevated glucose resolves and he does not develop diabetes. His kidney continues to function well, and he says that despite a few challenges that come with being a posttransplant patient, "I feel better than I have in years."

Intracranial Regulation

Case Study 76

Name_____ Class/Group_____ Date_____

▶ Scenario

L.C. is a 78-year-old man with a 3-year history of Parkinson disease (PD). He is a retired engineer, married, and living with his wife in a small farming community. He has 4 adult children who live close by. Since his last visit to the clinic 6 months ago, L.C. reports that his tremors are "about the same" as they were. However, further questioning reveals that he feels his gait is a little more unsteady and his fatigue is slightly more noticeable. L.C. is also concerned about increased drooling. Among the medications L.C. takes are carbidopa-levodopa 25/100 mg (Sinemet) and pramipexole (Mirapex) 0.5 mg, each three times daily. On the previous visit the Sinemet was increased from 2 to 3 times daily. He reports that he has become very somnolent with this regimen and that his dyskinetic movements appear to be worse just after taking his carbidopa-levodopa (Sinemet).

1. What is PD?

2. What is parkinsonism?

3. What are the clinical manifestations of PD? Underline the symptoms L.C. has mentioned.

4. L.C.'s wife asks you, "How do the doctors know he really has Parkinson disease? They never did a lot of tests on him." How is PD diagnosed?

5. L.C. asks, "Why don't they give me a dopamine pill? Wouldn't that just fix everything?" Why is oral dopamine not a replacement therapy?

6. Why is levodopa given in combination with carbidopa?

7. Why did L.C.'s dyskinetic movements appear to be worse just after taking carbidopa-levodopa? What changes to his medication therapy may be needed?

8. Because L.C. takes Sinemet, what serious adverse effect should you assess for in him?
   a. Suicidal thoughts
   b. Permanent hearing loss
   c. Steven-Johnson syndrome
   d. Spontaneous tendon rupture

9. L.C.'s wife asks, "They can do surgery for everything else. Why can't they do some kind of surgery to fix Parkinson disease?" How would you describe the surgical treatments available for patients with PD?

After examining L.C., the provider decides not to hospitalize him but to decrease the dosage of Sinemet. He tells L.C. and his wife that he thinks L.C. is likely experiencing some advancement in his disease and says that it is time for some changes in L.C.'s care. The provider looks at you and asks you to coordinate the "usual referrals."

10. What interprofessional team members would be involved in L.C.'s care and how?

11. What factors do you need to take into consideration when helping L.C. with these referrals?

12. L.C. is reporting an increase in drooling, and you are concerned about his ability to swallow. What further assessment could you perform to determine whether L.C. is at immediate risk for aspirating?

13. What are 3 nutrition interventions that should be implemented for L.C.?

14. Because L.C. is reporting that his gait is more unsteady, there is an increased risk for falls. Which suggestion could you offer to diminish this risk?
a. Only use a wheelchair to get around
b. Use a bag or backpack to carry objects
c. Stand as upright as possible and use a walker
d. Keep the feet close together while ambulating

15. What are 3 suggestions you can make to L.C. to help manage fatigue?

 16. You are giving instructions to L.C. and his wife about ambulating safely. You determine that they understand the directions if they say that L.C. will:
a. Schedule his PT appointments in the evening
b. Sit on a large, soft sofa with supportive pillows
c. Use a step stool to obtain difficult-to-reach items
d. When rising from a seat, rock back and forth to start moving

17. As L.C.'s case manager, identify 5 things that you would need to assess to determine whether L.C. could be cared for in his home.

CASE STUDY OUTCOME

L.C. starts a multifaceted speech, OT, and PT program for persons with Parkinson disease. After 8 weeks, his gait is steadier and he is using several strategies to manage his fatigue and drooling.

Case Study **77**

Name _____ Class/Group _____ Date _____

▶ Scenario

N.T., a 79-year-old woman, arrives at the emergency department with expressive aphasia, left facial droop, left-sided hemiparesis, and mild dysphagia. Her husband states that when she awoke that morning at 0700, she stayed in bed, saying she had a mild headache over the right temple and was feeling weak. He went and got coffee, then thinking it was unusual for her to stay in bed, went back to check on her. He found she was having trouble saying words and had a left-sided facial droop. When he helped her up from the bedside, he noticed weakness in her left hand and leg and brought her to the emergency department. Her medical history includes atrial fibrillation, hypertension, and hyperlipidemia. A recent cardiac stress test was normal, and her blood pressure is under good control. N.T. is currently taking amiodarone, amlodipine (Norvasc), aspirin, simvastatin (Zocor), and lisinopril (Zestril). The provider suspects N.T. is having an acute cerebrovascular accident (CVA).

1. What role do diagnostic tests play in evaluating N.T. for a suspected CVA?

2. Explain how knowing the type of CVA is an important factor in planning care.

3. Which factor in N.T.'s history is the most likely contributor to her having a CVA and why?

4. The *primary* factor influencing the manifestations of a CVA is the:
    a. Area of the brain affected
    b. Speed of onset of the CVA
    c. Amount of brain tissue affected
    d. Type of CVA the patient experienced

5. What are the common manifestations of a CVA?

6. How should you position N.T.?

7. Outline the focused assessment you need to obtain.

CASE STUDY PROGRESS

Your assessment findings are as follows: VS are 164/98, 94, 24, 97.2° F (36.2° C), Sao_2 94% on room air. Her lungs are clear, and she is alert and oriented. She is able to follow simple commands, has PERRL with intact extraocular movements, and no vison loss. Her facial movements are asymmetrical, with left-sided droop-ing. Speech is slightly slurred, although it remains intelligible. She is unable to move her left arm and leg; sensation is intact. There is no ataxia; however, she is experiencing some visual and tactile neglect of the left side.

8. Complete the National Institutes of Health Stroke Scale (NIHSS) scores for each of N.T.'s symptoms.

Symptom	Score
Alert	
Knows month and age	
Able to follow commands	
Extraocular movements (EOMs) intact	
No visual loss	
Partial left facial paralysis	
Left leg no movement	
Left arm no movement	
No ataxia	
Sensation intact	
Moderate aphasia	
Neglect of left side	
TOTAL SCORE	

9. Based on your scoring, what level of CVA did N.T. experience?

10. There are a number of manifestations of a CVA. Match the description of various losses with the term describing the loss:

_____ A. Alexia	1. Total inability to communicate
_____ B. Wernicke aphasia	2. Difficulty articulating words
_____ C. Dysarthria	3. Inability to perform purposeful movements in the absence of motor problems
_____ D. Apraxia	4. Sentences contain words that are irrelevant or non-existent
_____ E. Agraphia	5. Loss of the ability to read
_____ F. Agnosia	6. Inability to recognize familiar objects
_____ G. Global aphasia	7. Loss of the ability to write

CASE STUDY PROGRESS

A noncontrast CT scan confirms the diagnosis of a thrombolytic CVA. The provider writes the orders shown in the chart.

Chart View

Physician's Orders

IV 0.9% NaCl at 75 mL/hr
Activase (tPA) per protocol
Stat CBC, PT/INR, CPK isoenzymes
Neurologic assessment every hour
Obtain patient weight
VS every hour
O_2 at 2 L per nasal cannula (NC)
NPO until swallowing evaluation

11. Outline a plan of care for implementing these orders.

12. Which interventions can you delegate to the UAP? Select all that apply.
   a. Obtaining N.T.'s weight
   b. Obtaining a manual BP per protocol
   c. Initiating O_2 therapy by nasal cannula
   d. Assisting N.T. in repositioning every 2 hours
   e. Performing N.T.'s neurologic checks every hour

13. What is the purpose of monitoring the CK isoenzyme levels?

14. The instructions on the tPA vials read to reconstitute with 50 mL of sterile water to make a total of 50 mg/50 mL (1 mg/mL). The hospital protocol is to infuse 0.9 mg/kg over 60 minutes with 10% of the dose given as a bolus over 1 minute. N.T. weighs 143 pounds. What is the amount of the bolus dose, in both milligrams and milliliters, you will give in the first minute? What is the amount of the remaining dose you will need to give?

15. Contraindications for beginning fibrinolytic therapy include which of the following? Select all that apply.
   a. Systolic BP of 150
   b. Worsening neurologic status
   c. Major surgery in the last 14 days
   d. Platelet count of less than 100,000 (100 x 10^9/L)
   e. Blood glucose of less than 50 mg/dL (2.8 mmol/L)
   f. Currently on warfarin with an INR of 1.4
   g. History of myocardial infarction 3 months ago

16. What are your responsibilities during the administration of Activase (tPA)?

17. What signs and symptoms would alert you to the possible presence of an intracerebral hemorrhage during the tPA infusion?

CASE STUDY PROGRESS

N.T. is admitted to the neurology unit. A second CT scan 24 hours later reveals a small CVA in the right hemisphere. She is placed on aspirin, amiodarone, amlodipine (Norvasc), clopidogrel (Plavix), simvastatin (Zocor), and lisinopril (Zestril).

18. During the first 24 hours after Activase (tPA), the primary concern is controlling N.T.'s:
   a. Glucose level
   b. Blood pressure
   c. Cardiac rhythm
   d. Oxygen saturation

19. Why was N.T. placed on clopidogrel (Plavix) post-CVA?

20. Because N.T. had a thrombolytic infusion, how many hours had to pass before starting any anticoagulant or antiplatelet drugs?

21. Is there any benefit from continuing simvastatin?

22. While assessing N.T., you note the following findings. Which one is unrelated to the CVA?
   a. Lethargy
   b. Headache
   c. Lumbar pain
   d. Blurred vision

23. As you walk into the nurses' station, the charge nurse is coordinating the swallowing evaluation, including a modified barium swallow study and referral for a speech-language pathologist (SLP). Give the rationale for these orders.

24. If N.T.'s deficits are temporary, how long might it take before they completely reverse?

CASE STUDY OUTCOME

After spending 1 week on the neurology unit, N.T. is discharged to a rehabilitation center for continued therapy. Though she is still experiencing some mild deficits, she is able to go home after 6 weeks.

Case Study 78

Name_____ Class/Group_____ Date_____

▶ Scenario

T.H. is a 55-year-old man with an 8-month history of progressive muscle weakness. Initially, he tripped over things and seemed to drop everything. He lost interest in activities because he was always exhausted. He sought medical care when his speech became slurred and he started to drool. During the initial evaluation, the provider noted frequent, severe muscle cramps, muscle twitching, and inappropriate, uncontrollable periods of laughter. After undergoing a series of tests, T.H. was diagnosed with amyotrophic lateral sclerosis (ALS). He is upset and bewildered about a disease that he has "never even heard of." You are a home health nurse who is seeing T.H. for the first time.

1. How would you explain ALS to T.H.?

2. Who gets ALS?

3. How common is ALS?

4. What are the early manifestations of ALS?

5. What do patients with multiple sclerosis, myasthenia gravis, and ALS have in common?
   a. Each is caused by a deficiency of essential neurotransmitters
   b. Patients will experience a complete recovery after several months
   c. The diseases place the patient at higher risk for respiratory complications
   d. Manifestations include hyperactive deep tendon reflexes and muscle twitching

6. T.H. has many questions. He asks you, "How long can I expect to live?" How should you respond?

7. T.H. asks, "Will I lose my mind?"

8. T.H. then asks, "Are there any treatments for this?"

9. T.H. thinks a moment, then says, "How is the doctor even sure this is what I have?" What is your response?

10. As part of this initial visit, you will begin to coordinate care with speech, occupational, respiratory, and physical therapists, as well as a dietitian and a psychologist. Describe the role that each of these professionals will play in T.H.'s treatment.

11. Which actions will support communication among T.H.'s care providers? Select all that apply.
   a. Maintaining one central medical record
   b. Designating the physician as the team leader
   c. Having open communication among team members
   d. Holding periodic team conferences to communicate goals
   e. Inviting T.H. and his caregiver to take part in team conferences

12. You hold a family meeting to recruit adequate help for the caregiver—in this case, T.H.'s wife. Why is this important?

13. What are some suggestions you can give T.H.'s wife to help her reduce caregiver strain?

14. How would you *best* determine whether T.H.'s wife was experiencing caregiver strain?
   a. Ask how well T.H. thinks his spouse is caring for him
   b. Assess the caregiving situation and health of T.H. and his wife
   c. Evaluate his wife for any new symptoms of anxiety and depression
   d. Determine whether his wife feels overwhelmed by her responsibilities

15. T.H. asks you, "How will the end probably come for me?" What should you tell him?

16. T.H. wants to know whether he "has to be put on a breathing machine." What factors will you take into consideration when deciding what to tell him?

17. Which legal document should T.H. formulate to describe his wishes about being placed on a "breathing machine"? Give your rationale.
   a. Living will
   b. Living trust
   c. Standard will
   d. Health care power of attorney

CASE STUDY OUTCOME

T.H. stays at home and you continue to visit him weekly for the next 20 months. After aspirating, he develops pneumonia and after deciding not to be placed on mechanical ventilation, passes away surrounded by his family.

6 Intracranial Regulation

Case Study 79

Name_____ Class/Group_____ Date_____

▶ Scenario

J.G. is a 34-year-old woman who underwent an emergency cesarean delivery after a prolonged labor, during which she had a sudden change in neurologic functioning and had a tonic-clonic (grand mal) seizure. After delivery, J.G. had 2 more seizures and demonstrated dyskinesia, resulting in frequent falls when ambulating. She was diagnosed with a basal ganglion hematoma with infarct and started on phenytoin (Dilantin). Once the seizure disorder appeared to be under control, she was transferred to a rehabilitation facility for evaluation and 2 weeks of intensive physical therapy (PT). She is now home. She still has occasional falls but has had no seizures. She is receiving PT 3 times a week in her home. As case manager for J.G.'s health maintenance organization, you make a home visit with her and her family for evaluation of long-term follow-up care.

1. A seizure is not a disease in itself but a symptom of a disease. What is the term for chronically recurring seizures?

2. Does J.G. have epilepsy?

3. In addition to the brain injury, what are some other possible conditions that could be contributing to J.G.'s lowered seizure threshold?

4. What is the pathophysiology of a seizure?

5. J.G. had tonic-clonic, or grand mal, seizures. Describe this type of seizure.

6. They ask how phenytoin (Dilantin) works in preventing seizures. How would you respond?

7. What factors are considered when determining which seizure medication a patient should take?

8. J.G. tells you she is having trouble remembering to take her medication. Why does this concern you?

9. What are some strategies you could suggest to J.G. and her husband to help her with remembering to take the phenytoin?

10. You check the chart and note that J.G.'s last phenytoin level was 12.7 mcg/mL (50.3 mcmol/L). What action do you expect based on this level?
   a. Because this level is on the border of therapeutic, notify the neurologist.
   b. This level is dangerously high, and an immediate reduction in dose is necessary.
   c. J.G. is at immediate risk for a seizure so she should go to the emergency department.
   d. Because this level is within normal limits, J.G. would continue therapy as prescribed.

11. J.G. asks, "Will my blood levels stay under control as long as I take my medicine?" How would you answer her question?

12. J.G.'s husband asks if the phenytoin could harm his wife in any way. What general information would you review with them about phenytoin?

13. J.G. says that because she has not had a seizure since she was in the hospital, she questions how long she will have to continue taking the phenytoin. Which is your best response?
a. "Your seizures are cured only as long as you take the medication."
b. "This medication might need to be continued for the rest of your life."
c. "This medication can be stopped after you are seizure free for 6 months."
d. "This medication will have to be taken only when you are experiencing stress."

14. J.G.'s husband asks you what he should do if she has a seizure at home. What should you teach him?

15. Her husband states that he is afraid for J.G. to take care of the baby. What would you say to him?

16. What aspects of the home environment do you need to inspect and why?

 17. Describe safety measures you can teach J.G. that will minimize her risk of injury should she have a seizure.

 18. You would determine further teaching is needed regarding modifying their home environment to reduce J.G.'s risk of falling if J.G. or her husband states:
   a. "The decorative rugs are all going to be put into storage."
   b. "We will put some nonskid strips in the shower in the master bath."
   c. "We will keep the stairway free of clutter and turn the light on as needed."
   d. "J.G. will need some new socks to wear so she is not going barefoot indoors."

CASE STUDY OUTCOME

J.G. continued on the phenytoin for 14 months, and then she chose to stop taking it so she could have another child. She had no further seizures until after she delivered her next child, at which time she experienced a grand mal seizure. She resumed the phenytoin and has remained seizure-free.

Case Study 80

Name_____ Class/Group_____ Date_____

▶ Scenario

J.B. is a 58-year-old retired postal worker who has been on your floor for several days receiving plasma-pheresis every other day for myasthenia gravis. About a year ago, J.B. started having difficulty chewing and swallowing, diplopia, and slurred speech, at which time he was placed on pyridostigmine (Mestinon). Before this admission he had been relatively stable. His other medical history includes hypertension controlled with metoprolol (Lopressor) and glaucoma treated with timolol (ophthalmic preparation). Recently J.B. had a sinus infection and was treated with ciprofloxacin (Cipro). On admission, J.B. was unable to bear any weight or drink fluids through a straw. There have been periods of exacerbation and remission since admission.

Chart View

Vital Signs	
Blood pressure	170/68
Heart rate	118
Respiratory rate	32
Temperature	101.8° F (38.8° C)

1. You note that the UAP has just entered these vital signs into J.B.'s record. What is your immediate concern and why?

2. What action do you need to take based on this concern?

3. What other assessment findings would support this complication being present?

4. What is the physiologic difference between a cholinergic crisis and myasthenic crisis?

5. What medical treatment do you anticipate for J.B.?

6. What is your nursing priority at this time?

7. Based on this priority, what nursing interventions do you need to perform?

 8. Which actions do you need to implement to give edrophonium safely? Select all that apply.
   a. Have IV atropine sulfate readily available.
   b. Place J.B. on continuous cardiac monitoring.
   c. Initiate precautions to prevent excessive bleeding.
   d. Give an as-needed antiemetic drug before injection.
   e. Monitor for any changes in his level of consciousness.

9. J.B.'s wife asks you, "What may have caused my husband to get worse, and why does he keep having these episodes?" What explanation should you give her?

CASE STUDY PROGRESS

J.B.'s condition improves after receiving edrophonium and IV gamma globulin. Two days later, after he is stable, you sit down to discuss discharge plans with J.B. and his wife.

10. J.B.'s wife tells you she does not have a lot of information about myasthenia gravis (MG) and she would like to know more about it. What should you tell her?

11. They ask you to explain what to expect in terms of symptoms as his illness progresses. What should you tell them?

12. J.B.'s wife asks, "How do they know my husband has myasthenia gravis?" What should you tell her about how MG is diagnosed?

13. J.B.'s wife asks why he received plasmapheresis. Which statement best describes the purpose of this procedure? Plasmapheresis:
   a. replaces affected blood with unaffected blood.
   b. decreases the production of antireceptor antibodies.
   c. reduces inflammation by infusing immunoglobulins.
   d. removes circulating abnormal antibodies from the blood.

14. J.B. wants to know when he will be able to go home. How will you respond?

 15. J.B.'s wife asks you what information they will need before he goes home. What do you need to teach J.B. about taking pyridostigmine?

16. Outline other points you need to teach J.B. and his wife about managing myasthenia gravis.

17. You teach J.B. and his wife that the most effective means of preventing myasthenic and cholinergic crises is:
   a. Doing all errands early in the day
   b. Eating three large, well-balanced meals
   c. Taking medications at the same time each day
   d. Doing muscle-strengthening exercises twice a day

18. How will you know that your teaching has been effective?

19. What community resources might J.B. and his wife find helpful?

CASE STUDY OUTCOME

J.B. and his wife thank you for taking the time to sit down with them. They state that although they know they have a lot to deal with, and it won't be easy, they feel that they are better prepared to cope with myasthenia gravis having the information you shared.

Case Study **81**

Name_____ Class/Group_____ Date_____

▶ **Scenario**

Z.O. is a 3-year-old boy with no significant medical history. He is brought into the emergency department by the emergency medical technicians after experiencing a seizure that lasted for 3 minutes. His parents report no previous history that might contribute to the seizure. On questioning, they state that they have noticed that he has been irritable, has had a poor appetite, and has been clumsier than usual over the past 2 to 3 weeks. Z.O. is admitted for diagnosis and treatment for a suspected brain tumor. A magnetic resonance imaging (MRI) scan of the brain shows a 1-cm mass in the posterior fossa region of the brain, and Z.O. is tentatively diagnosed with a cerebellar astrocytoma. The tumor appears to be contained, and the treatment plan will consist of a surgical resection, with a definitive diagnosis determined by histologic examination of tissue obtained during surgery. The type of tumor and grading will determine further treatment.

1. What are common presenting symptoms of a brain tumor? Select all that apply.
   a. Pallor
   b. Ataxia
   c. Diarrhea
   d. Seizures
   e. Vomiting with eating
   f. Headaches, especially on awakening

2. Explain the reason that a brain tumor can cause the signs and symptoms listed in Question #1.

3. Outline a plan of care for Z.O., describing at least 2 nursing interventions that would be appropriate for managing fluid status, providing preoperative teaching, facilitating family coping, and preparing Z.O. and his family for surgery.

CASE STUDY PROGRESS

Z.O. returns to the pediatric intensive care unit after surgery. He is arousable but cannot answer questions. His pupils are equal and reactive to light. He has a head dressing covering the entire scalp with small amount of serosanguinous drainage. His IV is intact and infusing as ordered through a new central venous line. His breath sounds are equal and clear, and SpO_2 is 98% on room air. You get him settled in his bed and leave the room.

Chart View

Postoperative Orders

Vital signs every 15 minutes × 4, and then every 15 to 30 minutes until stable
Contact surgeon for temperature less than 36° C or over 38.5° C (96.8° F to 101.3° F)
Maintain NPO until fully awake; may offer clear liquids as tolerated
Maintain Trendelenburg position
Reinforce bandage as needed
Neuro checks every 8 hours
Elbow restraints if needed

4. You check the postoperative orders written by the resident, which are listed in the chart. Which orders are appropriate, and which would you question? State your rationale.

5. You return to the room later in the shift to check on Z.O. Which assessment findings would cause concern? Select all that apply and explain your answers.
   a. Facial edema
   b. Heart rate 120
   c. Decreased responsiveness
   d. Blood pressure 90/55
   e. Increased clear drainage on dressing

6. Discuss some of the emotional issues Z.O.'s parents will experience during the immediate postoperative period.

7. Which actions are appropriate ways to assist the family during this time? Select all that apply.
   a. Reassure them that everything will be fine.
   b. Tell them you understand how they are feeling.
   c. Ensure that they have as much privacy as possible.
   d. Encourage them to talk about their feelings, if they can.
   e. Remind them that they need to care of themselves to be able to care for their child.
   f. Ask them if they would like to talk with the hospital chaplain and/or social worker.

CASE STUDY PROGRESS

The health care team will create a treatment plan for Z.O. This plan will outline what types of treatments will be used, how often they will be administered, and the expected length of treatment. It will be customized based on Z.O.'s overall health, age, cancer type, and stage of cancer. The team will meet daily to weekly to update the ongoing treatment plan.

8. Which health care team members would you expect to be included in this interdisciplinary team? Select all that are appropriate and explain why you think they should be included.
   a. Pharmacist
   b. Oncologist
   c. Neurologist
   d. Hematologist
   e. Neurosurgeon
   f. General surgeon
   g. Oncology social worker
   h. Charge nurse and/or nurse caring for Z.O.
   i. Oncology nurse practitioner/clinical nurse specialist

6 Intracranial Regulation

CASE STUDY PROGRESS

Z.O.'s wound and neurologic status are monitored, and he continues to improve. He is transferred to the oncology service on postoperative day 7 for initiation of chemotherapy.

9. Outline a plan of care that addresses common risks secondary to chemotherapy, describing at least 2 nursing interventions that would be appropriate for managing risks for infection, bleeding, dehydration, altered growth and nutrition, altered skin integrity, and body image.

10. The unlicensed assistive personnel (UAP) is in the room caring for Z.O. Which safety observations would you need to address? Explain your answer.

    a. UAP assists Z.O. out of bed to prevent a fall.

    b. UAP encourages Z.O. to use a soft toothbrush for oral care.

    c. UAP applies the disposable probe cover to the rectal thermometer.

    d. UAP applies hand gel before and after assisting Z.O. to the restroom.

CASE STUDY PROGRESS

On day 10, after initiation of chemotherapy, you receive the lab results shown in the chart.

Chart View

Laboratory Test Results

Hemoglobin (Hgb)	12.5 g/dL (125 g/L)
Hematocrit (Hct)	36%
White blood cells (WBCs)	7.5×10^3 cells/mm³
Red blood cells (RBCs)	4.0 million/mm³ (4×10^{12}/L)
Platelets	$80{,}000 \times 10^3$/mm³ (80×10^9/L)
Albumin	2.5 g/dL (3.6 mcmol/L)
Absolute neutrophil count (ANC)	75/mm³ (0.0075×10^9/L)

---

11. Which lab results are you concerned about, and why?

12. Z.O. has a 5-year-old sister. She has been afraid of visiting at the hospital because her "brother might die." Discuss a preschooler's concept of death and strategies to help cope with the illness of a sibling.

Postoperatively, Z.O. completed his initial course of chemotherapy in the hospital. He completed the cancer protocol he was treated under and was in remission with follow-up monitoring every 3 months. Four months later, he is experiencing new symptoms, including behavior changes and regression in speech and mobility. After extensive diagnostic testing, it is determined that his tumor has recurred.

13. Before the health care team decides on the new treatment goals and how to achieve them, what are some of the questions/issues you think should be addressed with the parents?

14. After a long discussion with Z.O.'s parents, the health care team suggests hospice care. List at least 4 of the goals of hospice care for this patient and family.

15. Pain control, supplemental nutrition and hydration, and resuscitation are common ethical dilemmas nurses face when caring for terminally ill children. Complete the following chart, describing the common reasons for providing and withholding care for Pain Control, Supplemental Nutrition and Hydration, and Resuscitation.

Rationale for Providing Care	Rationale for Withholding Care
Pain Control	
Supplemental Nutrition and Hydration (IV, Enteral Feeding)	
Resuscitation	

CASE STUDY OUTCOME

Z.O. dies at home just before his fourth birthday. The hospice nurse and chaplain help the family by providing support and comfort for all family members and assistance in dealing with funeral arrangements. In addition, they offer the family ongoing bereavement resources and services.

Case Study 82

Name_____ Class/Group_____ Date_____

▶ Scenario

J.H. is a 5-week-old infant brought to the emergency department (ED) by his mother, who speaks little English. Her husband is at work. The mother is young and appears frightened and anxious. Through a translator, Mrs. H. reports that J.H. has not been eating, sleeps all of the time, and is "not normal."

1. What are some of the obstacles you need to consider, recognizing that Mrs. H. does not speak or understand English well?

2. You perform your primary assessment and question Mrs. H. with a translator. Which findings are abnormal and need to be reported? Select all that apply and state rationale.
   a. High-pitched cry
   b. Pupils equal and +3
   c. Heart rate: 85
   d. Positive Babinski reflex
   e. Refusal of PO intake per mother
   f. Anterior fontanel palpable and tense
   g. Temperature 36° C (96.8° F) rectally

3. Place an X where you would assess the Babinski reflex on an infant.

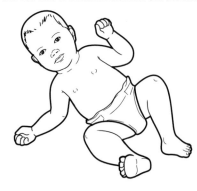

CASE STUDY PROGRESS

J.H. is admitted to the medical unit with the diagnoses of meningitis and rule out sepsis. The ED physician gives the orders shown in the chart.

Chart View

Emergency Department Orders

CBC with differential
Blood culture
CMP
UA
Cerebrospinal fluid (CSF) for culture, glucose, protein, cell count (after lumbar puncture)
Ceftriaxone (Rocephin) 260 mg IV now (loading dose)
Ampicillin 400 mg IV now and then every 6 hrs
Acetaminophen 50 mg per rectum for irritability X 1 dose
D5W 0.45% NS to infuse at 15 mL/hr

4. Prioritize the order of your interventions, with 1 being your first action and 7 being your last action.

_____1. Administer ceftriaxone and Ampicillin
_____2. Place IV
_____3. Straight catheterization for urine specimen
_____4. Place on contact isolation and droplet precautions
_____5. Assist with lumbar puncture
_____6. Administer acetaminophen
_____7. Obtain blood culture, CMP

5. You have a difficult time placing the IV line, and the physician writes an order to give the ceftriaxone IM while you wait for the vascular access team to place the IV. Name the appropriate site for an IM injection for an infant.

6. Before administering the ceftriaxone and Ampicillin, you verify the dose with another RN. The therapeutic range is for Rocephin 100 mg/kg loading dose and then 80 to 100 mg/kg daily. The therapeutic range for Ampicillin is 200 to 400 mg/kg/day in 4 divided doses with a maximum daily dosage of 12 g/day. J.H. weighs 3.5 kg. Is the loading dose ordered for Rocephin safe? Is it therapeutic? Is the ordered dose for Ampicillin, if given every 6 hours, safe and therapeutic? Show your work.

6 Intracranial Regulation

7. Interpret J.H.'s lab findings, and explain the rationale for abnormal results.

Chart View

Laboratory Test Results

Urinalysis

pH	7.2
Color	Clear
Leukocytes	Negative

Blood Tests

Hct	32%
HgB	10.5 g/dL (105 g/L)
WBC	22,000 cells/mm^3 (22 x 10^9/L)
Sodium	136 mEq/L (136 mmol/L)

---

8. Interpret the CSF findings. Would you suspect bacterial or viral meningitis? Why?

Chart View

Cerebrospinal Fluid Analysis

CSF	Clear
Gram stain	Pending
Protein	300 mg/dL (elevated) (3.0 g/L)
Leukocytes (cell count)	1030 (elevated)
Glucose	40 mg/dL (decreased) (2.2 mmol/L)

---

9. What are the most common bacterial pathogens in this age group?

CASE STUDY PROGRESS

J.H. is diagnosed with *Escherichia coli* meningitis. His medical care plan will include 21 days of antibiotic therapy with ceftriaxone. You are developing his nursing plan of care.

10. Outline a plan of care for J.H., describing at least 2 nursing interventions that would be appropriate for managing pain and infection, maintaining hydration, assisting with increased intracranial pressure (ICP), and teaching to review with his parents.

CASE STUDY PROGRESS

Mrs. H., through her translator, asks you what could have caused her baby to be sick, given that he had an immunization when he was born. She asks whether he should get "more shots" so this won't happen again. You reinforce to Mrs. H. that infants have immature immune systems, and they are vulnerable to infections until they have been fully immunized. Mrs. H. asks when J.H. will get more shots and what will they be.

11. According to the CDC immunization schedule, which immunizations will J.H. receive at 2 months? You can refer to the current immunization schedules posted at www.cdc.gov/vaccines/schedules/downloads/child/0-18yrs-child-combined-schedule.pdf
   a. Hib
   b. IPV
   c. OPV
   d. MMR
   e. DTaP
   f. Hep B
   g. Varicella
   h. Rotavirus
   i. Pneumococcal conjugate (PCV13)

12. What is the effect of hospitalization on J.H.'s growth and development?

13. J.H. is being discharged after 3 weeks of IV antibiotic therapy. What educational topics will be important to discuss with J.H.'s parents when he is discharged?

14. You are providing developmental teaching to Mrs. H. with a translator. Which milestones would be appropriate to anticipate at 2 months? Select all that apply.
   a. Coos and gurgles
   b. Develops a social smile
   c. Able to purposely reach for toys
   d. Able to roll from stomach to back
   e. Able to see an object 4 to 5 feet away

CASE STUDY OUTCOME

J.H. is discharged to home with his parents. He will continue antibiotics by mouth for 1 week and receive a home health visit for infant care follow-up. The parents are to return him to his primary care provider in 1 week or call with any concerns.

Case Study **83**

Name_____   Class/Group_____   Date_____

▶ Scenario

You admit L.M., a 2-month-old girl with a history of hydrocephalus and ventriculoperitoneal (VP) shunt placement 1 month earlier. Her parents report that she has been more irritable than usual, and for the past 3 days she has fed poorly and has had emesis 5 or 6 times every day.

1. Explain the pathophysiology of hydrocephalus and cerebrospinal fluid (CSF) imbalance.

2. Explain how the placement of a VP shunt helps the patient.

CASE STUDY PROGRESS

You get L.M. settled on the unit and promptly perform her admission assessment.

3. A nursing student is assisting you with L.M.'s admission. Assessment of growth and development is an important part of patient assessment. Which of the nursing student's statements is correct?
   a. "We should not see any head lag."
   b. "L. should be able to focus on objects that are near."
   c. "We will assess her anterior fontanel because it should be closed."
   d. "I do not need to do a frontal occipital circumference measurement because her sutures have fused."

4. Your assessment includes the following findings. Indicate the abnormal findings with a * and state the possible rationale for each.

System	Assessment and Vital Signs	If Abnormal, State Rationale
Weight	4.5 kg	
Neurologic	Irritable, awake, and fussy; difficult to console	
	FOC: 44 cm, "increased 2 cm from measurement yesterday" per mother	
	Anterior fontanel slightly bulging	
	Unable to palpate posterior fontanel	
	Pupils equal and reactive	
	Shunt observed and palpated lightly behind (L) ear, no warmth, tenderness or drainage	
Respiratory	Bilateral breath sounds equal and clear	
	Spo$_2$ 95% on room air	
	Respiratory rate: 40	
Cardiovascular	Rectal temperature: 38.8° C	
	Heart rate (HR): 182	
	Blood pressure (BP): 111/70	
	Pulses 2+ and equal bilaterally	
Gastrointestinal	Positive bowel sounds	
	Emesis during examination	
	Last feeding 6 hours ago	
Genitourinary	Last urine output 2 hours ago	
Musculoskeletal	Moves all extremities well	
	Head lag noted	
Skin	Diaper rash noted	
	Abdominal incision with well approximated edges, no warmth, tenderness, or drainage	

5. The doctors order a CT scan and lumbar puncture with a cell count, culture, Gram stain, glucose, and protein run on the CSF. What is the rationale for each procedure?

CASE STUDY PROGRESS

It is determined that the VP shunt is infected and must be temporarily removed. L.M. is taken to surgery to have a left extraventricular drain (EVD) placed. She returns to your unit in stable condition. You get her settled back into her room and perform an assessment. You note that her EVD is intact and draining CSF. The dressing is clean and dry and intact under a sterile dressing.

6. True or False: The position of the EVD should be maintained at the level of the external auditory meatus (tragus). Explain your answer.

Chart View

Medication Administration Record (MAR)

Acetaminophen 15 mg/kg PO q4-6hr prn
Morphine sulfate 0.05 mg/kg IV q4hr prn
Enalapril (Vasotec) 5 mcg/kg PO q24hr
Cefotaxime 150 mg/kg/day IV in divided doses q8hr
Baclofen (Lioresal) 10 mg/kg/day PO q8hr
Ondansetron (Zofran) 0.1 mg/kg IV now

7. Which medications are appropriate for L.M.'s diagnosis? Select all that apply and state the rationale for the ones you chose. Then, give a reason for those you feel are not appropriate.

8. You are preparing to give the first dose of antibiotic that is ordered. Referring to L.M.'s medication administration record, calculate the amount of the antibiotic that you will administer per dose. Show your work.

9. L.M. is very fussy, and you decide to medicate her for pain. Calculate the amount of morphine L.M. will receive for pain per dose (do not round). Then calculate the amount you will draw up for the required dose, and mark the syringe appropriately (round to hundredths/two decimal places). The morphine is available in an injection solution of 2 mg/mL.

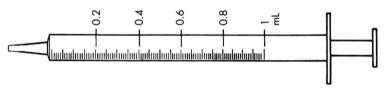

10. Which task can be appropriately delegated to the UAP?
    a. Changing the dressing on the surgical site
    b. Obtaining and charting a complete set of vital signs
    c. Performing the every-2-hour neurologic check
    d. Instructing the parents on changes in neurologic status

11. In which position should L.M. be placed immediately postoperatively unless ordered otherwise by the surgeon?
    a. Flat, left side-lying
    b. Flat, right side-lying
    c. Supine, Trendelenburg
    d. Supine, head of bed (HOB) 45 degrees

12. What points will you address while teaching the parents about the EVD system?

CASE STUDY PROGRESS

Several days later, L.M.'s mother is changing L.M.'s diaper and she tells you that she is worried because L.M. has started having diarrhea recently, and it is getting worse.

13. Based on the medications that L.M. is receiving, what is the most likely cause of the diarrhea? What is a possible concern you should consider, and what should your care plan include?

CASE STUDY PROGRESS

L.M. responds well to the antibiotics, and her shunt is internalized 2 weeks later. She is released from the hospital after observation for 2 days.

14. While you are giving your discharge instructions, L.M.'s mother states that she normally gives L.M. 1 mL of acetaminophen (Tylenol Elixir), 160 mg/5 mL, and asks whether this is the correct dose. L.M.'s current weight is 4.5 kg and the therapeutic range of acetaminophen dosage is 10 to 15 mg/kg PO q4-6hr. Which statement is most accurate?

    a. "Tylenol should not be given to a child her age."

    b. "This is a safe amount; you should continue to give that dose every 4 hours."

    c. "You should give 1.4 to 2.1 mL every 4 to 6 hours based on her current weight."

    d. "You can continue to give her that amount; you can give her a dose every 2 hours."

 15. When giving discharge instructions for this 2 month old, which guidelines/practices would help decrease the risk for a medication error occurring at home? Select all that apply. Then, give your rationale for why each answer is either appropriate or not.

    a. L.M. may receive up to 6 doses of acetaminophen per day as needed.

    b. Ask the pharmacist to give you an oral syringe to give the medication to L.M.

    c. Give L.M. 1.4 to 2.1 mL every 4 to 6 hours as needed, which is based on her weight at this time

    d. You should give L.M. 2 mL every 4 to 6 hours as needed, which is based on her weight at this time.

    e. Give parents detailed medication instructions, such as demonstration and return demonstrations, and picture-based-dosing instructions.

CASE STUDY OUTCOME

L.M. returns for her postoperative checkup 2 weeks later and is playful and alert. The neurologist will continue to monitor her closely with follow-up visits.

Intracranial Regulation

6 Intracranial Regulation

Case Study **84**

Name_____ Class/Group_____ Date_____

▶ Scenario

The charge nurse tells you that you will be admitting a 1-hour-old infant, Baby Girl R., to the neonatal intensive care unit (NICU) with a myelomeningocele that was discovered in utero. Her aunt and father arrive shortly after her admission while the mother remains at the local medical center recovering from a cesarean delivery.

1. What is the rationale for doing a cesarean delivery for babies with myelomeningocele?

CASE STUDY PROGRESS

While you are getting vital signs, the father tells you that he has been trying to research myelomeningocele on the Internet, but he is still confused, especially about the difference between myelomeningocele and meningocele.

2. Using lay terms, what would you tell the father about the pathophysiology of myelomeningocele? What is the difference between myelomeningocele and meningocele?

3. After your discussion with the family, which of the father's statements would indicate a need for more teaching?
   a. "My baby will need to lie on her stomach in her incubator."
   b. "I need to wash my hands carefully to prevent spread of germs."
   c. "My baby will probably not require surgery until she is a year old."
   d. "My baby's malformation can also be referred to as *spina bifida cystica*."

4. The father asks questions about the infant's condition but does not look at his newborn. Which statements are correct? Select all that apply.
    a. People grieve for the loss of a "normal newborn" differently.
    b. Most new fathers are not interested in looking at their newborns.
    c. It is apparent that he does not care about his newborn's condition.
    d. This is an abnormal reaction for a parent of a child born with a very visible physical defect.
    e. Even though the myelomeningocele was diagnosed in utero, seeing the congenital anomaly or physical defect on his infant is very difficult.

CASE STUDY PROGRESS

R. is in an open warmer. You document the information shown in the chart.

Chart View

Admission Data	
Blood pressure	67/33
Pulse	173
Respirations	52
Axillary temperature	37.1° C (98.8° F)
Spo$_2$	95%
Weight	3.5 kg
Frontal occipital circumference (FOC)	35 cm

5. Which assessment and monitoring data are abnormal for a 1-hour-old infant? Select all that apply.
    a. Acrocyanosis
    b. Bilateral clubfeet
    c. Breath sounds clear
    d. Fontanelles soft and flat
    e. Pupils 2 cm, brisk reaction
    f. Sleepy, squirms and fusses during pupil check
    g. No reaction when pulse oximeter is placed on right foot
    h. Pulses 2+ and capillary refill time less than 2 to 3 seconds

6. You are carefully assessing the sutures and fontanelles. True or False: The posterior fontanel is joined by the temporal and parietal bones.

7. Explain the rationale for each order in the table.

Orders	Rationale
1. Open warmer	
2. Place in Trendelenburg position, prone	
3. Use appropriate positioning aids such as diaper rolls, pads, pressure-reducing mattress	
4. Maintain sterile gauze/sponges with normal saline (NS) or lactated ringers to Telfa-covered sac and monitor q2-4hr	
5. Place peripheral IV with $D_{10}W$ at 15 mL/hr	
6. Administer IV antibiotics as ordered.	
7. NPO	
8. Keep clean padding under diaper area; check frequently	
9. Assess for urine output every 2 to 4 hours; if none, assess for retention	
10. Clean intermittent catheterization (CIC) as needed	
11. Measure FOC every shift	
12. Physical therapy (PT) consultation	
13. Orthopedic consultation	
14. Maintain latex-free environment	

CASE STUDY PROGRESS

The next day Baby Girl R. is taken to the operating room. The anesthesiologist orders cefazolin (Ancef) 140 mg IV to be given 30 minutes before the surgery begins.

8. You add 10 mL of sterile water to the 1-g vial for a concentration of 100 mg/1 mL. Calculate how many milliliters you will draw up for this dose. Shade in the dose on the syringe.

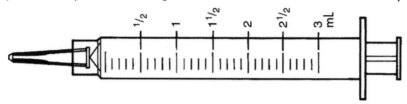

CASE STUDY PROGRESS

Postoperatively, the postanesthesia care unit (PACU) nurse tells you Baby Girl R. did well during surgery and is ready to return to your unit. When she arrives, you and the unlicensed assistive personnel start putting on the monitors. R.'s father is present, and he asks you to give the baby some pain medication. The open warmer starts alarming because the infant's skin temperature is reading 35° C (95° F). You look to see whether the temperature probe has fallen off. You see that it is still on, but you notice that the suture from surgery is no longer intact. The oxygen monitor reads 71% saturation with an accurate waveform, and the pulse oximeter probe is correctly placed. The respiratory rate is 25 and heart rate is 102.

9. Which of the issues should you address first? Give rationale.

CASE STUDY PROGRESS

Baby Girl R.'s condition stabilizes. Her temperature is 36.7° C (98.1° F) per skin probe. Respiratory rate and heart rate improve and her Spo_2 is 98% on ¼ L of oxygen per minute via nasal cannula. The surgeon is at the bedside and opts to return her to the OR for revision of the incision.

Two nights later, you are caring for Baby Girl R. In report, you hear that the parents really want to hold their baby, but they have not yet done so because they are afraid of causing the suture to open again. They are currently at the bedside, and the infant is due for a feeding.

10. How can you help the parents become comfortable with holding their baby?

11. When you take the bottle into the room, you notice a growth chart next to the bed tracking the FOC measurement at least once per shift. Baby Girl R.'s FOC has increased to 36 cm. Using the appropriate WHO (World Health Organization) growth chart (www.who.int/childgrowth/standards/second_set/cht_hcfa_girls_p_0_13.pdf?ua=1) is the following statement True or False? The FOC is close to the 95th percentile and can be monitored less frequently because this is a normal finding. (Explain your answer.)

CASE STUDY PROGRESS

Discharge teaching is an essential part of Baby Girl R.'s care. Teaching and preparation of the family have been done since the diagnosis in utero and are ongoing issues.

12. Which topics would be important to include in discharge teaching for Baby Girl R.? Select all that apply.
   a. Positioning
   b. Skin care and wound care
   c. Specialized feeding technique
   d. Maintenance of the Foley catheter
   e. Comfort measures and pain control
   f. Importance of multidisciplinary follow-up
   g. Signs and symptoms of when to call the physician
   h. Range-of-motion (ROM) exercises as appropriate per PT
   i. Appropriate stimulation such as sitting in an infant seat or swing

CASE STUDY OUTCOME

Baby Girl R. is followed closely in the Level 2 nursery/NICU. She stabilizes and is able to be discharged to home in 2 weeks with intensive discharge teaching and close multidisciplinary follow-up.

Case Study 85

Name_____ Class/Group_____ Date_____

▶ **Scenario**

You are the nurse on a medical unit taking care of a 50-year-old man, A.A., who was admitted 18 hours ago with peptic ulcer disease secondary to suspected chronic alcoholism. You enter A.A.'s room and find him having a generalized convulsive (tonic-clonic) seizure.

1. What is your immediate concern for A.A.?

2. List 5 things you would do in order of priority.

3. Given A.A.'s history, state 3 possible causes for his tonic-clonic seizure.

CASE STUDY PROGRESS

The rapid response team is called, and the provider gives the orders shown in the chart.

Chart View

Medication Administration Record

Thiamine (vitamin B_1) 100 mg IM now
50% glucose, 1 50-mL IV bolus now
Lorazepam (Ativan) 4 mg IV now over 2 to 5 minutes

4. Indicate the expected outcome for A.A. associated with each medication.

5. In what order would you give A.A.'s medications? Give your reason.

_____ Thiamine (Vitamin B$_1$)

_____ Glucose

_____ Lorazepam (Ativan)

6. List your primary concern when giving lorazepam intravenously.

 7. The lorazepam is supplied in a single-use vial. How many milliliters will A.A. receive? Shade in the dose on the syringe.

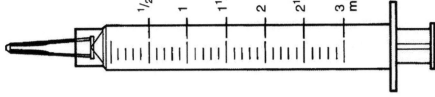

8. What assessments do you need to make during his ongoing seizure activity?

A.A.'s seizure activity does not subside. The provider orders an additional 4 mg of IV lorazepam without effect. Twenty minutes has now elapsed since you initially found A.A. having seizure activity.

9. What is the significance of this time lapse?

10. Define status epilepticus.

11. The provider decides to administer propofol (Diprivan) and intubate A.A. to support his airway. What is propofol? Why is it being given to A.A.?

12. The provider also orders a phenytoin 15 mg/kg IV loading dose at a rate of 50 mg/min. What is the reason for giving A.A. phenytoin?

13. A.A. weighs 143 pounds. How much phenytoin will you administer?

14. As you prepare to administer the phenytoin, you see that A.A. has D$_5$W infusing at 75 mL/hr. Why does this concern you, and what are your options?

15. You accompany A.A. as the rapid response team transfers him to the ICU. During the transport, his seizure activity ceases. Using SBAR, what information will you provide to the ICU nurse?

16. What are the main complications of status epilepticus that the nurse will monitor for?

17. Describe the assessment A.A. needs over the next few hours.

18. Identify nursing interventions that are appropriate for A.A. since the seizure activity has subsided.

CASE STUDY OUTCOME

A.A.'s seizure is successfully treated with lorazepam and phenytoin, and he has no further seizure activity. After his acute care needs are resolved, A.A. decides to enter a detoxification program on discharge. He successfully completes the program and remains free of drug and alcohol use.

Case Study 86

Name_____ Class/Group_____ Date_____

▶ Scenario

T.W. is a 22-year-old man who fell 50 feet (15 meters) from a chairlift while skiing and landed on hard-packed snow. He is now at the emergency department (ED) with spinal cord injury (SCI) with paraplegia from a suspected T5-T6 fracture.

Chart View

Physician's Orders

Insert indwelling urinary catheter
ECG monitoring
Immobilize the cervical spine
Oxygen at 4 L per nasal cannula
Neurologic assessment every hour
Apply warming blankets as needed

1. Describe a plan for implementing these orders.

2. What are the nursing priorities at this time?

3. Which assessment would you complete first?
   a. Auscultating breath sounds
   b. Testing the peripheral reflexes
   c. Determining pupil response to light
   d. Assessing ability to move the extremities

4. What other interventions would likely be done by the ED nurse?

5. Awareness of the prehospital management of a SCI is critical to T.W.'s ultimate neurologic outcome. What actions will the nurse take to ensure this goal is met?

6. T.W. anxiously asks, "With this broken back, am I going to be paralyzed for life or can it be reversed?" How would you respond?

CASE STUDY PROGRESS

The diagnosis of the fracture is confirmed, and T.W. is transferred from the ED to the surgical intensive care unit (SICU). Although T.W.'s injury is at a level at which independent respiratory function is expected, he experiences low oxygen saturation levels and is intubated and placed on mechanical ventilation. The provider states that this is because of spinal shock. He has a central venous catheter (CVC) inserted for medication administration. T.W.'s medication list includes pantoprazole 40 mg IV bid, propofol (Diprivan) 10 mcg/kg/min continuous IV infusion, and enoxaparin 30 mg SubQ every 12 hours.

7. How would you explain spinal shock to T.W.'s family and why T.W. needs mechanical ventilation?

8. Indicate the reason T.W. is receiving each medication.

9. T.W. weighs 158 pounds. The pharmacy-supplied infusion bottle reads "propofol 500 mg/ 50 mL." At how many milliliters per hour would you set the infusion pump? (Round to the nearest hundredth.)

10. After the CVC is inserted, T.W. has a STAT portable chest x-ray examination. Why?

CASE STUDY PROGRESS

T.W. is taken to surgery 48 hours after the accident for spinal stabilization. He spends 2 additional days in the SICU and 5 days in the neurology unit and now is in the rehabilitation unit. He continues to have paralysis of his lower extremities. Shortly after the transfer, T.W. turns on his call light and asks for medication for headache. As you walk into the room, you immediately note that T.W.'s face is flushed and he is profusely sweating.

11. What complication do you suspect T.W. is experiencing and why?

12. What further assessment data do you need to collect?

13. What interventions do you need to perform for T.W.?

14. What could happen if autonomic dysreflexia (AD) is left untreated?

15. After your prompt intervention, T.W.'s AD resolves and you need to document what happened. Write an example of a documentation entry describing this event.

CASE STUDY PROGRESS

After spending 6 weeks in acute care, T.W. is transferred to the rehabilitation unit for interprofessional, intensive therapy. The interprofessional team will address the complex effects of SCI, including paraplegia, respiratory disorders, bowel and bladder function, as well as emotional and psychological issues related to T.W.'s adjusting to a new way of life.

16. What members of the interprofessional team would likely be involved in his care?

17. What are realistic functional goals for T.W.?

18. Part of rehabilitation care includes teaching T.W. how to manage his continuous urinary drainage system. What would this teaching include?

19. What outcome parameters would you use to determine whether efforts to promote urinary excretion have been effective?

20. T.W. is experiencing some spasticity of the lower extremities. What should be included in the plan of care to prevent developing contractures of the lower extremities?

21. T.W. has special dietary needs, and the registered dietitian is part of developing an optimal diet for T.W. Describe the components of this diet.

22. T.W. will be taught bowel-training techniques. What will this teaching include?

23. T.W. is concerned whether he will ever be able to have sex again. What would you tell him, and what are some possible referrals?

24. While assisting T.W. with his morning hygienic care, he states, "Why would anyone want to live like this? No woman will ever want me. I just wish you would have let me die." How would you initially respond?
a. "You wish you would have died?"
b. "Tell me why you are talking like this."
c. "Let's finish your bath and then we can talk."
d. "I know this is hard now, but things will work out."

CASE STUDY OUTCOME

Although his rehabilitation was slow the first few years, he eventually progressed to the point that he was independent in all activities of daily living. He lives in his childhood home, which required some accessibility modification, and is periodically struggling with depression and anger.

Case Study **87**

Name_____ Class/Group_____ Date_____

▶ Scenario

J.R. is a 28-year-old man who was doing home repairs. He fell from the top of a 6-foot stepladder, striking his head on a rock. He experienced a momentary loss of consciousness. By the time his neighbor got to him, he was conscious but bleeding profusely from a laceration over the right temporal area. The neighbor drove him to the emergency department of your hospital. As the nurse, you immediately apply a cervical collar, lay him on a stretcher, and take J.R. to a treatment room.

1. What steps will you take to assess J.R.?

2. List at least 6 components of a neurologic examination.

3. What types of injuries may J.R. have sustained?

4. Differentiate between primary and secondary head injury.

5. What complication common to each of these diagnoses concerns you most?

6. Why is this complication clinically important?

7. Name at least 6 findings that would indicate this complication is occurring.

8. Which one is the most sensitive indicator of neurologic change?

CASE STUDY PROGRESS

You complete your neurologic examination and find the following: Glasgow Coma Scale (GCS) score of 15; pupils equal, round, reactive to light; and full sensation intact. J.R. complains of a headache and is somewhat drowsy. His vital signs are 120/72, 114, 30, 98.7° F (37.1° C), and Spo$_2$ 94%. As the radiology technician performs a portable cross-table lateral cervical spine x-ray examination, J.R. begins to speak incoherently and appears to drift off to sleep.

9. What are the next actions you will take?

CASE STUDY PROGRESS

While waiting for the provider to arrive, J.R. becomes unresponsive to verbal stimuli. The right pupil is larger than the left and does not respond to light. J.R. responds to painful stimuli in the manner shown in the illustration.

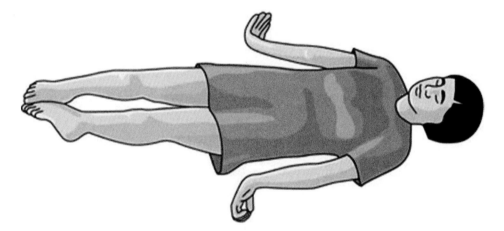

10. What is this response called and what does it signify?

11. Calculate J.R.'s GCS score. Describe the clinical implications of this score.

12. What is the most likely cause of the change in J.R.'s neurologic status?

13. What are your immediate nursing priorities?

14. What immediate actions will you take?

15. His vital signs are now 160/72, 64, 10, 98.7° F (37.1° C), and Spo$_2$ 94%. What is your concern and why?

CASE STUDY PROGRESS

The provider arrives and gives the orders shown in the chart.

Chart View

Physician's Orders

Insert indwelling urinary catheter
Insert nasogastric tube to continuous low wall suction
Intubate: Vent settings assist-control 16, V$_T$ 900 mL, Fio$_2$ 0.5, PEEP (positive end-expiratory pressure) 3 cm
IV fluid 0.9% normal saline at 100 mL/hr
160 grams Mannitol IV STAT over 30 minutes
Phenytoin 1360 mg IV STAT over 30 minutes, then 100 mg IV every 8 hours
STAT CT scan
STAT labs: CBC, CMP, UA, type and cross, PT/INR and PTT, ABGs, toxicology screen

16. Outline a plan for implementing these orders.

17. What is mannitol, and why is it being given to J.R.?

18. What is the expected outcome associated with administering phenytoin to J.R.?

CASE STUDY PROGRESS

J.R. goes to radiology for a CT scan, which shows a large epidural hematoma on the right with a hemispheric shift to the left. He is taken straight to the operating room for evacuation of the hematoma. While he is in surgery, J.R.'s family arrives with their chaplain. They ask if they can anoint J.R. and pray over him.

19. How should you respond?

CASE STUDY PROGRESS

Postoperatively J.R. is admitted to the neurologic ICU.

20. What assessment indicators will be closely monitored in J.R.?

21. An appropriate nursing intervention for J.R. to promote cerebral tissue perfusion is:
   a. Avoiding passive range-of-motion exercises
   b. Repositioning him every 4 to 6 hours, using logrolling
   c. Limiting endotracheal suctioning to no longer than 15 seconds
   d. Clustering nursing activities so he has periods of uninterrupted rest

22. The best way to position J.R. is to:
   a. Elevate the head of the bed to 30 degrees
   b. Keep him flat with his hips slightly flexed
   c. Place him on the right side with his head flexed
   d. Turn his head from side-to-side to decrease aspiration risk

23. Name 4 independent nursing interventions that would be used to control environmental stimuli during the first 48 postoperative hours.

24. What measures will be used to prevent J.R. from developing hyperthermia? Why are these important?

25. What outcome criteria would determine whether the independent nursing measures for J.R. were effective?

CASE STUDY OUTCOME

J.R. has lingering effects several months after his accident. He has frequent headaches, tires easily, and is sensitive to light. Neurologically, he is "normal," though he has yet to return to work. Still, he feels lucky. "I'm still alive. If I would not have had that terrible cut, I may have died."

Case Study **88**

Name_____ Class/Group_____ Date_____

▶ Scenario

C.J. is a 48-year-old violinist in the local symphony. Before the performance this evening, she told a friend that she was experiencing what she called "the worst headache I've ever had" and that she had taken two extra-strength acetaminophens, but they "didn't touch my headache." During the performance, she stopped playing, reached up, grasped her head, and then fell unconscious. When the paramedics arrived, she was intubated and an IV line was started with normal saline.

On arrival at the emergency department, she has a Glasgow Coma Scale (GCS) score of 3. Her husband reports a history of hypertension and states she recently quit taking her medication because it made her feel tired. She is trying to quit smoking and is down to a half pack of cigarettes per day. She drinks alcohol socially on weekends and has a remote history of cocaine use. He says that she was complaining of worsening, intermittent headaches for the past few weeks.

1. Describe C.J.'s neurologic presentation that equates with a GCS score of 3.

2. The provider immediately suspects a subarachnoid hemorrhage (SAH). Why?

CASE STUDY PROGRESS

After CT angiography is done, C.J. is diagnosed with a massive grade V SAH. She is transported to the intensive care unit for close monitoring. She is ventilator dependent, is unresponsive to verbal or painful stimuli, and has no physical movement. Her husband, mother, and children are at her bedside; several relatives and friends are in the waiting area.

3. What is a SAH?

4. What are common causes of an SAH?

5. What are C.J.'s risk factors for a SAH?

6. Describe a patient with a grade V SAH.

7. What common complications of SAH would you anticipate?

8. What is the likely goal of treatment for C.J.?

9. Treatment of SAH can include surgery, embolization, medications, and watchful waiting. What factors are considered in determining treatment?

Chart View

Physician's Orders

   Nimodipine 60 mg every 4 hours per NG tube for systolic BP >140
   0.9% normal saline at 100 mL/hr
   Labetalol 10 mg IV over 2 minutes q1hr for systolic BP greater than 140
   Acetaminophen 650 mg q6hr for temperature greater than 101.0° F (38.3° C)
   Insulin aspart (NovoLog) SubQ per sliding scale every 6 hours

10. Identify the expected outcome associated with each treatment C.J. is receiving.

11. Name 4 independent nursing interventions that would be used to control environmental stimuli during the next 24 hours.

12. How would you position C.J.?

13. What assessment indicators will be closely monitored in C.J.?

14. Describe how you would support C.J.'s family during this time.

After C.J. has been in the ICU for 12 hours, the provider decides to begin testing C.J. to determine whether she is clinically brain dead.

15. What is brain death?

16. What are the general criteria for declaring a patient clinically brain dead?

17. It is determined that C.J.'s condition meets the criteria, and she is declared legally brain dead. She had previously indicated her willingness to be an organ donor, and her husband agrees to honor her wishes. C.J.'s husband asks you to explain the donation process. How will you explain it to him?

18. While you are waiting for the transplant team to arrive, you are working to maintain C.J.'s hemodynamic stability. Which parameter would indicate your efforts are successful? Give your rationale.
    a. Urine output of 40 mL/hr
    b. Cardiac index less than 2.4 L/min
    c. Mean arterial BP is greater than 50
    d. Left ventricular ejection fraction greater than 30%

CASE STUDY OUTCOME

C.J.'s family received several letters from donors. Each acknowledges that they will not forget their kindness, nor C.J.'s memory. C.J.'s family appreciated receiving these letters, which help them with their grief over her death.

Metabolism and Glucose Regulation

Case Study 89

Name_____ Class/Group_____ Date_____

▶ Scenario

L.L., a 28-year-old house painter, has been too ill to work for the past 3 days. When he arrives at the emergency department with his girlfriend, he seems alert but acutely ill, with an average build and a deep tan over the exposed areas of skin. He reports headaches, joint pain, a low-grade fever, cough, anorexia, and nausea and vomiting, especially after eating any fatty food. L.L. describes vague abdominal pain that started about the same time as the other problems. He says he has been using "a lot of Tylenol" for his pain. His past medical history reveals he has no health problems, is a nonsmoker, and drinks "a few" beers each evening to relax. Vital signs are 128/84, 88, 26, 100.6° F (38.1° C); awake, alert, and oriented × 3; moves all extremities × 4 with complaints of aching pain in his muscles; very slight scleral jaundice present; heart and breath sounds clear and without adventitious sounds; bowel sounds positive × 4 quadrants; abdomen soft and palpable without distinct masses. L.L. mentions that his urine has been getting darker over the past 2 days and he has been feeling a little "itchy."

1. Underline the assessment findings that concern you.

2. Your institution uses electronic charting. Based on the health history and assessment described in the scenario, document your findings.
   ☐ Neurologic:

   ☐ Respiratory:

   ☐ Cardiovascular:

   ☐ Gastrointestinal:

   ☐ Genitourinary:

   ☐ Musculoskeletal:

   ☐ Skin:

   ☐ Pain:

CASE STUDY PROGRESS

L.L. has key signs of hepatitis. The provider admits him to the medical unit and orders lab work to help identify the precise problem.

3. Which key diagnostic tests will determine exactly the type of hepatitis present?

Chart View

Laboratory Test Results

Indirect bilirubin	1.6 mg/dL (27.4 mcmol/L)
Total bilirubin	2.3 mg/dL (39.3 mcmol/L)
Albumin	3.8 g/dL (5.5 mcmol/L)
Total protein	6.5 g/dL (65 g/L)
ALT	66 units/L
AST	52 units/L
LDH	245 units/L
ALP	176 units/L (3.0 mckat/L)
PT/INR	12 seconds/1.06
aPTT	32 seconds
Urine urobilinogen	1.6 IU/L
Anti-HAV	Negative
Anti-HCV	Negative
HBsAg	Positive
Anti-HBc	Positive
IgM anti-HBc	Positive
Anti-HBs	Negative

4. Interpret L.L.'s lab results.

5. What is the difference between the hepatitis B surface antigen (HBsAg) and the hepatitis B surface antibody (HBsAb)?

6. For each characteristic below, name whether it describes hepatitis A *(A)* or hepatitis B *(B)*.

   _____a. Fecal-oral transmission

   _____b. Transmitted by sharing needles

   _____c. Transmitted by blood transfusions

   _____d. Vaccination is a three-shot series

   _____e. Illness is usually mild, similar to a flulike infection

   _____f. Symptoms include anorexia, nausea, vomiting, fever, fatigue, and jaundice

7. What factors in his history could have compounded the increased ALT levels?

8. How will you explain to L.L. the likely progression of his disease?

9. Is L.L. contagious? What precautions would you take while he is in the hospital?

10. What will you do to help ease L.L.'s itching? State 5 interventions.

11. What type of diet will you teach L.L. to follow?

7 Metabolism Regulation

12. Which new assessment finding, if present, would concern you *most*?
   a. Irritable and disoriented
   b. Mild abdominal tenderness
   c. Guaiac-negative diarrheal stools
   d. Easily fatigued when ambulating

CASE STUDY PROGRESS

L.L. is ready for discharge in a few days, and he confides to you that he feels so "guilty" about having hepatitis and endangering his girlfriend and family. L.L. lives at home with his parents and four younger siblings. The youngest is 4 years old. He tells you he was at a party and did not think the one-time needle use could hurt him. He hopes his family is not too afraid to have him return home.

13. What action will you take?

 14. He asks how to prevent giving hepatitis to his family. What specific instructions will you give?

15. Given L.L.'s lifestyle, what specific patient teaching points must you emphasize?

CASE STUDY OUTCOME

L.L. remained ill for about 2 months after discharge. The provider did a liver biopsy, which showed some damage to the liver. He did not give his girlfriend hepatitis; her titers were adequate from prior immunization. L.L. continued to refrain from alcohol and substance use and followed a healthy lifestyle. Three years later, he is doing well.

Case Study **90**

Name_____ Class/Group_____ Date_____

▶ Scenario

D.G., 57 years old, is admitted to your unit for observation from the emergency department (ED) with the diagnosis of cirrhosis with possible hepatic encephalopathy. He is lethargic, appears cachectic, and is mildly combative when aroused. He is jaundiced, with a notably distended abdomen. He is receiving an IV infusion of D_5 ½ NS.

1. Briefly discuss the pathophysiology of cirrhosis.

2. What are the common causes of cirrhosis?

3. How is hepatic encephalopathy related to cirrhosis?

CASE STUDY PROGRESS

Chart View

Admission Orders

IV D$_5$ ½ NS with 20 mEq KCl at 75 mL/hr
Insert indwelling urinary catheter to gravity drainage
Bed rest
Lactulose 30 mL orally daily
Rifaximin 550 mg orally twice daily
Spironolactone 100 mg orally twice daily
Abdominal ultrasound in a.m.
Vitamin K 10 mg/day IV × 3 doses; change to PO when alert and able to swallow
CBC with differential, BMP, liver function tests, PT/INR and aPTT, serum ammonia (NH$_3$) now and
    in a.m.
2-Gram sodium diet when alert and able to swallow
Call for any signs of bleeding; systolic BP <100; diastolic BP <50; or pulse >120

4. What do you need to do for D.G., and what can you delegate to the UAP?

5. What is the reason for routinely assessing D.G. for bleeding?

6. What assessment findings would indicate the presence of bleeding?

7. Indicate the expected outcome associated with each of the medications he is receiving.

8. What is the rationale for placing him on a low-sodium diet?

CASE STUDY PROGRESS

While you are getting D.G. settled, you continue your assessment.

Neurologic: PERRL; moves all extremities, but is sluggish, pulling away during assessment; follows commands sporadically.

CV: Pulse is regular without adventitious sounds. All peripheral pulses are palpable at 3+ bilaterally; 3+ pitting edema in lower extremities.

Respiratory: Breath sounds clear but diminished in all lobes; musty breath.

GI: Tongue and gums are beefy red and swollen. Abdomen moderately distended, firm, and slightly tender. Bowel sounds positive × 4.

GU: Foley to gravity drainage, with 75 mL dark amber urine past 2 hours.

Skin: Mild jaundice. Skin appears thin and dry. Numerous spider angiomas on upper abdomen with several dilated veins across abdomen. Several ecchymoses on lower extremities.

VS: 120/60, 104, 32, 99.1° F (37.3° C), Spo_2 90%. Ht. 74 in (188 cm); wt. 145 lb (65.8 kg).

9. What is the significance of the spider angiomas, dilated abdominal veins, peripheral edema, and distended abdomen?

10. How would you further assess the distended abdomen? What is the clinical name for and the significance of your findings?

11. In what position should you place D.G? Write a brief rationale for your response.
   a. Supine
   b. Fowler's
   c. Right side-lying
   d. Left lateral recumbent

7 Metabolism Regulation

12. What objective findings concern you about his nutritional assessment and why?

13. Why is D.G.'s breath musty?

14. Which of D.G.'s assessment findings are consistent with hepatic encephalopathy?

15. Which assessment findings, if present, would indicate a deterioration of D.G.'s condition?
   a. Frequent diarrhea
   b. Nausea and vomiting
   c. Increased urine output
   d. Development of asterixis

16. What is asterixis?

CASE STUDY PROGRESS

Chart View

Laboratory Results

Potassium	3.4 mEq/L (3.4 mmol/L)
Alanine transaminase (ALT)	146 units/L
Aspartate transaminase (AST)	207 units/L
Alkaline phosphatase (ALP)	154 units/L
Total bilirubin	3.6 mg/dL (61.6 mcmol/L)
Albumin	2.1 g/dL (3.0 mcmol/L)
Total protein	5.3 g/dL (53 g/L)
Ammonia	155 mcg/dL (111.0 mcmol/L)
PT/INR	16 seconds/1.6

17. Interpret D.G.'s lab results.

18. You begin to develop D.G.'s care plan. It is imperative to prevent bleeding when caring for a person with cirrhosis. List 4 specific interventions you will take to reduce D.G.'s bleeding risk.

19. Falls are particularly dangerous for someone in his situation. Why?

20. What measures will you implement to promote optimal skin integrity?

21. You identify the nursing problem "excess fluid volume." Which is the *best* short-term goal for D.G.? D.G. will:
   a. Have a decrease in abdominal girth
   b. Maintain his ordered fluid restriction
   c. Select low-sodium foods from the diet menu
   d. Have no further weight gain before discharge

22. Describe 5 interventions that will help improve D.G.'s nutritional status.

23. What interprofessional referrals might you initiate and why?

CASE STUDY OUTCOME

D.G. develops an upper GI bleed during his third hospital day. After 24 days, including a week in the intensive care unit, he is discharged to a rehabilitation facility. He had been employed as a loading dock worker; unfortunately, his health never recovers to the point where he can return to work.

Case Study 91

Name_____ Class/Group_____ Date_____

▶ Scenario

Y.L., a 34-year-old Southern Asian woman, comes to the clinic with chronic fatigue, increased thirst, constant hunger, and frequent urination. She denies any pain, burning, or low-back pain on urination. She tells you she has a vaginal yeast infection that she has treated many times with over-the-counter medication. She works full time as a clerk in a loan company and states she has difficulty reading numbers and reports, resulting in her making frequent mistakes. She says, "By the time I get home and make supper for my family, then put my child to bed, I am too tired to exercise." She reports her feet hurt; they often "burn or feel like there are pins in them." She has a history of gestational diabetes and reports following a traditional eating pattern, which is high in carbohydrates.

In reviewing Y.L.'s chart, you note she last saw the provider 6 years ago after the delivery of her last child. She has gained considerable weight; her current weight is 173 pounds (78.5 kg). Today her BP is 152/97, and a random plasma glucose level is 291 mg/dL (16.2 mmol/L). The provider suspects she has developed type 2 diabetes mellitus (DM) and orders the lab studies shown in the chart.

Chart View

Laboratory Test Results

Fasting glucose	184 mg/dL (10.2 mmol/L)
Hemoglobin A_{1c} (A_{1C})	8.8%
Total cholesterol	256 mg/dL (6.6 mmol/L)
Triglycerides	346 mg/dL (3.91 mmol/L)
Low-density lipoprotein (LDL)	155 mg/dL (4.01 mmol/L)
High-density lipoprotein (HDL)	32 mg/dL (0.83 mmol/L)
Urinalysis (UA)	+ glucose, − ketones

1. Interpret Y.L.'s lab results.

7 Metabolism Regulation

2. Identify 3 methods used to diagnose DM.

3. Describe the major pathophysiologic difference between type 1 and type 2 DM.

4. Name 6 risk factors for type 2 DM. Underline those that Y.L. has.

CASE STUDY PROGRESS

Y.L. is diagnosed with type 2 DM. The provider starts her on metformin (Glucophage) 500 mg, glipizide (Glucotrol) 5 mg, orally each day at breakfast and atorvastatin 20 mg orally at bedtime. She is referred to the dietitian for instructions on starting a 1200-calorie diet using an exchange system to facilitate weight loss and lower blood glucose, cholesterol, and triglyceride levels. You are to provide teaching about pharmacotherapy and exercise.

5. How can you incorporate Y.L.'s cultural preferences as you develop her teaching plan?

6. What is the reason for starting Y.L. on metformin and glipizide?

7. Outline the teaching you need to provide to Y.L. about oral hypoglycemic therapy.

8. What do you teach Y.L. to do if she becomes ill with the flu or viral illness?

9. You determine she understands your teaching about treating hypoglycemia if she states, "If my blood sugar is low, I should first have:
   a. an apple with milk."
   b. peanut butter sandwich."
   c. fruit juice or regular soda."
   d. crackers with cheese slices."

10. What benefits should Y.L. receive from exercising?

11. What do you need to teach Y.L. about exercise?

12. Besides the dietitian, what interprofessional and community referrals may be appropriate for Y.L.?

CASE STUDY PROGRESS

Y.L. comments, "I've heard many people with diabetes lose their toes or even their feet." You take this opportunity to teach her about neuropathy and foot care.

13. Which symptoms that Y.L. reported today led you to believe she has some form of neuropathy?

14. What other findings in Y.L.'s history increased her risk for developing neuropathy?

15. What would you teach Y.L. about neuropathy?

16. Because Y.L. has symptoms of neuropathy, placing her at risk for foot complications, you realize you need to instruct her on proper foot care. Outline what you will include when teaching her about proper diabetic foot care.

17. What monitoring will Y.L. need for nephropathy and retinopathy?

CASE STUDY OUTCOME

Y.L. returns to the clinic 6 weeks later. Her BP is 130/78 and fasting glucose level is 153 mg/dL (8.5 mmol/L). She says she has not had any episodes of tingling in her toes or blurred vision lately. She did meet with the diabetic educator. She is making changes to her eating, has started walking, and is happy to have lost 6 pounds (2.7 kg).

Case Study **92**

Name_____ Class/Group_____ Date_____

▶ **Scenario**

You are working as a registered nurse (RN) in a large women's clinic. Y.L., a 28-year-old Asian woman, arrives for her regularly scheduled obstetric appointment. She is in her 26th week of pregnancy and is a primigravida. After examining the patient, the nurse-midwife tells you to schedule Y.L. for an oral glucose tolerance test (OGGT). You review Y.L.'s chart and note she is 5 feet, 3 inches (160 cm) tall and weighs 143 pounds (65 kg). Her prepregnancy body mass index (BMI) was 25. Her father has type 2 diabetes mellitus (DM), and both paternal grandparents had type 2 DM. You enter the room to talk to Y.L.

1. What is the purpose of an oral glucose tolerance test?

2. When is an OGGT performed?

3. What instructions would you provide Y.L. about the test?

CASE STUDY PROGRESS

Y.L.'s 1 hour OGTT test is positive, and she returns to the clinic the next day for a 3-hour (100 g) glucose tolerance test. The results are listed next.

Chart View

Laboratory Test Results: 3 hour (100 g) OGTT

Time of Test	Value	Normal Range
0730	109 mg/dL (6.0 mmol/L)	Less than 95 mg/dL (5.3 mmol/L)
0830	213 mg/dL (11.8 mmol/L)	Less than 180 mg/dL (10.0 mmol/L)
0930	162 mg/dL (9.0 mmol/L)	Less than 155 mg/dL (8.6 mmol/L)
1030	156 mg/dL (8.7 mmol/L)	Less than 140 mg/dL (7.8 mmol/L)

4. Interpret the results of Y.L.'s test.

5. Y.L. is diagnosed with gestational diabetes mellitus (GDM). What is GDM?

6. List 5 risk factors for GDM. Place a star next to those risk factors that Y.L. has.

CASE STUDY PROGRESS

Medical nutrition therapy is the primary treatment for the management of GDM. Because treatment must begin immediately, you call the dietitian to come see Y.L. You also schedule Y.L. to meet with other members of the DM management team later in the week.

7. What is the goal of medical nutrition therapy?

8. Describe the usual diet used in treating GDM.

9. Why is medical nutrition therapy for a woman with GDM higher in fat and protein than for a woman who is not pregnant?

10. Women with GDM cannot metabolize concentrated simple sugars without a sharp rise in blood glucose. Name 5 examples of simple sugars you would teach Y.L. to limit.

11. Complex carbohydrates (CHOs) do not cause a rapid rise in blood glucose when eaten in small amounts. Identify 5 foods from this group.

CASE STUDY PROGRESS

During the meeting with the dietitian, Y.L. gives a diet history that is high in noodles and white rice with little protein. She informs the dietitian she is lactose intolerant but can have dairy products occasionally in small portions.

12. Is it important that Y.L. take a calcium supplement along with her prenatal vitamins?

CASE STUDY PROGRESS

You provide teaching about monitoring her blood glucose levels and watch as Y.L. checks her own blood glucose with the glucometer.

13. Y.L. is instructed to check her fasting blood glucose first thing in the morning and 2 hours after every meal. What are the purposes of this request?

14. Which blood glucose levels are considered abnormal for Y.L.? Select all that apply.
   a. Fasting glucose 60 mg/dL (3.3 mmol/L)
   b. Fasting glucose 88 mg/dL (4.9 mmol/L)
   c. Fasting glucose 100 mg/dL (5.6 mmol/L)
   d. 2 hour post-meal glucose 119 mg/dL (6.6 mmol/L)
   e. 2 hour post-meal glucose 150 mg/dL (8.3 mmol/L)

15. Y.L. is instructed to complete ketone testing using the first-voided urine in the morning. What is the reason for this request?

16. You review what to do if she develops hypoglycemia, and then ask her to "teach back" to you what she has learned about what to do. Which statement by Y.L. reflects a correct understanding of treatment of a blood glucose below 60 mg/dL (3.3 mmol/L)?

a. "I will call my doctor immediately."
b. "I will eat a meal and check it again in an hour."
c. "I will drink a cup of orange juice mixed with sugar."
d. "I will drink half a cup of regular soda, and recheck it in 15 minutes.

17. Y.L. asks whether having gestational diabetes will hurt her baby. How would you respond?

18. At the end of the visit, you need to evaluate your teaching. Which statement made by Y.L. indicates that clarification is necessary?

a. "I should immediately report any ketones in my urine."
b. "I will stay on the diabetic diet described by the dietitian."
c. "I will monitor my glucose levels at least four times each day."
d. "I need to stop exercising because I will need more carbohydrates."

19. Y.L. states that she plans to have another child soon and asks you if she will develop GDM with that pregnancy. Select the best response:

a. "No, there is no further risk for development of GDM if you get pregnant again."
b. "Yes, once you develop GDM during a pregnancy, you will develop it with any future pregnancies."
c. "If you lose weight and do not eat any sweets before your next pregnancy, you will not develop GDM again."
d. "There is a risk for recurrence of GDM in the next pregnancy. Let your health care provider know that you had GDM with this pregnancy."

CASE STUDY OUTCOME

Y.L. safely delivers an 8 pound 9-ounce (3884 gram) baby boy at 39 weeks without complications. She is monitored closely for her GDM during the postpartum period.

Case Study **93**

Name_____ Class/Group_____ Date_____

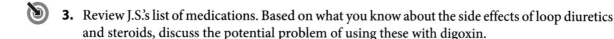

▶ Scenario

You are working with a home care agency. One patient in your caseload is J.S., a 66-year-old man with chronic obstructive pulmonary disease (COPD) related to cigarette smoking. He has been on home oxygen, 2 L oxygen by nasal cannula, for a few years. About 5 months ago, he started on chronic oral steroid therapy. His current medications include albuterol (Proair HFA) inhaler, fluticasone/salmeterol (Advair), prednisone, digoxin (Lanoxin), atenolol, aspirin, and furosemide.

1. On the way to J.S.'s home, you make a mental note to check him for signs and symptoms of Cushing syndrome. Why?

2. Differentiate between Cushing syndrome and Cushing disease.

3. Review J.S.'s list of medications. Based on what you know about the side effects of loop diuretics and steroids, discuss the potential problem of using these with digoxin.

4. Differentiate between the glucocorticoid and mineralocorticoid effects of prednisone.

5. How would your assessment change if J.S. were taking a glucocorticoid that had significant mineralocorticoid activity?

6. You need to assess J.S. for signs and symptoms of an infection. Why?

7. What signs and symptoms of infection do you assess for in J.S.? Select all that apply.
a. Pain
b. Fever
c. Palpitations
d. Loss of function
e. Localized edema
f. Unusual drainage

8. You plan to ask him about the presence of gastric discomfort, vision, and joint pain. Why?

CASE STUDY PROGRESS

Your assessment includes the following findings.

9. Determine whether each finding is attributable to J.S.'s COPD or possible Cushing syndrome. Place an *L* beside the symptoms consistent with COPD and a *C* next to those consistent with Cushing syndrome.
a. _____ Barrel chest
b. _____ Full-looking face (moon face)
c. _____ BP 180/94
d. _____ Pursed-lip breathing, especially when patient is stressed
e. _____ Striae over trunk and thighs
f. _____ Bruising on both arms
g. _____ Acne
h. _____ Diminished breath sounds throughout lungs
i. _____ Truncal obesity with thin extremities
j. _____ Supraclavicular and posterior upper back fat

You call the provider with J.S.'s assessment. The provider believes J.S. has developed Cushing syndrome and decides to change the prescription for prednisone from 10 mg daily to 10 mg given on alternate days.

10. Explain the reason for this change.

11. Discuss the possible consequences of suddenly stopping prednisone therapy.

12. You reinforce with J.S. the importance of taking prednisone at breakfast. Why?

13. Cushing syndrome can affect memory. Patients can easily forget what medications have been taken, especially when there are several different medications and some are taken on alternating days. List 3 ways you can help J.S. remember to take his medications as prescribed.

14. J.S. states his appetite has increased but he is losing weight. He reports trying to eat, but he gets short of breath and cannot eat any more. How would you address this problem?

15. Realizing J.S. is susceptible to infection, you review with him ways to reduce the risk for infection. Discuss 4 points to include.

16. In addition to ways to reduce the risk for infection, what other information do you want to stress to J.S. at your visit? Select all that apply.
   a. Increase intake of foods high in sodium.
   b. Weigh yourself first thing in the morning.
   c. Take vitamin and electrolyte supplements as prescribed.
   d. Notify the provider if your pulse is lower than 60.
   e. Take the furosemide first thing in the morning and again at bedtime.
   f. Call the provider if your weight increases more than 2 to 3 pounds (1 to 1.5 kg) in 1 day.

CASE STUDY OUTCOME

At your next visit, J.S.'s respiratory status is unchanged. Although most of the symptoms of Cushing syndrome remain despite the decrease in the dose of the prednisone, you are pleased that his blood pressure is lower, measuring 150/82.

Case Study 94

Name_____ Class/Group_____ Date_____

▶ Scenario

You are working in a community outpatient clinic where you perform the intake assessment on R.M., a 38-year-old woman who is attending graduate school and is very sedentary. Her chief complaint is overwhelming fatigue that is not relieved by rest. She is so exhausted that she has difficulty walking to classes and trouble concentrating when studying. She reports a recent weight gain of 15 pounds (6.8 kg) over 2 months without clear changes in her dietary habits. Her face looks puffy, she has experienced excessive hair loss, and her skin is dry and pale. She says she has general body aches and pains with frequent muscle cramps and constipation. You note she is dressed inappropriately warmly for the weather.

Chart View

Vital Signs (VS)

Blood pressure (BP)	142/84
Heart rate	52
Respiratory rate	12
Temperature	96.8° F (36° C)

1. Compare her VS with those of a healthy person her same age.

2. List 8 general questions you might ask R.M. to help determine what is going on.

3. What are some potential causes for R.M.'s symptoms?

4. As part of your screening, describe how you would begin to determine whether any of these conditions explain R.M.'s symptoms.

5. What diagnostic tests are appropriate for R.M., and why?

Chart View

Laboratory Test Results

Thyroid-stimulating hormone (TSH)	20.9 mU/L (2–10 mU/L)
Thyrotropin-releasing hormone (TRH)	18.8 ng/dL (2–10 ng/dL)
T$_3$	24 mU/L (70–205 ng/dL)
Free T$_4$	0.2 ng/dL (0.8–2.4 ng/dL)

6. Interpret R.M.'s lab results.

7. The practitioner affirms a diagnosis of hypothyroidism. With this diagnosis, what other signs and symptoms would you want to assess for in R.M.?

8. What is the most common cause of primary hypothyroidism?
   a. Thyroidectomy
   b. Acute thyrotoxicosis
   c. Hashimoto's thyroiditis
   d. Radioactive iodine exposure

 9. The practitioner prescribes levothyroxine (Synthroid) 1.7 mcg/kg body weight per day. Now, R.M. weighs 130 pounds. What should be her daily dose of levothyroxine in milligrams? How would her prescription read?

10. What teaching will you provide R.M. about levothyroxine?

11. What should you teach R.M. about preventing myxedema coma?

12. What other general teaching issues will you address with R.M. about hypothyroidism?

13. Which statements show R.M. understands your teaching about hypothyroidism and taking levothyroxine? Select all that apply.
   a. "It may take several weeks before I feel better."
   b. "The best time to take my medicine is ½ hour before breakfast."
   c. "If my heart rate is over 100, I will hold my medication until it is back below 100."
   d. "I will be able to discontinue my medication after the symptoms are under control."
   e. "I will come in when needed so my blood levels can be checked to make sure the medicine is working."

14. Before R.M. leaves the clinic, she asks how she will know whether the medication is "doing its job." How long does it take to see effects of levothyroxine therapy?

15. Outline simple expected outcomes for R.M.

16. A few weeks later, R.M. calls the clinic saying she cannot remember whether she took her thyroid medication. What other data should you obtain, and what would you tell her?

17. Discuss 2 ways you can help R.M. remember to take her medication.

CASE STUDY OUTCOME

R.M. comes in 2 months later for a follow-up visit. You cannot believe she is the same person. She looks and walks as if she were 10 years younger. Her skin appears more radiant, and her hair looks much healthier. "You can't believe how different I'm feeling," she says. "I didn't know how bad off I was; I'm starting to live again."

Case Study **95**

Name_____ Class/Group_____ Date_____

▶ Scenario

You are working on the surgical floor and will be receiving a patient from the postanesthesia care unit. The nurse calls and gives the following report: C.P. is a 55-year-old woman who underwent a subtotal right thyroidectomy for papillary carcinoma. Estimated blood loss was 25 mL. Vital signs (VS) are 130/82, 80 to 90, 20, and SaO_2 94% on room air. She is receiving an IV infusion of D5.45NS at 100 mL/hr. She has received a total of 3 mg morphine sulfate IV push, and she is awake, but drowsy, and fully oriented. C.P.'s past medical history includes a total abdominal hysterectomy for fibroids and low-level radiation treatments to the neck 30 years ago for eczema. Both parents are living; her father had a myocardial infarction at 70 years of age; her mother has hypothyroidism but never had thyroid tumors.

1. Name the major risk factor that likely contributed to C.P. developing thyroid cancer.

2. What are the common manifestations of thyroid cancer?

3. What specific preparations will you make before C.P. arrives?

4. You receive C.P. from the recovery room. How will you focus your initial assessment, and why?

5. During your initial assessment, you document negative Chvostek and Trousseau signs. Describe data that would support this conclusion.

6. Which assessment findings may indicate C.P. has laryngeal nerve damage? Select all that apply.
a. Stridor
b. Hoarseness
c. Breathy voice
d. Circumoral numbness
e. Difficulty swallowing

7. Name 3 interventions to use to reduce the risk for postoperative swelling.

8. Besides laryngeal nerve damage, C.P. is at risk for other complications postoperatively. List 3 complications, and describe actions you would include in her plan of care related to each.

9. What interventions will you use to meet the outcome of controlling C.P.'s surgical pain?

10. After surgery, C.P.'s thyroid hormone levels are elevated. The provider orders propranolol 80 mg ER orally twice daily for "surgically induced thyrotoxicosis." Is this reaction expected after thyroid surgery, or did something go wrong during surgery? Explain.

11. What assessment findings would indicate that C.P. was experiencing thyrotoxicosis?

CASE STUDY PROGRESS

Eighteen hours after surgery, C.P. calls you into her room complaining of numbness around her mouth, tingling at the tips of her fingers, and jitteriness. She appears restless but denies any pain at the operative site. She can swallow and speak without difficulty.

12. What is your immediate concern and why?

13. What actions do you need to take based on this concern?

14. The provider orders you to give C.P. 1 gram of IV calcium gluconate over 15 minutes now, and then start an infusion of 2 grams of calcium gluconate in 500 mL D5W over 12 hours. After the bolus is complete, at what rate will you set the IV pump?

15. What precautions do you need to take while administering the calcium gluconate infusion?

CASE STUDY PROGRESS

Six hours after initiation of the calcium gluconate infusion, C.P. is no longer complaining of numbness around her mouth or tingling in her fingertips and toes. Chvostek and Trousseau signs remain negative.

Chart View

Laboratory Test Results

Serum calcium	7.4 mg/dL (1.85 mmol/L)
Ionized calcium	3.4 mg/dL (0.85 mmol/L)
Parathyroid hormone (PTH)	< 3.0 pg/mL (< 3.0 ng/L)

---

16. Has C.P.'s status improved or not? Defend your response.

CASE STUDY PROGRESS

C.P. is started on oral calcium gluconate. Her calcium levels stabilize within 24 hours and she recovers without further complications. Two days postoperatively, you are preparing her for discharge.

17. As part of your discharge instructions, what would you teach C.P.? Select all that apply.
   a. Keep her head raised while sleeping for 3 to 4 days
   b. The importance of keeping follow-up medical appointments
   c. Not to return to work until her thyroid hormone level is normal
   d. Cover her incision with clothing or sunscreen when she is in the sun
   e. Proper care of the incision and signs of infection to report to the provider
   f. To avoid foods containing iodine because they increase her risk for recurrent cancer

CASE STUDY OUTCOME

Two years later, C.P. began having dysphagia with pain on the left side of her throat. The remaining thyroid tissue was surgically removed after finding the cancer had reoccurred. Postoperatively she underwent 12 weeks of radiation treatment, which left her with some permanent voice changes. She is still cancer free 1 year later.

Case Study **96**

Name_____ Class/Group_____ Date_____

▶ Scenario

You work in the diabetes mellitus (DM) center at a large teaching hospital. The first patient you meet is K.W., a 35-year-old Hispanic woman, who was just released from the hospital 2 days ago after being diagnosed with type 1 DM.

Nine days ago, K.W. went to see the provider after a 1-month history of frequent urination, thirst, severe fatigue, blurred vision, and some burning and tingling in her feet. She attributed those symptoms to working long hours at the computer. Her random glucose level was 410 mg/dL (22.8 mmol/L). The next day her lab values were as follows: fasting glucose 335 mg/dL (18.6 mmol/L), A_{1c} 8.8%, cholesterol 310 mg/dL (8.03 mmol/L), triglycerides 300 mg/dL (3.39 mmol/L), HDL 25 mg/dL (0.65 mmol/L), LDL 160 mg/dL (4.14 mmol/L), ratio 12.4, and creatinine 0.9 mg/dL (80.0 mcmol/L). Her body mass index was 29.6 with a BP 160/96. She was admitted to the hospital for control of her glucose levels and the initiation of insulin therapy with carbohydrate counting. After discharge, K.W. has been referred to you for diabetes education. You are to cover four areas: pharmacotherapy, glucose monitoring, basic nutrition therapy, and exercise.

1. What is the overall teaching goal with a patient newly diagnosed with type 1 DM?

2. What assessments do you need to make before starting your session?

3. K.W. was started on sliding scale lispro (Humalog) four times daily and glargine (Lantus) insulin at bedtime. What are the significant differences between the two therapies?

4. K.W. says she knows people who "only take 2 shots" because they are on NPH and regular insulin and wants to know why she cannot do that. Explain the advantages of using the glargine (Lantus) and lispro (Humalog) insulin regimen.

5. Outline important content to include about pharmacologic therapy.

6. What specific points would you include about managing insulin therapy? Select all that apply.
   a. Store unused insulin in the freezer.
   b. The insulin can be used if it is yellow but not expired.
   c. Administer the lispro (Humalog) within 15 minutes of eating.
   d. Ideally, the glargine (Lantus) should be administered at bedtime.
   e. Always administer the injections in the same, easy-to-reach location.
   f. The current vial of lispro (Humalog) can be kept at room temperature for 1 month.
   g. Two injections will be needed to administer lispro (Humalog) and glargine (Lantus).

7. What is the best way to determine whether K.W. can safely self-administer insulin?
   a. Having her describe the process step-by-step
   b. Evaluating her A_{1C} levels and daily glucose logs
   c. Observing her draw up and administer an insulin dose
   d. Asking her to rate her confidence in her ability to give a self-injection

8. Outline important content to review about self blood glucose monitoring.

9. K.W. states her diet is mostly fast foods, and the foods cooked at home are high in starch and fat. Her mealtimes often vary from day to day because of her work schedule. What is CHO (carbohydrate) counting, and why would this method work well for K.W.?

10. Outline important points to cover about a basic nutrition plan with CHO counting.

11. K.W. states that she currently does not exercise at all. What benefits will K.W. receive from taking part in an exercise program?

12. What do you need to teach K.W. about safe exercise?

7 Metabolism Regulation

13. What can you and other members of the health care team do to help her deal with her condition and follow the treatment plan?

14. What evaluative parameters could you use to determine whether your teaching with K.W. was effective?

CASE STUDY PROGRESS

K.W. calls the clinic several days later says she has "the flu." She says she has been nauseated and vomited once during the night. She has had two loose stools. On questioning, she states that she does have a few chills and might have a low-grade fever but does not have a thermometer to check her temperature. She did not check her glucose level this morning or take her insulin because she has "not eaten."

15. Describe the instructions that you need to give K.W. about managing illness and DM.

16. Outline how you will document the phone call with K.W.

CASE STUDY OUTCOME

In her mid-forties, K.W. began to show signs of diabetic nephropathy. At age 55, she was becoming increasingly fatigued upon mild physical exertion, felt nauseated most of the time, and had increased swelling in her ankles. She began hemodialysis; however, she died 9 months later from a myocardial infarction.

Case Study **97**

Name_____ Class/Group_____ Date_____

▶ Scenario

K.B. is a 65-year-old man admitted to the hospital after a 5-day episode of "the flu" with symptoms of dyspnea on exertion, palpitations, chest pain, insomnia, and fatigue. K.B. was diagnosed with Graves' disease 6 months ago and placed on methimazole (Tapazole) 15 mg/day. His other past medical history includes heart failure and hypertension requiring antihypertensive medications; however, he says that he has not been taking these medications on a regular basis. Vital signs (VS) are: 150/90, 124 irregular, 20, 100.2° F (37.9° C). Admission assessment findings are: height 5 ft, 8 in (173 cm); weight 132 lb (60 kg); appears anxious and restless; loud heart sounds; 1+ pitting edema noted in bilateral lower extremities; diminished breath sounds with fine crackles in the posterior bases. K.B. begins to cry when he tells you he recently lost his wife; you notice someone has punched several more holes in his belt so he could tighten it.

Chart View

Laboratory Test Results

Hemoglobin (Hgb)	11.8 g/dL (118 g/L)
Hematocrit (Hct)	36%
Erythrocyte sedimentation rate (ESR)	48 mm/hr
Sodium	141 mEq/L (141 mmol/L)
Potassium	4.7 mEq/L (4.7 mmol/L)
Chloride	101 mEq/L (101 mmol/L)
Blood urea nitrogen (BUN)	33 mg/dL (11.78 mmol/L)
Creatinine	1.9 mg/dL (168 mcmol/L)
Free thyroxine (T_4)	14.0 ng/dL (180 pmol/L)
Triiodothyronine (T_3)	230 ng/dL (353 nmol/L)

1. Which of K.B.'s assessment findings represent manifestations of hypermetabolism?

2. Interpret K.B.'s lab results.

3. You go to assess K.B. What other data do you need to obtain because he has Graves' disease?

Chart View

Physician's Orders

    Propranolol (Inderal) 20 mg PO q6hr
    Dexamethasone 10 mg IV q6hr
    Methimazole (Tapazole) 15 mg/day twice daily
    Verapamil (Calan SR) 120 mg/day PO
    Furosemide 80 mg IV push now, then 40 mg/day IV push
    Diet as tolerated
    Stat ECG and echocardiogram
    Up ad lib
    IV of D5W at 125 mL/hr
    Daily weights with intake and output (I&O)

---

4. The resident on call writes admission orders. Which will you question, and why?

5. What role does methimazole have in treating Graves' disease?

6. Describe 4 priority problems that will guide K.B.'s nursing care.

7. What measures can you use to promote K.B. receiving adequate rest?

Later in your shift, you note that K.B. is extremely restless and disoriented to person, place, and time. VS are 174/82, 180 and irregular, 32 and labored, 104° F (40° C). His ECG shows atrial fibrillation.

8. What is likely happening with K.B.? Give your rationale.

9. What actions do you need to take first?

10. You need to call the resident regarding K.B.'s status. Using SBAR, what will you report?

The resident evaluates K.B. and determines he is in thyroid crisis. New orders are shown in the chart.

Chart View

Physician's Orders

Oxygen at 2 L per nasal cannula
Stat ABGs, BNP, and cardiac enzymes
Digoxin 0.25 mg IV push now, then 0.125 mg IVP q8hr × 2 doses
Diltiazem bolus dose of 0.25 mg/kg IV; after 15 minutes, give a second dose of 0.35 mg/kg IV for heart rate greater than 140
Increase methimazole to 15 mg PO q6hr
Hydrocortisone 50 mg IV push q6hr
Absolute bed rest
Acetaminophen 650 mg PO q6hr prn for temperature over 100° F (37.8° C)

11. Describe how you would care for K.B. in the next hour.

 12. How many total milliliters of diltiazem will you give for the first dose? How many for the second, if needed?

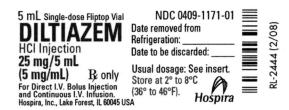

13. What is your primary nursing goal at this time?

14. Describe 6 interventions you will perform over the next few hours based on this priority.

15. Why was K.B. at risk for developing thyroid storm?

16. Identify 3 outcomes that you expect for K.B. as a result of your interventions.

CASE STUDY PROGRESS

After several hours of treatment, K.B.'s condition stabilizes. The resident discusses two treatment options with K.B. and his family: radioactive iodine (RAI) therapy and subtotal thyroidectomy.

17. K.B. is fearful of radiation treatment and asks you for your opinion. How would you respond?

 18. K.B. decides to receive RAI. During pretreatment instructions, the family asks whether he will be radioactive and what precautions they should take. Outline important guidelines for teaching K.B. and his family about home precautions.

19. Amid all this, you remain concerned about K.B.'s bereavement after the loss of his wife. How would you address this issue?

 20. K.B. does have some exophthalmos and is experiencing periodic photophobia and dry eyes. What should you include in teaching him how to manage these problems? Select all that apply.
a. Always wear sunglasses when outside.
b. Report any changes in vision to the provider.
c. Use artificial tears to provide moisture as needed.
d. Tape the eyes closed at night with nonallergenic tape.
e. Apply warm compresses to the eyes if they are irritated.

21. Which statement shows K.B. understands the discharge instructions?
    a. "I will take this medication on a full stomach."
    b. "If I get a sore throat, ice chips should help me feel better."
    c. "I should see an improvement in my symptoms by tomorrow."
    d. "I will follow the precautions for 2 weeks to keep my family safe."

CASE STUDY OUTCOME

Six months later, K.B.'s heart rate, blood pressure, and thyroid hormone levels are within normal limits. He has gained 14 lbs (6.4 kg) and has started walking in the mornings without any dyspnea. He says he has started to do woodworking and has been doing some volunteer work at the senior center.

Case Study **98**

Name_____ Class/Group_____ Date_____

▶ **Scenario**

You are working in an outpatient clinic when a mother brings in her 20-year-old daughter, C.J., who has type 1 diabetes mellitus (DM) and has just returned from a trip to Mexico. She has had a 3-day fever and diarrhea with nausea and vomiting. She has been unable to eat and has tolerated only sips of fluid. Because she was unable to eat, she did not take her insulin as directed. You note C.J. is unsteady, so you take her to the examining room in a wheelchair. While helping her onto the examination table, you note her skin is warm and flushed. Her respirations are deep and rapid, and her breath is fruity and sweet smelling. C.J. is drowsy and unable to answer your questions. Her mother states, "She kept telling me she's so thirsty, but she can't keep anything down."

1. List 5 pieces of additional information you need to obtain from C.J.'s mother.

2. Describe the pathophysiology of diabetic ketoacidosis (DKA).

CASE STUDY PROGRESS

C.J.'s mother tells you the following:

"Blood glucose monitor has been reading 'high.'"

"C.J. has had sips of ginger ale, but that's all."

"She has been vomiting about every other time she drinks."

"When she first got home, she went [voided] a lot, but yesterday she hardly went at all, and I don't think she has gone today."

"She went to bed early last night, and I could hardly wake her up this morning. That's why I brought her in."

Chart View	
Vital Signs	
Blood pressure	90/50
Heart rate	124
Respiratory rate	36 and deep
Temperature	101.3° F (38.5° C) (tympanic)
Laboratory Test Values	
Glucose	677 mg/dL (37.6 mmol/L)
Potassium	6.3 mEq/L (6.3 mmol/L)

3. Interpret C.J.'s VS and lab results, relating them to the pathophysiology.

4. Explain the reason for C.J.'s other presenting signs and symptoms.

5. The decision is made to transport C.J. by ambulance to the local emergency department (ED). C.J.'s mother realizes that C.J. is more acutely ill than she thought. She leaves the room and begins to cry. How would you handle this situation?

6. After assessing C.J., the ED resident on call writes the following orders. Review each order. Mark an *A* if the order is appropriate; mark an *I* if inappropriate. For each order you mark as *I*, explain why it is inappropriate, and correct the order.

1. _____ 1000 mL lactated Ringer's IV stat
2. _____ 36 units NPH (Humulin N) and 20 units regular (Humulin R) insulin subQ now
3. _____ CBC with differential; CMP; blood cultures × 2 sites; clean-catch urine for UA and C stool for ova and parasites, *Clostridium difficile* toxin, and C serum lactate, ketone, and osmolality; ABGs on room air
4. _____ 1800-calorie, carbohydrate-controlled diet
5. _____ Bed rest
6. _____ Acetaminophen 650 mg rectal suppository q4hr as needed
7. _____ Furosemide 60 mg IV push now
8. _____ Urinary output every hour
9. _____ VS every shift

7. List 5 other collaborative interventions that C.J. needs and the reason for using each.

8. Which ABG results would you expect to see in C.J.?
a. pH 7.40, Pao_2 88, $Paco_2$ 34, HCO_3 23
b. pH 7.48, Pao_2 90, $Paco_2$ 30, HCO_3 28
c. pH 7.27, Pao_2 90, $Paco_2$ 50, HCO_3 20
d. pH 7.26, Pao_2 94, $Paco_2$ 23, HCO_3 18

9. When C.J. is attached to the cardiac monitor, what would you expect to see on the ECG tracing?
a. Peaked P waves and a shortened PR interval
b. Presence of a U wave and ST segment depression
c. Tall, peaked T waves and widened QRS complexes
d. Narrow QRS complexes and shortening of the QT interval

CASE STUDY PROGRESS

All orders have been corrected and therapies started. C.J. receives fluid resuscitation and sliding-scale insulin drip via infusion pump. After several hours, her latest lab findings are as shown in the chart.

Chart View

Laboratory Test Results

Na	149 mEq/L (149 mmol/L)
K	3.0 mEq/L (3.0 mmol/L)
Cl	119 mEq/L (119 mmol/L)
Total CO_2	21 mEq/L (21 mmol/L)
BUN	12 mg/dL (4.28 mmol/L)
Creatinine	1.2 mg/dL (106 mcmol/L)
Glucose	307 mg/dL (17 mmol/L)

10. Based on C.J.'s lab results, what changes in her IV fluids would you anticipate, and why?

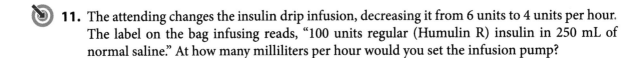

11. The attending changes the insulin drip infusion, decreasing it from 6 units to 4 units per hour. The label on the bag infusing reads, "100 units regular (Humulin R) insulin in 250 mL of normal saline." At how many milliliters per hour would you set the infusion pump?

12. What is the rationale behind using an infusion pump for the insulin drip?

13. True or False? A second registered nurse or physician must verify the IV infusion rate for the insulin dose change. State your rationale.

CASE STUDY OUTCOME

C.J. continues to improve and is discharged from the hospital 3 days later. Her mother and she agree to attend an outpatient class offered by the diabetes education department to assist C.J. with better managing her diabetes.

Case Study **99**

Name_____   Class/Group_____   Date_____

> ► **Scenario**

T.R. is a 19-year-old college freshman who lives in the honors dormitory. His friend finds him wandering aimlessly about the campus appearing pale and sweaty. He engages T.R. in conversation and walks him to the campus medical clinic, where you are on duty. The friend explains to you how he found T.R. and says T.R. is "diabetic" and takes insulin. T.R. is not wearing a medical warning tag. It is 1020.

1. What do you think is going on with T.R.?

2. What is the first action you would take?

3. Which assessment findings would support the premise that T.R. is experiencing a hypoglycemic reaction?
   a. Extreme thirst and nausea
   b. Nervousness and tachycardia
   c. Hypertension with bounding pulses
   d. Fruity breath with deep, rapid respirations

4. If no glucose meter were available, would you treat T.R. on the assumption he is hyperglycemic or hypoglycemic? Explain your reasoning.

5. It is 1025. T.R.'s glucose reading is 50 mg/dL (2.8 mmol/L). What should your next action be?

6. When you enter the room to give the juice, T.R. is not responsive enough to drink the juice safely. What should you do?

7. T.R.'s breathing rate is 16 and he has a pulse of 112 and regular. Because outpatient resources vary, describe your next actions if (1) your clinic is well equipped for emergencies or (2) your clinic has no emergency supplies.

CASE STUDY PROGRESS

A few minutes after administering 2 mg subcutaneous glucagon, T.R. begins to awaken. He becomes alert and asks where he is and what happened to him. You orient him and then explain what has transpired.

8. What questions would you ask to find out what precipitated this event?

9. What further action do you need to take at this time?

10. At 1045, you recheck T.R.'s glucose and the reading is 64 mg/dL (3.6 mmol/L). His vital signs are 120/72, 18, 92. Has his status improved or not? Defend your response.

11. What would your next action be?

12. At 1110, you recheck T.R.'s glucose and the reading is 104 mg/dL (5.8 mmol/L). What should you do now?

CASE STUDY PROGRESS

T.R. tells you he took 35 units glargine (Lantus) insulin and 12 units of regular (Humulin R) insulin at 0745. He says he was late to class, so he just grabbed an apple on the way.

13. Based on this information, why did T.R. experience this episode of hypoglycemia?

14. Based on your knowledge of the types of insulin T.R. is receiving, when would you expect T.R. to experience a hypoglycemic reaction?

15. T.R. says he had a few similar episodes recently. He treated them by eating a candy bar. He says he is on a 2000-calorie, carbohydrate-controlled diet but has been checking his blood glucose levels every "couple of days" only. What common mistake in previously treated episodes of hypoglycemia did T.R. make?

16. He goes on to say he has had "a little bit much to drink at a few of the parties he has been to" on the weekends. What effect does alcohol have on blood glucose?

17. What should you teach T.R. about alcohol consumption and managing his diabetes?

18. List 4 additional points you would stress in a teaching plan with T.R.

19. You tell T.R. to check his blood glucose at 1230 then eat lunch at the normal time. You determine that he understands your teaching regarding averting hypoglycemia if he states:
   a. "I need to eat within 30 minutes of taking the regular insulin."
   b. "If I am too sick to eat, I will not take any insulin until I feel better."
   c. "Only certain kinds of alcoholic drinks will affect my blood glucose levels."
   d. "I will exercise just before eating and taking insulin so I do not get cramps."

20. Write a sample documentation note for the encounter with T.R.

CASE STUDY OUTCOME

T.R. follows up with you in 1 week to discuss how he has been managing his meals and insulin dosing. He states he feels that he has been doing a better job with eating meals at regular times and shows you the log from his new diabetes tracking app. You congratulate him on his progress and decide together that meeting weekly will help T.R. manage his diabetes while adjusting to college life.

Case Study 100

Name_____ Class/Group_____ Date_____

▶ Scenario

B.K. is a 63-year-old woman who is admitted to the step-down unit from the emergency department (ED) with nausea, vomiting, and epigastric and left upper quadrant abdominal pain that is severe, sharp, and boring and radiates through to her mid back. The pain started 24 hours ago and awoke her in the middle of the night. B.K. is a divorced, retired sales manager who smokes a half-pack of cigarettes daily. The ED nurse reports that B.K. is anxious and demanding. B.K. denies using alcohol. Her vital signs are as follows: 100/70, 97, 30, 100.2° F (37.9° C) (tympanic), SpO_2 88% on room air and 92% on 2 L of oxygen by nasal cannula (NC). She is in normal sinus rhythm. She is under the care of the hospitalist service. She has no primary care provider and has not seen a physician "in years."

The ED nurse giving you the report states that the admitting diagnosis is acute pancreatitis of unknown etiology. An abdominal ultrasound showed "no cholelithiasis, gallbladder wall thickening, or choledocholithiasis. The pancreas was not well visualized due to overlying bowel gas." An abdominal CT is scheduled for the morning. Admission labs have been drawn; a clean-catch urine specimen was sent to the lab, and the urine was dark in color.

1. What are the usual causes of pancreatitis?

2. What other information do you need from the ED nurse before you assume responsibility for B.K.'s care?

CASE STUDY PROGRESS

Chart View

Medication Administration Record

Esomeprazole 40 mg IV push daily
Metoclopramide 10 mg IV push every 6 hrs
Metronidazole 500 mg IV piggyback every 8 hrs
Morphine sulfate 5 mg IV push every 4 hrs as needed
Ondansetron 4 mg IV push every 6 hrs as needed

3. Indicate the expected outcome associated with each medication she is receiving.

4. Which admission order would you question?
   a. Clear liquid diet
   b. IV 0.9% NS at 150 mL/hr
   c. Bed rest with bathroom privileges.
   d. CBC with differential, BMP, amylase, and lipase now

5. What preparation is needed for B.K.'s CT scan?

CASE STUDY PROGRESS

You complete your admission assessment and note the following abnormalities: B.K. is restless and alert, lying on her right side in a semi-fetal position. Assessment findings are as follows: Skin is cool, diaphoretic, and pale with poor skin turgor; mucous membranes are dry. ECG shows sinus tachycardia, rate 106, heart sounds without murmurs or rubs. Peripheral pulses are palpable at 1+ in four extremities. Respiration rate 24, but unlabored on 2 L O_2/NC with Spo_2 90%. Breath sounds are extremely diminished in lower left lobe (LLL) posteriorly—otherwise, clear to auscultation throughout. She complains of nausea and is having dry heaves. Bowel sounds are hypoactive throughout. Abdomen is distended, firm, and tender in a diffuse fashion to light palpation, with guarding noted. The admission chest x-ray report reads, "moderate pleural effusion in the left lower lobe."

6. Your institution uses electronic charting. Based on the assessment given, document your findings.

☐ Neurologic

☐ Respiratory

☐ Cardiovascular

☐ Gastrointestinal

☐ Genitourinary

☐ Musculoskeletal

☐ Skin

☐ Psychosocial

☐ Pain

7. Based on your assessment, what is your nursing priority right now?

8. Name 3 interventions you would initiate based on this priority.

9. Besides giving as-needed medications, what other interventions would help with B.K.'s pain management?

10. B.K. turns on her call light. Despite the nausea, she complains of thirst and demands something to drink. Her orders indicate "NPO, except sips and chips." What is your response to her request? What might help her?

Chart View

Admission Laboratory Test Results

Lipase	3000 units/L
Amylase	2000 units/L
ALP	350 units/L (6 μkat/L)
ALT	90 units/L (1.53 μkat/L)
AST	150 units/L (2.55 μkat/L)
Total bilirubin	2.0 mg/dL (34.2 μmol/L)
Albumin	3.0 g/dL (4.35 μmol/L)
BUN	24 mg/dL (8.57 mmol/L)
Creatinine	1.4 mg/dL (124 mcmol/L)
WBC count	17,500/mm³ (17.5 x 109/L)

11. Which lab results support a diagnosis of pancreatitis?

12. Which lab results are the most important to monitor in acute pancreatitis? Why are they significant?

13. What do the BUN and creatinine tell you about her renal function and volume status?

14. Why are the WBCs elevated?

CASE STUDY PROGRESS

B.K. eventually falls asleep and seems to be sleeping peacefully. Several hours later, you hear an alarm on her pulse oximeter and enter her room to investigate. You find B.K. moaning softly; her oximeter reads 87%.

15. What will you do next?

16. B.K.'s respirations become increasingly labored. You perform a quick assessment, with findings as follows: Lung sounds absent in the LLL and very diminished in the right lower lobe. You percuss a dull thud over the left lung up to the scapula tip. On percussion, you hear resonance over the entire right lung. What is the significance of your findings?

CASE STUDY PROGRESS

The provider orders a stat chest x-ray examination, which shows a significant pleural effusion developing in the LLL, with extension into the lower portion of the upper lobe.

17. Based on the evolving pleural effusion with evidence of decompensation, the provider decides to perform a thoracentesis to remove fluid. What are your responsibilities regarding this procedure?

7 Metabolism Regulation

CASE STUDY PROGRESS

The provider removed 200 mL of slightly cloudy serous fluid. Antibiotics were adjusted to provide broad-spectrum coverage for an upper respiratory tract infection until culture and sensitivity results are returned. B.K. is resting quietly with oxygen at 3 L per NC, and her respirations are unlabored and regular. Her SpO$_2$ reads 96%.

It is now 72 hours after B.K.'s admission, and her lab test results show improvement. An abdominal CT scan is completed and shows "a moderately severe pancreatitis, but no local fluid collection or pseudocysts. No ileus or evidence of neoplasia was noted." BUN is 9.0 mg/dL, and creatinine is 1.0 mg/dL. She has adequate urinary output. Her IV fluids are decreased to 75 mL/hr. Her amylase and lipase levels are decreasing toward normal levels. The provider writes an order to advance B.K.'s diet from clear to full liquids.

18. How would you know if B.K. was not tolerating the advancement in her diet?

19. If B.K. does not tolerate the advancement in diet, what physiologic need should be addressed at 72 hours?

CASE STUDY OUTCOME

Three days later, B.K.'s pain is under control with oral pain medications. The provider advances her diet to "low-fat/low-cholesterol" and writes orders to discharge that evening if she tolerates the advancement in diet, which she does.

20. What will you include in your discharge teaching with B.K.?

21. Which statement shows that your teaching about dietary instructions was effective?
   a. "I must eat six, small meals a day."
   b. "I need to eliminate all protein from my diet."
   c. "Avoiding greasy and fried foods is important."
   d. "It is okay for me to drink coffee, tea, and soda."

CASE STUDY OUTCOME

At her one-week follow-up appointment, B.K. relates that finding foods that she can eat has been the greatest challenge but that overall, she feels better. She says she is irritated with her friends, who assume this happened because she is secretly drinking. She has not resumed smoking. She says she does not want this to happen again because it has been a "really, really bad experience."

Immunity

Case Study **101**

Name_____ Class/Group_____ Date_____

▶ **Scenario**

C.Z. is a 37-year-old woman who was diagnosed with rheumatoid arthritis 3 years ago. Her current medications include naproxen 500 mg twice daily, methotrexate 20 mg once weekly, and folic acid 1 mg daily. She says she has improved on this plan but has persistent joint pain and swelling in her hands and feet, with some lingering fatigue. She came to the clinic today because her family recently moved to the area and she needs to establish a relationship with a new primary care provider. She is married with 2 school-aged children and was just hired part-time as a cashier at a local department store.

1. Describe the pathophysiology of rheumatoid arthritis (RA).

2. RA and osteoarthritis have some common symptoms but have different causes, progression, and treatment. Place an "R" next to the statements that describe RA and an "O" next to those that describe osteoarthritis.
   1. _____ Develops over weeks to months
   2. _____ Localized disease with variable, progressive course
   3. _____ Morning stiffness lasts 1 hour to all day
   4. _____ Pain improves with joint use
   5. _____ Age of onset is generally over 40 years
   6. _____ Joint effusions are common
   7. _____ Typically affects small joints first
   8. _____ Fever, fatigue, and loss of energy may occur
   9. _____ Pain worsens with joint use

3. What are the long-term systemic complications of RA?

4. What are the overall goals of collaborative care for a patient with RA?

5. Outline the history information you need to obtain from C.Z.

CASE STUDY PROGRESS

C.Z. says her symptoms started suddenly. She stated, "she woke up one morning and was so weak she could barely get out of bed or walk." Over the next few days she started to hurt and feel stiff all over, making it hard to sit, stand, or lay down without pain. She lost her appetite and noticed some hair loss. After having lab testing, the previous provider told her she had RA and started her on her current medications. Recent x-rays showed some bone erosion in her right wrist and 3 metacarpophalangeal (MCP) joints of her right hand. She denies any family history of RA or other autoimmune disorders and has had no hospitalizations except for childbirth.

6. What other signs of RA do you need to assess for when performing her assessment?

CASE STUDY PROGRESS

C.Z.'s physical assessment was unremarkable except that her left and right index and middle PIP joints were slightly tender and swollen with limited range of motion. Her vital signs were 120/78, 74, 16, 98.2° F (36.8° C). Her height is 5 ft, 5 in (165 cm), and she weighs 170 lbs (77 kg).

Chart View

Laboratory Results

C-reactive protein (CRP)	2.7 mg/dL (25.7 nmol/L) (normal: < 1.0 mg/dL [<9.5 nmol/L])
Erythrocyte sedimentation rate (ESR)	38 mm/hr (normal: 0–20 mm/hr)
Rheumatoid factor (RF)	344 (negative or titer <1:17)
ANA	26 mmol/L (negative at 1:40 dilution)

7. Explain the significance of C.Z.'s lab results.

8. The provider decides to start C.Z. on the immunomodulator etanercept 50 mg SC weekly via autoinjector and orders a tuberculin (TB) test and chest x-ray. What is the reason for performing a TB test and chest x-ray?

9. What teaching do you need to provide about etanercept therapy?

CASE STUDY PROGRESS

You ask C.Z. how having RA has affected her life. She states that she used to be a very active person, but now she must be careful about how much she does each day because she has noted that too much activity triggers increased fatigue and pain.

10. Name 3 priority nursing problems you need to address with C.Z.

11. Describe the teaching you would provide C.Z. about physical activity.

12. What would you review with C.Z. to meet the expected outcome of protecting joints from stress?

13. What suggestions can you make to C.Z. about managing fatigue?

14. After teaching C.Z. to use heat and cold therapy to relieve symptoms, you determine teaching has been effective when she states:
   a. "Taking a warm shower can help ease morning stiffness."
   b. "Cold therapy can be applied for 30 minutes to relieve joint stiffness."
   c. "I can use heat therapy for 20 minutes to relieve the symptoms of an acute flare."
   d. "When my joints are swollen, a heating pad for 10 to 15 minutes can relieve the pain."

15. You are concerned with C.Z.'s psychological status. Write a nursing outcome addressing this issue and identify independent nursing actions you would implement.

16. What interprofessional referrals may benefit C.Z.?

17. What assessment data would you use to determine whether C.Z.'s condition is improving?

18. Using a SOAP format, write a sample documentation entry for this encounter.

CASE STUDY OUTCOME

After switching to etanercept, C.Z. noticed a substantial improvement in joint pain and swelling. She decided to continue with this regimen and began an exercise program under the supervision of PT. By implementing the recommendations made by the provider, PT, OT, and you, she says she is has less fatigue and finding it easier to "make it through each day."

Case Study **102**

Name_____   Class/Group_____   Date_____

▶ Scenario

You are working in a community health clinic and you have just taken C.Q., a 38-year-old woman, into the consultation room. C.Q. has been divorced for 5 years, has two daughters (ages 14 and 16), and works full time as a legal secretary. She is here for her yearly routine physical examination. C.Q. states she is in a serious relationship, is contemplating marriage, and just wants to make certain she is "okay." No abnormalities were noted during C.Q.'s physical examination. Blood was drawn for routine blood chemistries and hematology studies; since she has never been tested, C.Q. agrees to a human immunodeficiency virus (HIV) test. The provider requests you perform a rapid HIV test, which is an antibody test. Within 20 minutes, the results are available and are positive.

1. Does a positive rapid HIV test mean that C.Q. has HIV? If it is negative, does it mean she does not have HIV?

2. What counseling do you need to offer to C.Q.?

CASE STUDY PROGRESS

C.Q. returns to the clinic 2 days later. The provider informs you that C.Q.'s Western blot test results confirm that she has HIV infection; he requests you be present when he talks to her. Before leaving C.Q.'s room, the provider requests that you give C.Q. verbal and written information about local support groups and help her call a friend to accompany her home this evening. She looks at you through her tears and states, "I can't believe it. J. is the only man I've had sex with since my divorce. He told me I had nothing to worry about. I can't believe he would do this to me."

3. C.Q.'s statement is based on 3 assumptions: (1) J. is HIV positive; (2) he intentionally withheld the information from her; and (3) he intentionally transmitted the HIV to her through unprotected sex. Based on your knowledge of HIV infection, how would you counsel C.Q.?

4. In addition to offering alternative explanations and exploring options, what is your most important role right now?

5. C.Q. asks you whether she has AIDS. What do you tell her?

6. Why is it a good idea for C.Q. to have someone she trusts take her home this evening?

7. C.Q. gives you the name and phone number of someone she wants you to call. You stay with her until she leaves with her friend. Has C.Q.'s right to privacy been violated? Explain why or why not.

CASE STUDY PROGRESS

C.Q. returns to the clinic 4 days later to discuss her diagnosis.

8. What are your goals for C.Q. at this time?

9. What additional lab tests would you anticipate for C.Q. and why?

10. C.Q. asks whether there is any treatment available. How would you respond?

11. The provider starts C.Q. on a regimen of tenofovir-emtricitabine (Truvada), darunavir (Prezista), and ritonavir (Norvir). What general information will you give C.Q. about antiretroviral therapy (ART) therapy?

12. C.Q. asks why she has to take so many drugs instead of a "big dose" of one drug. What would you tell her?

13. What other issues will you discuss with C.Q. at this visit?

8 Immunity

14. Review the general measures you will discuss with C.Q. to promote her overall health.

15. C.Q. asks if she must tell J. of her HIV status. Does she have a legal responsibility to inform him?

16. What reporting obligations does the clinic have?

17. Before C.Q. leaves the clinic, you recognize the need for further teaching when she says:
a. "Joining a support group can help me deal with my HIV diagnosis."
b. "I will not use any other medications without checking with my health care provider."
c. "If my viral load becomes undetectable, I will not have to worry about transmitting HIV to someone else."
d. "If my skin turns yellow, I have unusual muscle pain or feel dizzy or weak, I will call the provider immediately."

CASE STUDY OUTCOME

Two weeks later, C.Q. visits the office and asks to speak to you in private. She thanks you for talking to her the day she received the news of her diagnosis. She tells you that J. confessed to her that he has hemophilia and tested positive for HIV after having been infected through contaminated recombinant factor VIII products. He was afraid to tell her about his diagnosis because she might leave him. C.Q. tells you that she is angry with J. They are going through counseling and the wedding is "off" at the moment.

Case Study **103**

Name_____ Class/Group_____ Date_____

▶ **Scenario**

K.D. is a 56-year-old man who has been living with human immunodeficiency virus (HIV) infection for 6 years. He had been on antiretroviral therapy (ART) with a regimen of tenofovir and emtricitabine (Truvada), with darunavir and cobicistat (Prezcobix). He stopped taking his medications 4 months ago because of depression. The appearance of purplish spots on his neck and arms persuaded him to make an appointment with his provider. At the provider's office, K.D. stated he was feeling fatigued and having occasional night sweats. He said he had been working long hours and skipping meals. Other than the purplish spots, the remainder of K.D.'s physical examination findings was within normal limits. The doctor took 3 skin biopsy specimens and obtained a chest x-ray examination, tuberculin test, and lab studies, including a CBC, CD4 T-cell count, and viral load.

Over the next week, K.D. developed a nonproductive cough and increasing dyspnea. Last night, he developed a fever of 102° F (38.9°C) and was acutely short of breath, so his partner brought him to the emergency department. He was admitted with probable *Pneumocystis jiroveci* pneumonia (PJP), which was confirmed with bronchoalveolar lavage examination under light microscopy. K.D.'s CD4 T-cell count is 175 cells/μL and viral load 35,230 copies/μL. K.D. is on nasal oxygen, IV fluids, and IV trimethoprim-sulfamethoxazole. His current VS are 138/86, 100, 30, 100.8° F (38.2° C) and SpO$_2$ 92%.

1. What is the importance of CD4 T-cell and viral load counts?

2. What is PJP?

3. The skin biopsies return a diagnosis of Kaposi sarcoma (KS). What is KS?

4. What is the significance of K.D. developing KS and PJP in light of the CD4 count?

5. K.D. has been seropositive for several years. What factors might have influenced his development of PJP and KS?

6. Name 4 problems you must manage at this time with K.D.

7. What type of isolation precautions do you need to use when caring for K.D.?
   a. Droplet
   b. Contact
   c. Standard
   d. Airborne

8. What immediate complication is K.D. at risk for experiencing?

9. To detect this complication, what will be the focus of your ongoing assessment?

10. Why was K.D. placed on trimethoprim-sulfamethoxazole? What major side effects do you need to monitor for in K.D.?

11. What aspects of K.D.'s care can you delegate to the licensed practical nurse (LPN)? Select all that apply.
 a. Providing instructions about a high-calorie, high-protein diet
 b. Administering first dose of IV trimethoprim-sulfamethoxazole
 c. Repositioning K.D. and having him deep breathe every 2 hours
 d. Developing a plan of care to improve K.D.'s oxygenation status
 e. Reinforcing teaching with K.D. about good hand washing techniques
 f. Monitoring K.D.'s pulse oximetry readings and reporting values under 95%

12. K.D. has 20 KS lesions on his neck, upper chest, and both upper arms, all of which are closed and painless. How will you care for these lesions?
 a. Keep each lesion covered with a clear, transparent dressing.
 b. Place sterile, saline-soaked gauze over each lesion twice daily.
 c. Keep the lesions dry, cleaning the affected areas gently as needed.
 d. Apply topical antibiotic ointment twice daily to the affected areas.

13. Because of compromised immune function, K.D. is at risk for developing other opportunistic infections. List 5 infections.

14. Outline the assessment you need to perform to determine whether these problems are present.

15. What interventions can you use to help K.D. in managing his depression?

16. Recognizing that K.D. has multiple posthospital needs, you begin discharge planning. What type of assessment do you need to complete as part of K.D.'s discharge planning?

8 Immunity

17. What other health care team members might you involve in K.D.'s discharge planning?

K.D. is responding well to treatment for PJP and plans are being made for discharge. He will receive follow-up care at the outpatient clinic and soon begin radiation treatments for the KS. His ART regimen is changed to a fixed-dose combination regimen with emtricitabine-tenofovir-efavirenz (Atripla).

18. K.D. is kept on trimethoprim-sulfamethoxazole (Bactrim) 2 tablets once daily. He asks why he has to keep taking Bactrim "since the pneumonia is gone." How would you respond?

19. What is the reason that K.D. receives combination ART therapy with emtricitabine-tenofovir-efavirenz (Atripla)?
   a. Combination ART is only effective when CD4-positive T-cell counts are below 200/μL
   b. Giving the drugs in a single pill reduces the incidence of cross-resistance between drugs
   c. Using smaller doses of three different drugs reduces the incidence of side effects of each drug
   d. Combination ART inhibits viral replication in different ways and decreases the chance of drug resistance

 20. How can you help K.D. take Atripla as prescribed?

21. What ongoing lab monitoring will K.D. need?

22. K.D. was taught about disease transmission and safer sex and encouraged to maintain moderate exercise, rest, and dietary habits when he was first diagnosed with HIV infection. Give at least 3 additional topics to stress with K.D. before he goes home.

CASE STUDY OUTCOME

K.D. took the Atripla as prescribed and was happy that after 3 months of therapy, his CD4 T-cell count was up to 403 cells/µL. The KS lesions have declined in number and size with the ART and radiation therapy. He says his partner and he are dealing with his fatigue., Overall, he says he feels better and taking the diagnosis of HIV "more seriously" by doing more to stay healthy.

8 Immunity

Case Study **104**

Name_____ Class/Group_____ Date_____

 Scenario

M.M., a 46-year-old male, presents to the emergency department (ED) after being stung 3 times by bees while doing yard work. He said he initially had localized pain and swelling but was not concerned because he has no prior history of an allergic reaction with previous stings. About 15 minutes after the stings, he began to feel dizzy and short of breath. He went inside and his girlfriend, seeing he had developed hives and was having some trouble breathing, drove him the 15 minutes to the ED.

1. What other information do you need to obtain?

2. What should be included as part of M.M.'s primary survey?

CASE STUDY PROGRESS

Chart View

Physical Assessment

VS: 100/60, 112, 32, SpO$_2$ 93% on RA, 98.8° F (37.1° C)

HEENT: No periorbital edema. Mild edema of lip and tongue. PERRLA. States he has metallic taste in mouth.

CV: Moderate wheezing with minimal retractions in all fields. AP S1, S2; regular.

Neuro: GCS 15. Drowsy. Full movement in all extremities. Reports dizziness.

GI: Soft, nontender, + BS ×4. Denies nausea and abdominal pain.

Skin: Generalized urticarial rash with flushing. Reports pruritus. Bee sting sites present on left hand and forearm; foreign body seen in left-hand sting site.

M.M. denies any history of allergies. He has mild hypertension that is controlled with furosemide 40 mg orally every morning.

8 Immunity

3. What is most likely happening with M.M.?

4. What assessment findings led you to making this conclusion?

5. What is the immediate priority with M.M.?

6. How would you remove the stinger?

8 Immunity

CASE STUDY PROGRESS

Chart View

Provider's Orders

Oxygen to maintain saturation ≥95%
Epinephrine 0.5 mg IM now, repeat in 15 minutes if needed
Diphenhydramine 50 mg IV now
Hydrocortisone 200 mg IV now
IV fluid bolus 1000 mL of 0.9% normal saline over 1 hour

7. Outline a plan for implementing these orders.

8. What is the reason for giving each of the ordered medications and the fluid bolus?

9. How many milliliters of epinephrine will you give per dose?

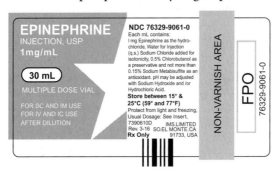

10. What type of oxygen should you apply?

11. Describe the ongoing assessment you need to perform for M.M.

12. As you continue to assess M.M., which 3 findings would *most* concern you and why?
   a. Wheezing
   b. Hoarseness
   c. High-pitched cough
   d. Abdominal cramping
   e. Nausea and vomiting
   f. Joint swelling and arthralgia

13. How would you decide whether to give a repeat epinephrine dose?

14. What other nursing interventions would you implement for M.M.?

15. M.M.'s girlfriend asks you why he is reacting now, since he has been stung several times before and nothing had happened. How would you respond?

CASE STUDY PROGRESS

M.M. rapidly begins to respond to the medications and does not need a second dose of epinephrine. The urticaria are resolving, his vital signs normalize, and his lungs sounds are clear. He must stay in the ED for another 3 hours for observation. Your designated shift time is over and the incoming nurse assigned to care for M.M. has arrived at the bedside to receive report.

 16. Outline the SBAR you need to give the nurse assuming responsibility for M.M.

17. The provider writes prescriptions for an epinephrine autoinjector and an oral prednisone 5-day dose pack, with instructions for M.M. to take over-the-counter oral diphenhydramine. What is an Epinephrine autoinjector and when is one used?

18. What teaching do M.M. and his girlfriend need about using an epinephrine autoinjector?

19. What teaching does M.M. need to reduce the risk for further stings?

8 Immunity

20. After teaching M.M. what to do if he has a bee sting reaction again, the nurse determines that teaching was effective if he states: (Select all that apply)
    a. "The best place to administer the injection is in my stomach."
    b. "I should only give myself an injection if I have difficulty breathing."
    c. "I will not put my fingers or hand over the orange tip of the injector."
    d. "My girlfriend needs to call 911 after I use the Epinephrine autoinjector."
    e. "I need to take an antihistamine before using the Epinephrine autoinjector."

21. Why would M.M. need to return to the ED?

CASE STUDY OUTCOME

After being observed in the ER for 3 hours, M.M. reports that he feels as if he is back to normal. His vital signs have remained stable and his lung sounds are clear. He was discharged home with instructions to follow up with an allergist to identify the cause of the anaphylaxis.

Case Study 105

Name_____ Class/Group_____ Date_____

▶ Scenario

D.W. is a 29-year-old married woman with three children under 5 years of age. She saw her provider 7 months ago with intermittent fatigue, joint pain, low-grade fever, and unintentional weight loss. Her provider noted small, patchy areas of vitiligo and a scaly rash across her nose, cheeks, back, and chest at that time. Lab studies showed D.W. had a positive antinuclear antibody (ANA) titer, positive anti-dsDNA test, positive anti-Sm test, elevated C-reactive protein (CRP) and erythrocyte sedimentation rate (ESR), and decreased C3 and C4 serum complement. Joint x-ray films showed joint swelling without joint erosion. D.W. was diagnosed with systemic lupus erythematosus (SLE). Initial treatment consisted of hydroxychloroquine (Plaquenil), prednisone, and naproxen sodium, and ice packs. D.W. responded well and the steroid was tapered and stopped. She was told she could follow up every 6 months unless her symptoms became acute. D.W. resumed her job in medical billing at a large geriatric facility.

1. What is the significance of each of D.W.'s lab findings?

2. Using the mnemonic SOAP BRAIN MD, how is SLE diagnosed?

3. What priority problems would be addressed in D.W.'s care plan at the time of diagnosis?

CASE STUDY PROGRESS

Twenty-eight months after diagnosis, D.W. seeks out her provider, saying that she has increased fatigue and puffy hands and feet. D.W. reports that she has been working longer hours because of the absence of two co-workers who are on maternity leave.

Chart View

Laboratory Test Results

Sodium	129 mEq/L (129 mmol/L)
Potassium	4.2 mEq/L (4.2 mmol/L)
Chloride	119 mEq/L (119 mmol/L)
Total CO_2	21 mEq/L (21 mmol/L)
Blood urea nitrogen (BUN)	34 mg/dL (12.1 mmol/L)
Creatinine	2.6 mg/dL (230 mcmol/L)
Glucose	123 mg/dL (6.8 mmol/L)
Urinalysis	2+ protein, 2+ hematuria

4. Which lab findings concern you, and why?

5. The goal of therapy in lupus nephritis is to normalize or prevent the loss of renal function. To reach this goal, what additions to D.W.'s care can you anticipate?

 6. The provider orders cyclophosphamide 100 mg/m²/day orally in two divided doses. D.W. weighs 140 lbs (63.5 kg) and is 5 feet, 4 inches (163 cm) tall. How much will she receive with each dose?

7. What key points should you include in a teaching plan about cyclophosphamide therapy?

CASE STUDY PROGRESS

D.W. is seen in the immunology clinic twice monthly during the next 3 months. Although her condition does not worsen, her BUN and creatinine remain elevated. While at work one afternoon, D.W. begins to feel dizzy and develops a severe headache. She reports to her supervisor, who has her lie down. When D.W. starts to become disoriented, her supervisor calls 911, and D.W. is taken to the hospital. D.W. is admitted for probable lupus cerebritis related to acute exacerbation of her disease.

8. What other findings indicative of central nervous system involvement should you assess for in D.W.?

 9. What protective measures need to be instituted at this time?

10. In caring for D.W., which care activities can be delegated to the UAP? Select all that apply.
   a. Monitoring D.W.'s BUN and creatinine levels
   b. Counseling D.W. on seizure safety precautions
   c. Assisting D.W. with personal hygiene measures
   d. Assessing D.W.'s neurologic status every 2 hours
   e. Measuring D.W.'s blood pressure (BP) every 2 hours
   f. Emptying the urine collection device and measuring the output

CASE STUDY PROGRESS

The provider orders pulse therapy with methylprednisolone 125 mg IV every 6 hours and plasmapheresis once daily.

 11. What major complications associated with immunosuppression therapy will D.W. have to be monitored for?

12. D.W. asks about what plasmapheresis does and why it might help her feel better. How you would respond?

Chart View

Vital Signs	
BP	80/43
Pulse rate	118
Respiratory rate	18
Temperature	97.2° F (36.2° C)

13. D.W. returns to the floor after the plasmapheresis. The UAP reports D.W.'s vital signs to you. Based solely on her vital signs, what could be happening with D.W. and why?

14. You go to assess D.W. What do you need to include in your assessment?

15. D.W. is complaining of dizziness and is slightly diaphoretic but denies any headache, nausea, or paresthesia. What do you immediately suspect is occurring and why?

16. You need to call the provider regarding D.W.'s status. Using SBAR, what would you report to the provider?

17. What do you expect your care of D.W. will include over the next 2 to 3 hours?

18. What outcome criteria would support that D.W.'s condition is stabilizing?

19. You note that D.W.'s husband is visiting her. You enter the room to ask whether they have any questions. D.W.'s husband states, "I have tried to tell her that she cannot go back to work. Sure, we need the money, but the kids and I need her more. I'm afraid that this lupus has weakened her whole body and it will kill her if she goes back to work. Is that right?" How should you respond to his concerns?

CASE STUDY OUTCOME

D.W.'s condition stabilizes with fluids and plasmapheresis and she can be discharged 6 days later. With the addition of cyclophosphamide to her regimen, her condition improves and she experiences no further episodes of cerebritis. Her husband and she decide that she is not going to return to work so she can focus on her health and family.

8 Immunity

Case Study 106

Name _____ Class/Group _____ Date _____

► Scenario

You are directly admitting a 30-year-old woman, J.L., to your telemetry unit with the diagnosis of status post-cardiac transplantation and fever of unknown origin. She was healthy until the birth of her only child at 27 years of age. She developed idiopathic cardiomyopathy after childbirth and 7 months ago underwent cardiac transplantation. Her endomyocardial biopsies have been negative for signs of rejection; her last one was 3 weeks ago. She is on a regimen of baby aspirin, multivitamins, mycophenolate mofetil (CellCept), tacrolimus (Prograf), nifedipine (Procardia), and metolazone (Zaroxolyn). The UAP reports her VS as 130/78, 104, 20, 101.7° F (38.7° C).

1. Admitting has assigned J.L. to a semiprivate room. Her roommate is on day 4 of IV antibiotic treatment for pneumonia and now has a near normal white blood cell (WBC) count. Is this an appropriate assignment?

2. Fever is a sign of 2 major complications of organ transplantation. What are they?

3. Why is J.L. receiving mycophenolate mofetil (CellCept) and tacrolimus (Prograf)?

4. How will her being on immunotherapy influence your assessment?

5. Compare and contrast the signs and symptoms of organ rejection and sepsis that you need to assess for in J.L.

CASE STUDY PROGRESS

While you are performing your admission assessment, J.L. tells you she urinates frequently because of "that Zaroxolyn." She mentions she has experienced burning with urination for the past 2 days. You decide to collect a urine specimen for lab analysis in addition to ordered blood cultures, a complete blood count (CBC), and a basic metabolic panel (BMP).

6. What are possible causes of the burning? What type of urine specimen should you obtain?

Chart View

Urinalysis (UA)

Color and appearance	Yellow, cloudy
WBCs	12
RBCs	≤2
Glucose	Negative
Ketones	Negative
Nitrates	Positive
Bacteria	≥100,000 colonies

7. Interpret J.L.'s UA results.

CASE STUDY PROGRESS

J.L.'s BUN and creatinine are within normal limits, and the CBC shows WBCs 11,000/mm³. Pending blood and urine culture results, the provider believes a urinary tract infection (UTI) is the reason for J.L.'s symptoms and orders IV levofloxacin 500 mg every 12 hours.

8. What are your primary nursing concerns for J.L. at this time?

9. Considering J.L.'s UTI and her immunosuppressed status, what other interventions should you implement when caring for J.L.?

10. Identify 3 expected outcomes for J.L. as a result of your interventions.

CASE STUDY PROGRESS

Thirty-six hours later, preliminary results of J.L.'s blood and urine cultures are available. The blood cultures show no growth.

Chart View

Urine Culture and Sensitivity (C&S)

Staphylococcus aureus	≥100,000 colonies
Amoxicillin	R
Ceftriaxone	R
Ciprofloxacin	R
Clindamycin	R
Doxycycline	S
Levofloxacin	R
Trimethoprim-sulfa	R
Vancomycin	S

11. Interpret J.L.'s urine C&S results.

12. What action do you need to take?

13. Describe the transmission-based precautions you need to begin for J.L.

CASE STUDY PROGRESS

The provider changes J.L. to IV vancomycin 500 mg every 8 hours and sends her to interventional radiology for placement of a peripherally inserted central catheter (PICC). Her first dose of vancomycin arrives from the pharmacy just as J.L. returns to the floor.

14. What other information do you need to know before you begin the vancomycin?

 15. What interventions do you need to implement to safely administer vancomycin? Select all that apply.
   a. Hold the infusion if J.L. complains of tinnitus.
   b. Obtain a trough level 6 hours after each infusion.
   c. Monitor urine output, BUN, and creatinine levels.
   d. Anticipate replacing the PICC line every 48 hours.
   e. Administer each infusion over a minimum of 1 hour.
   f. Assess for the onset of hypertension during the infusion.

CASE STUDY PROGRESS

After 7 days, J.L. shows a positive response to antibiotic therapy, and she is preparing for discharge. She will continue her prehospital drug regimen, with the addition of 3 weeks of sulfamethoxazole 800 mg/trimethoprim 160 mg (Bactrim DS) PO twice daily.

16. Which statement indicates J.L. understands your teaching about Bactrim?
    a. "I will drink at least eight glasses of fluid per day."
    b. "I should wait 2 hours after taking this medicine before I eat."
    c. "I will notify the health care provider if my hands and feet become numb."
    d. "This drug may make me dizzy, so I should not do an activity that requires alertness."

17. While you are talking with J.L., she tells you that her husband's parents gave her son a pet cat. She jokingly says, "They gave me the work! My husband is going to have to help. I'm not up to looking after a cat, too." What job does her husband need to do, and why?

18. Because of her remark, you decide to reinforce teaching regarding things J.L. can do to protect herself from infection. List 6 points you will include.

19. What information would you review with J.L. about the signs and symptoms of infection and when to seek treatment?

CASE STUDY OUTCOME

J.L. did not experience any further episodes of urinary infection. However, her next 2 biopsies showed acute rejection. Both episodes were treated with methylprednisolone boluses. She developed steroid-induced diabetes requiring treatment with insulin.

Cellular Regulation

Case Study 107

Name_____ Class/Group_____ Date_____

▶ Scenario

R.T. is a 64-year-old man who went to his primary care provider's office for a yearly examination. He initially reported having no health problems; however, on further questioning, he admitted to having some fatigue, abdominal bloating, and intermittent constipation. His physical examination findings were normal except for stool positive for occult blood. He had a complete blood count with differential, basic metabolic panel, and carcinoembryonic antigen (CEA) testing and was referred to a gastroenterologist for a colonoscopy. Colonoscopy revealed a 5-cm mass in the sigmoid colon, which was diagnosed as adenocarcinoma of the colon. A distant metastatic workup is negative, and R.T. is undergoing a laparoscopic sigmoidectomy with anastomosis.

1. What is a risk factor?

2. Name 6 risk factors for colon cancer.

3. Outline the American Cancer Society's current evidence-based screening procedures for persons at average risk for developing colon cancer.

4. What are the warning signs of colon cancer? Underline those that R.T. has.

5. What is CEA? How does it relate to the diagnosis of colon cancer?

6. Shade in the area of the colon that will be removed during R.T.'s surgery.

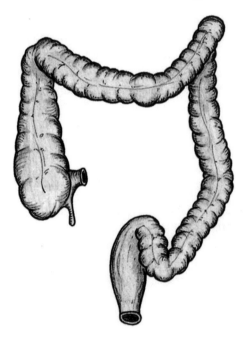

Modified from Potter, P.A., Perry, A.G., Stockert, P., & Hall, A.: Basic Nursing, ed. 7, St. Louis, 2011, Mosby.

9 Cellular Regulation

7. The preoperative chart includes detailed instructions for a clear liquid diet, bowel preparation regimen with polyethylene glycol, and prescriptions for neomycin and metronidazole tablets. What is the purpose of taking neomycin and metronidazole?

8. What are some suggestions you can make to help R.T. successfully complete the bowel preparation?

9. Describe the rest of your preoperative teaching for R.T. and his family.

CASE STUDY PROGRESS

R.T.'s surgical course is uneventful, and he is discharged after 5 days. Based on the final pathology report, his cancer is designated stage IIIB. The cancer had spread to the muscle layer of the colon wall with 9 lymph nodes being positive. Four weeks after surgery, R.T. is scheduled to begin 6 months of adjuvant chemotherapy.

10. Current chemotherapy protocols include varying doses of fluorouracil and leucovorin alone or in combination with oxaliplatin or irinotecan. The purpose of leucovorin is to:
   a. Rescue healthy cells from the toxic effects of methotrexate
   b. Improve R.T.'s nutritional status by supplementing vitamin intake
   c. Reduce the incidence of renal failure associated with methotrexate
   d. Help the methotrexate be more effective by inhibiting cancer cell mitosis

11. Discuss the major toxicities and side effects associated with fluorouracil and leucovorin.

12. When prioritizing R.T.'s plan of care, which effects are the most serious?

 13. When R.T.'s white blood cell count begins to drop, which is the **most** important means to teach him to protect himself from infection?
   a. Brushing and flossing his teeth after meals and before bed
   b. Having someone else clean the litterbox of all household pets
   c. Staying away from people who are visibly sick or have a cold
   d. Washing his hands often, especially after using the restroom and before eating

14. Develop a teaching plan for R.T. focusing on the common effects of diarrhea and nausea and vomiting.

15. What would you teach R.T. to do to help manage fatigue? Select all that apply.
   a. Accept assistance as needed.
   b. Limit the number of daily visitors.
   c. Avoid napping throughout the day.
   d. Encourage exercise to maintain his strength.
   e. Plan activities for periods when he has the most energy.
   f. Encourage him to do activities in small amounts and rest between activities.

16. R.T. shows he understands the adverse effects of methotrexate when he says:
   a. "I should take ibuprofen if I have a mild headache or joint pain."
   b. "If I develop a bad rash, there is no need to worry. This is normal."
   c. "Coffee and black tea are good choices to help me maintain my fluid intake."
   d. "If I have any chills or unusual pain, I need to let my doctor know immediately."

CASE STUDY OUTCOME

After completing chemotherapy, R.T. remains cancer-free. He undergoes regular colonoscopies and walks every day. He does have some problems with chronic diarrhea and manages his symptoms through diet and medications.

9 Cellular Regulation

Case Study **108**

Name_____ Class/Group_____ Date_____

▶ Scenario

You are a home health nurse seeing for the first time P.C., a 64-year-old divorcee diagnosed with small cell lung cancer about 1 year ago. P.C. was treated with radiation and chemotherapy; however, her oncologist recently informed her that her cancer is not curable because it has spread to her bones and liver. The focus of her treatment will now be primarily palliative. She is confused and somewhat bewildered. She vaguely remembers the term *palliative treatment* from the discussion of her situation with her oncologist but does not know what it means.

1. How would you describe palliative treatment?

2. Describe the assessment you need to perform now.

3. Palliative care is delivered by an interprofessional team. What team members would likely be involved in P.C.'s care and how?

P.C. confides that she has not formally written down her wishes concerning the types of treatments she would or would not want. You recommend she complete advance directives, including a living will and a medical durable power of attorney form.

4. How would you describe the purpose of these documents to her?

5. What health care decisions are considered in these documents?

6. How are advance directives formalized?

7. P.C. states that she is confused and has mixed feelings about her health care wishes right now. She asks, "If I fill out a living will, can I change my mind down the road?" How should you answer this question?

8. As P.C. becomes more frail and incoherent, how will these documents guide her treatment?

CASE STUDY PROGRESS

You inform P.C. that one of your roles will be to help with the symptom control as her illness progresses. P.C. relates that her primary goal is to be able to spend time with family and friends. You begin with pain control because it has a powerful effect on quality of life.

9. What interventions will you use to help her be as pain free as possible?

10. Because her advancing lung cancer will likely result in respiratory distress, which interventions should you include in her plan of care? Select all that apply.
   a. Perform a respiratory assessment at each visit.
   b. Administer low-dose morphine sulfate if vital signs are adequate.
   c. Maintain room at a warm temperature and have blankets available.
   d. Have her space activities and rest as needed in a position of comfort.
   e. If oxygen saturation falls below 90% on room air, begin oxygen at 2 L.

11. Why is P.C. at risk for impaired skin integrity?

12. Realizing that loss of appetite often accompanies the dying process, describe how you can maintain P.C.'s oral nutrition and hydration.

13. Toward the end of your visit, P.C. looks at you and says, "You know, I just really thought I had more time." The most appropriate response is:
   a. "Dying is a natural process; we will help you through it."
   b. "Your feelings are understandable; most people aren't ready to die."
   c. "Tell me more about what you mean when you say, 'I thought I had more time.'"
   d. "No one ever really knows when it is their time, even if they don't have cancer."

14. You are concerned with P.C.'s psychological status, particularly because she is expressing feelings of grief. Write a nursing outcome addressing this issue. Identify independent nursing actions that you would implement to provide her emotional support.

CASE STUDY OUTCOME

P.C. discusses her wishes with her family and completes the documents describing what she would like her plan of care to be over the rest of her life span. She dies peacefully 7 weeks later in her home, supported by her family and friends, on her terms.

Case Study **109**

Name_____ Class/Group_____ Date_____

▶ Scenario

A.B. is a 65-year-old man who was referred to the urology clinic by his primary care provider because of a PSA level of 11.9 ng/mL (11.9 mcg/L). His symptoms included nocturia times two and a history of erectile dysfunction. CBC, lipid profile, UA, and blood chemistry findings are all within normal limits. The prostate is slightly tender on examination. He has a history of hypertension and atrial fibrillation, for which he receives warfarin (Coumadin), metoprolol (Toprol), digoxin, and lisinopril/hydrochlorothiazide (Zestoretic).

1. A.B. wonders whether he has prostate cancer. What can you tell A.B. about his PSA level?

2. What are the common manifestations of prostate cancer?

3. Name 3 risk factors for prostate cancer.

4. A.B. is scheduled for a transrectal ultrasound (TRUS) of the prostate. What is the purpose of this test?

5. Based on the PSA and TRUS results, A.B. is scheduled for a transrectal prostate biopsy. He asks what he needs to do to prepare for this test. Explain what to expect during the procedure and the pre- and postprocedure teaching needed.

CASE STUDY PROGRESS

A.B.'s prostate biopsy is positive for cancer, with a Gleason score of 7. Chest x-ray, bone scan, and abdominal CT scan are all negative. He has discussed his diagnosis with the urologist. He is now thinking about his treatment options and asks you to answer some questions. He was told about his Gleason score but is not sure what this is.

6. What is a Gleason score?

7. The urologist discusses treatment options for prostate cancer with A.B. Describe 3.

CASE STUDY PROGRESS

After consulting with his urologist, A.B. has decided to have his prostate removed using a laparoscopic procedure. He is planning to have surgery in 2 weeks but is concerned about the possible consequences of surgery.

8. Identify the major immediate postoperative concerns for A.B.

9. Describe the 2 main long-term consequences of having a prostatectomy.

A.B. undergoes a laparoscopic radical prostatectomy and is an inpatient on the urology surgery unit.

10. Which initial postoperative orders are appropriate for A.B.? Select all that apply and correct the inappropriate answers.
   a. Up ad lib
   b. Docusate 100 mg PO daily
   c. Vital signs per hospital protocol
   d. Change indwelling catheter if clotting occurs
   e. Morphine 4 mg IV push q4hr as needed for pain
   f. Oxybutynin (Ditropan XL) 10 mg PO every morning
   g. Notify urologist if urinary output is less than 30 mL/hr

11. Which assessment findings would be of **most** concern in the first 24 hours after surgery?
   a. Reports of bladder spasms.
   b. The urine is light pink in color.
   c. A few blood clots are noted in the urine drainage bag.
   d. Bright red blood suddenly appears in the Foley catheter tubing.

12. Choose the type of catheter that you expect A.B. to have after surgery and explain the rationale for it.
   a. Catheter A
   b. Catheter B
   c. Catheter C

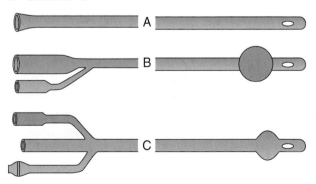

From Lewis SL, Dirksen SR, Heitkemper MM, et al: Medical-surgical nursing: assessment and management of clinical problems, *ed. 8, St. Louis, 2011, Mosby.*

13. What would be ordered if clotting of the irrigation system were to occur?

14. What interventions regarding the irrigation system can be delegated to the UAP?

15. At the end of the shift, 2535 mL were emptied from the drainage bag of the irrigation system. The amount of irrigant in the hanging bag was 3000 mL at the beginning of the shift. There was 1175 mL left in the bag 8 hours. What was the amount of actual urine output for the shift?

16. A.B. complains of bladder spasms and is given a dose of oxybutynin (Ditropan XL). The nurse will monitor for which adverse effects? Select all that apply.
   a. Diarrhea
   b. Dizziness
   c. Dry mouth
   d. Palpitations
   e. Watery eyes

17. Describe 5 areas to cover in a discharge teaching plan for A.B. before he goes home.

CASE STUDY OUTCOME

A.B. does not require any additional therapy after surgery. At his 6-month follow-up visit, he reports he can get an erection but has difficulty maintaining an erection for sexual relations. The urologist discusses erectile aids with A.B. After a failed trial of vasoactive medications, he chose penile injections, which are successful.

9 Cellular Regulation

Case Study **110**

Name_____ Class/Group_____ Date_____

▶ Scenario

You are a nurse working as a preoperative evaluation nurse. J.B., a well-known 62-year-old homeless man with a history of chronic alcohol use, comes to you before a left radical neck dissection with total laryngectomy and placement of a permanent tracheostomy to treat stage III hypopharyngeal cancer. He has a long history of tobacco use, poor diet, and no dental care. Over the past several months, he has experienced increasing shortness of breath, hoarseness, and odynophagia. A piriform sinus mass was found on bronchoscopy. The large mass extends and is fixed to the left true vocal cord. His chest x-ray film is normal except for changes related to chronic tobacco use. Past medical history includes reactive airway disease and hypertension. On examination, you find 1 palpable left-sided cervical node, which is firm and fixed.

1 Identify J.B.'s risk factors for cancer.

2 Name the warning signals listed on the American Cancer Society's list of warning signs of cancer. Underline those J.B. has.

3 Describe the surgical intervention J.B. will undergo.

4 J.B. has several important postoperative needs. Name 2 serious complications for which he is at risk.

5 What type of follow-up therapy is J.B. likely to undergo after his surgical wound heals?

6 You note placement of a percutaneous endoscopic gastrostomy (PEG) feeding tube is on the operative procedure list. Why is J.B. having a PEG tube placed?

7 Which point would you include in his preoperative teaching plan?
   a. "The head of your bed will be kept up at all times."
   b. "You will not be able to eat or drink for 7 to 14 days."
   c. "We will be encouraging you to whisper frequently after surgery."
   d. "You will have to avoid all coughing until the sutures are removed."

8 J.B. asks you, "How will I talk after the surgery?" Which is the best response?
   a. "Unfortunately, you will not be able to communicate orally ever again."
   b. "You will be able to speak again after the tracheostomy tube is removed."
   c. "If you work hard at speech therapy, you may regain some of your normal voice."
   d. "You won't be able to speak. There are some alternative means you can learn to use."

9 J.B. asks how he will be able to let the nurses know what he needs if he cannot talk. How will you respond?

10 J.B. has multiple medical needs that make discharge planning problematic. Describe how you could ensure he is not discharged into homelessness.

CASE STUDY PROGRESS

J.B. undergoes surgery. His postoperative course is complicated by pneumonia and poor wound healing. After being hospitalized for 6 weeks, he is discharged to a long-term care facility for training in esophageal speech and care while receiving external radiation therapy. He is scheduled to receive 2000 cGy to the head and neck 3 times weekly for the next 8 weeks.

11   What is esophageal speech? What primary advantage does it have for J.B.?

12   As J.B.'s nurse, which adverse effects of external radiation therapy would most concern you?

13   Outline independent nursing actions that will help J.B. in managing mucositis and xerostomia.

14 What instructions will you provide the UAP caring for J.B. regarding skin care? Select all that apply.
a. "Assist J.B. with selecting loose-fitting shirts."
b. "After his shower, apply lotion to the irradiated area."
c. "Dry the area with patting motions using a soft cloth."
d. "Make sure you thoroughly rinse away all of the soap."
e. "Remove the ink marked on his neck with a washcloth."
f. "He can have an ice pack applied to the red areas for 15 minutes."

 15 What interventions would you place in a plan of care to reduce J.B.'s risk for infection?

16 How can the nurse assist J.B. in combating fatigue during his treatment?

CASE STUDY OUTCOME

Despite radiation therapy, J.B.'s disease progresses, and he develops lung and brain metastases. He chooses to stay in the long-term care facility and dies from pneumonia 5 months later.

Case Study **111**

Name_____ Class/Group_____ Date_____

▶ Scenario

M.D. is a 50-year-old woman whose routine mammogram showed a 2.3- × 4.5-cm lobulated mass at the 3 o'clock position in her left breast. M.D. underwent a stereotactic needle biopsy and was diagnosed with invasive ductal carcinoma, estrogen and progesterone receptor positive, HER-2 negative. The staging workup was negative for distant metastasis. Her final staging was stage IIB. She had a modified radical mastectomy with axillary lymph node dissection. The sentinel lymph node and 4 of 16 lymph nodes were positive for tumor cells. An implanted port was placed during surgery.

1. What are the risk factors for breast cancer?

2. Describe the biopsy technique used to diagnose M.D.'s cancer.

3. Breast cancer is classified as noninvasive or invasive. Compare these terms.

4. Discuss the implications of a positive sentinel node.

5. What factors affect prognosis and treatment for breast cancer?

6. Is she a candidate for tamoxifen therapy? Explain your reasoning.

7. Surgical intervention is the primary treatment for breast cancer. Describe the surgical procedure that M.D. had.

8. Describe M.D.'s risk for lymphedema.

9. What actions will you teach M.D. to reduce her risk for developing lymphedema?

10. What are some community resources from which she may benefit?

CASE STUDY PROGRESS

Eight weeks after surgery, M.D. is now beginning a prescribed chemotherapy regimen of 6 cycles of CAF (cyclophosphamide, doxorubicin, and fluorouracil).

11. M.D. asks you why she has to have chemotherapy with so many drugs if the surgeon removed all the cancer. How would you respond?

12. Compare the drug actions of cyclophosphamide, doxorubicin, and fluorouracil.

13. Name the common side effects experienced by patients receiving the CAF regimen.

14. What information would you want to review with M.D. about the signs and symptoms of infection and when to seek treatment?

15. M.D. is ordered doxorubicin at 75 mg/m². Her height is 5 feet, 7 inches (170 cm), and her weight is 155 lbs (70.3 kg). Calculate the dose she will receive.

16. What ongoing assessment will you need to perform since M.D. is receiving doxorubicin?

17. M.D. is prescribed filgrastim (Neupogen) as part of her treatment regimen. You teach her filgrastim is used is to:
   a. Improve the number and function of neutrophils
   b. Help CAF be more effective in treating her cancer
   c. Replace abnormal cells in the bone marrow with normal cells
   d. Decrease the level of fatigue she will experience during treatment

18. You have finished teaching M.D. about the effects of CAF. You know that she understands instructions about cyclophosphamide (Cytoxan) when she says: (Select all that apply)
   a. "This medication should be taken with food."
   b. "I will drink 2000 to 3000 mL of fluids each day."
   c. "Taking this drug at nighttime will reduce nausea."
   d. "I will increase my intake of foods with potassium."
   e. "Urinating often will help decrease the risk for cystitis."

19. However, after reviewing with her how to manage alopecia, you determine further teaching is needed after she says:
   a. "I should go buy a wig now, before I start losing my hair."
   b. "Wearing a scarf or hat when outside will help to protect me."
   c. "My hair should begin to return 2 months or so after treatment ends."
   d. "I can prevent hair loss if I wash every other day with a gentle shampoo."

CASE STUDY PROGRESS

M.D. has now completed three cycles of CAF, with her last treatment 12 days ago. She comes to the emergency department with a 1-day history of fever, chills, and shortness of breath. On arrival, she is slightly confused and agitated. Vital signs are 100/60, 119, 26, 103.6° F (39.8° C), SpO_2 86% on room air. The chest x-ray examination shows diffuse infiltrates in the left lower lung consistent with pneumonia. Her basic metabolic panel is within normal limits, except the blood urea nitrogen (BUN) 28 mg/dL (10.0 mmol/L) and creatinine 1.6 mg/dL (141 mcmol/L).

Chart View

Complete Blood Count	
White blood cells (WBCs)	1200/mm³ (1.2 x 10⁹/L)
Neutrophils	34%
Segmented ("polys")	30%
Bands	4%
Lymphocytes	60%
Monocytes	3%
Eosinophils and basophils	2%
Hematocrit (Hct)	24.9%
Hemoglobin (Hgb)	8.7 g/dL (87 g/L)
Platelets	85,000/mm³ (85 x 10⁹/L)

20. Interpret M.D.'s lab results and explain the reason for any abnormal results.

21. Calculate M.D.'s absolute neutrophil count (ANC) and describe its significance.

22. What is your nursing priority at this time?

23. What is the single most important nursing intervention for a patient with an ANC below 500/mm^3?

24. When is neutropenia most likely to occur in a person receiving chemotherapy?

25. What type of isolation do you need to initiate for M.D.? Outline the guidelines for maintaining this type of isolation.

26. What collaborative care measures do you expect for M.D.?

27. What immediate nursing interventions do you need to take?

28. What actions do you need to take because M.D. had a left axillary lymph node dissection and why?

 29. The provider orders a 500-mL normal saline bolus now, with orders to infuse over 2 hours. You decide to use M.D.'s implanted port for IV access. After you access the port and connect the fluid, the infusion pump alarms that the line is occluded. What will you do?

CASE STUDY OUTCOME

M.D. is admitted to the intensive care unit, where she soon needs endotracheal intubation. She spends 3 days there receiving IV antibiotics and fluids with respiratory support. After she is extubated, she returns to the oncology unit, where she stays for a few more days before being discharged to home.

Case Study **112**

Name_____ Class/Group_____ Date_____

▶ Scenario

C.P. is a 71-year-old married farmer with a past medical history of hernia surgery in 2006 and prostate surgery in 2015 for BPH. C.P. has smoked for 40 years; for the past 3 years, he has smoked two to three packs per day. Two weeks ago, C.P. visited the local rural health clinic with a progressive cough and chest congestion. Despite a week of antibiotic therapy, C.P.'s condition continued to worsen; he experienced progressive dyspnea and productive cough, and he began to have night sweats. C.P. refused to be admitted to the hospital because "there's no one to look after the cows," but he agreed to go for a chest x-ray (CXR) study. The radiologist reads C.P.'s CXR film as "left hilar lung mass, probable lung cancer." C.P. is scheduled for a diagnostic fiberoptic bronchoscopy with endobronchial lung biopsy as an outpatient this morning to confirm the diagnosis.

1. What are the common manifestations of lung cancer? Underline those C.P. is experiencing.

2. True or false? Most cases of lung cancer are related to smoking. Explain your response.

3. What information does a fiberoptic bronchoscopy with endobronchial lung biopsy provide?

4. As the nurse who works with the pulmonologist, it is your responsibility to prepare C.P. for the fiberoptic bronchoscopy procedure. What will you include in your teaching plan?

5. What is your responsibility during and immediately after the bronchoscopy?

6. C.P. tolerates the procedure well. He returns to the office 4 days later to learn the test results. The pulmonologist tells C.P. and his wife that he has poorly differentiated oat cell lung cancer and explains that it is a very fast-growing cancer with a poor prognosis. This kind of lung cancer is directly related to C.P.'s history of smoking. What is your role at this time?

7. Define the concept of differentiation. What does *poorly differentiated* mean?

8. What are the common sites of lung cancer metastasis?

CASE STUDY PROGRESS

C.P. undergoes a metastatic workup and is found to have cancer in multiple lymph nodes, his liver, and sternum. The pulmonologist tells C.P. and his wife that surgery is not an option and schedules C.P. to begin combination chemotherapy.

9. Using simple terms, how would you explain combination chemotherapy and how it works to C.P. and his wife?

9 Cellular Regulation

10. C.P. says he doesn't know if he should undergo chemotherapy if he "isn't going to live anyway." What are 2 goals of administering chemotherapy to patients such as C.P.?

11. C.P.'s wife tells you she's heard that chemotherapy makes you really sick. Again, using simple terms, how would you explain chemotherapy side effects?

12. C.P. agrees to chemotherapy and is scheduled to receive cisplatin 60 mg/m² in 100 mL normal saline (NS) IV over 1 to 2 hours daily, and etoposide 200 mg in 250 mL NS IV over 1 to 2 hours daily, both during the first 3 days of each month. What is the nadir for each drug, and what implications does the nadir have for C.P.?

13. Based on your knowledge of the most common side effects of cisplatin and etoposide, describe the ongoing assessment C.P. will need.

14. List 8 interventions that should be incorporated into C.P.'s care plan to assist him with managing chemotherapy-induced nausea and vomiting.

15. Which statement indicates further teaching is needed about alopecia?
    a. "My hair will thin and start to fall out in 1 to 2 months."
    b. "I need to wear a hat or scarf when I am outside working."
    c. "The chemotherapy may cause me to lose all my body hair."
    d. "Washing my hair with a mild shampoo will prevent hair loss."

16. C.P. plans to continue to work the farm as long as possible and says his brother-in-law has promised to help him. C.P. needs to have a working understanding of how to balance his treatment with his work. You sit down with C.P. to plan a daily work, activity, and rest schedule to accommodate his treatments and side effects. List at least 3 points you would emphasize.

CASE STUDY PROGRESS

A month later, when C.P. returns for his second round of chemotherapy, he complains of shortness of breath, chest tightness, and palpitations. He looks exhausted. An electrocardiogram (ECG) reveals new-onset atrial fibrillation, and a CXR film suggests a large left lower lobe pleural effusion. C.P. is admitted to the hospital for supportive care. The pulmonologist performs a thoracentesis and drains 985 mL of fluid, immediately relieving most of C.P.'s dyspnea and chest discomfort.

Chart View

Laboratory Test Values

WBCs	2500/mm³ (2.5 x 10⁹/L)
RBCs	4.9 million/mm³ (4.9 x 10¹²/L)
Hemoglobin (Hgb)	12.7 g/dL (127 g/L)
Hematocrit (Hct)	37.6%
Platelets	152,000/mm³ (152 x 10⁹/L)
Sodium	131 mEq/L (131 mmol/L)
Potassium	4.2 mEq/L (4.2 mmol/L)
Chloride	90 mEq/L (90 mmol/L)

 17. What do these lab values indicate?

18. Describe 4 interventions you would implement to help C.P. manage dyspnea.

19. You assess C.P. 2 hours after the thoracentesis. Which information is important to report to the pulmonologist? CP has
    a. occasional chest pain when taking deep breaths.
    b. some burning and stinging at the thoracentesis site.
    c. a small amount of serosanguineous drainage on the dressing.
    d. a blood pressure of 90/50 and an increase in dyspnea.

20. C.P. tells you he does not want to live like this and that he would like to stop chemotherapy, but his pulmonologist wants him to continue with aggressive therapy. Discuss what role you can play in supporting him.

21. How do you feel about this in relation to his condition?

CASE STUDY OUTCOME

C.P. refuses the second round of chemotherapy and after his condition stabilizes, is discharged to home. He receives no further treatment and dies 3 weeks later with his wife at his side.

Case Study 113

Name_____   Class/Group_____   Date_____

▶ Scenario

H.J. is a 46-year-old man diagnosed with non-Hodgkin lymphoma (NHL) 4 months ago. He finished receiving his third of six chemotherapy courses 5 days ago. Yesterday morning, he was seen at his oncologist's office for malaise, muscle weakness, and palpitations. He had splenomegaly on examination. A computed tomography (CT) scan of the abdomen showed metastatic disease in the liver and spleen. He is admitted to the hospital with progressive disease.

Chart View

Basic Metabolic Panel (BMP)

Na	136 mEq/L (136 mmol/L)
K	6.1 mEq/L (6.1 mmol/L)
Cl	97 mEq/L (97 mmol/L)
CO_2	28 mEq/L (28 mmol/L)
Glucose	98 mg/dL (5.4 mmol/L)
Blood urea nitrogen (BUN)	54 mg/dL (19.28 mmol/L)
Creatinine	2.7 mg/dL (239 mcmol/L)
Ca	6.3 units/L
Total protein	5.4 g/dL (54 g/L)
Albumin	2.8 g/dL (4.0 mcmol/L)
Phosphorus	4.8 mg/dL (1.55 mmol/L)
Uric acid	20.7 mg/dL (1.23 mmol/L)
Total bilirubin	0.8 mg/dL (13.7 mcmol/L)
Alkaline phosphatase	172 units/L (2.87 µkat/L)
Aspartate transaminase (AST)	254 units/L (4.23 µkat/L)
Alanine transaminase (ALT)	74 units/L (1.23 µkat/L)
Lactate dehydrogenase (LDH)	214 IU/L (3.57 mckat/L)

1. Interpret H.J.'s admitting BMP panel.

2. Based on these values, which common oncologic emergency is H.J. experiencing?

3. Describe the pathophysiology of this condition.

4. What assessment findings related to this diagnosis would you expect in H.J.?

Chart View

Complete Blood Count (CBC)

White blood cells (WBCs)	1500/mm³ (1.5 x 10⁹/L)
Neutrophils	66%
Lymphocytes	16%
Monocytes	15%
Eosinophils	5%
Hemoglobin (Hgb)	8.3 g/dL (83 g/L)
Hematocrit (Hct)	23.6%
Platelets	21,000/mm³ (21 x 10⁹/L)

5. Based on his lab values, name 3 additional problems for which H.J. is at risk.

6. What are your nursing priorities right now?

Chart View

Medication Record

IV 0.9% saline at 150 mL/hr
100 mEq sodium bicarbonate in the first liter of IV fluid
Rasburicase 6 mg IV now
Allopurinol 500 mg twice daily orally
Furosemide 40 mg IV now then every 6 hours
Sodium polystyrene sulfonate 15 g orally every 6 hours
Aluminum hydroxide 2 caps orally with meals

CASE STUDY PROGRESS

The oncologist confirms a diagnosis of acute tumor lysis syndrome (TLS) and writes several orders for H.J.

7. What is the expected outcome associated with each medication H.J. is receiving?

8. After giving sodium polystyrene sulfonate, it is important for you to monitor H.J.'s:
   a. Urine output
   b. Bowel sounds
   c. Peripheral pulses
   d. Level of consciousness

9. What major complication of TLS is H.J. at risk for and why?

10. Name 3 signs and symptoms of this complication you will assess for in H.J.

11. List 4 independent nursing interventions that you would include in H.J.'s plan of care and the reason for each.

 12. The best way to prevent infection in a patient such as H.J. is
a. Giving prophylactic antibiotics
b. Placing him in reverse isolation
c. Limiting his intake of fresh fruits and vegetables with skins
d. Practicing good handwashing by all who are in contact with him

CASE STUDY PROGRESS

Twenty-four hours after admission, H.J.'s lab tests are repeated.

Chart View

Basic Metabolic Panel

Na	138 mEq/L (138 mmol/L)
K	4.8 mEq/L (4.8 mmol/L)
Cl	109 mEq/L (109 mmol/L)
CO_2	26 mEq/L (26 mmol/L)
Glucose	148 mg/dL (8.2 mmol/L)
BUN	34 mg/dL (12.14 mmol/L)
Creatinine	2.4 mg/dL (212 mcmol/L)
Ca	7.3 units/L (1.83 mmol/L)
Total protein	5.4 g/dL (54 g/L)
Albumin	2.8 g/dL (4.06 mcmol/L)
Phosphorus	3.8 mg/dL (1.23 mmol/L)
Uric acid	0.5 mg/dL (29.7 mcmol/L)
Total bilirubin	1.0 mg/dL (17.1 mcmol/L)
Alkaline phosphatase	96 units/L (1.6 µkat/L)
AST	49 units/L (0.8 µkat/L)
ALT	48 units/L (0.8 µkat/L)
LDH	224 IU/L (3.73 µkat/L)

13. Interpret H.J.'s lab results. Is his condition improving?

Because H.J.'s condition has stabilized, the oncologist orders another round of chemotherapy.

14. Because the TLS is just resolving, what interventions would you include in your plan of care?

 15. What precautions should you take when administering H.J.'s chemotherapy to reduce the risk for injury? Select all that apply.
   a. Independently verify the completeness of the drug order and infusion rate.
   b. Dispose of any equipment that held the drug in special biohazard containers.
   c. Scrub skin that comes into contact with the drug for 5 minutes with a surgical brush.
   d. Wear goggles, powdered gloves, and a disposable, fluid-resistant, long-sleeved gown.
   e. If using a peripheral site, place a disposable drape under the arm where the drug will be infused.
   f. Use a Luer-Lok connector to attach the drug tubing to the main IV line, using the IV port closest to H.J.

16. The UAP you are working with states she is unfamiliar with caring for patients receiving chemotherapy. What instructions do you give to the UAP to reduce her risk for injury?

17. Which tasks can you delegate to the UAP? Select all that apply.
   a. Giving IV fluids as prescribed
   b. Assisting H.J. with oral hygiene
   c. Practicing good hand washing technique
   d. Determining the need for antiemetic therapy
   e. Reporting the amount and type of oral fluid intake
   f. Taking vital signs and recording them every 4 hours

CASE STUDY OUTCOME

H.J. does not experience any acute kidney injury. He is discharged home 3 days later after finishing this round of chemotherapy. He will be following up with the oncologist in 1 week.

Case Study 114

Name_____ Class/Group_____ Date_____

▶ Scenario

R.M. is a 58-year-old woman with stage III ovarian cancer. Her initial treatment is an exploratory laparot-omy with a total abdominal hysterectomy, an ileocecal resection and anastomosis, omentectomy, and peritoneal biopsies. The postoperative CA-125 level is 69 units/mL. Family history analysis reveals a strong positive occurrence of breast and ovarian cancer. Her mother died of breast cancer at 56 years of age, and a maternal aunt died of ovarian cancer at 59. The oncologist recommends testing for the presence of the *BRCA1* and *BRCA2* genes and, if the results are positive, testing R.M.'s two daughters and son.

1. What is the association between cancer development and the *BRCA1* and *BRCA2* genes?

2. Discuss the pros and cons of genetic testing for cancer.

3. In reviewing R.M.'s family history, which factors are considered significant? Select all that apply. Defend your response.
   a. Aunt who died from ovarian cancer at age 59
   b. Mother who died from breast cancer at age 56
   c. Sister was diagnosed with cervical cancer at age 50
   d. Grandmother who died from gastric cancer at age 84
   e. Aunt was diagnosed with endometrial cancer at age 65

4. R.M. tests positive for the *BRCA2* gene. What implications does this have for her children?

5. Why is ovarian cancer usually stage III or IV when initially diagnosed?

R.M. begins a chemotherapy regimen of paclitaxel and cisplatin. After receiving the fourth course, she presents with shortness of breath, complaints of nausea, and early satiety with a recent weight loss of 10 lbs (4.53 kg). Her abdomen is distended, and her SpO_2 is 86% on room air. Her current CA-125 level is 328 units/mL. You are admitting her directly from the oncologist's office to the medical floor.

6. Explain the significance of R.M.'s CA-125 level.

7. Knowing the chemotherapeutic agents R.M. has received, what lab tests will you expect the oncologist to order?

8. You perform R.M.'s admission assessment. Which finding must be immediately reported to the oncologist?
   a. Dark, amber-colored urine
   b. A temperature of 100.3° F (37.9° C)
   c. Bleeding gums and mouth ulcerations
   d. Numbness in her lower legs bilaterally

9. R.M.'s chest x-ray film reveals bilateral pleural effusions. How do these relate to her underlying disease? How might they be treated?

After performing a thoracentesis, the oncologist orders a magnetic resonance imaging (MRI) scan of the chest, abdomen, and pelvis, which reveals a mass in the left lower quadrant and a malignant bowel obstruction. He immediately schedules R.M. for a tumor debulking and possible placement of an ostomy.

10. What does scheduling R.M. for a debulking procedure imply?
    a. After this surgery, R.M. will be cured of her cancer.
    b. R.M. has advanced disease and the prognosis is poor.
    c. Chemotherapy will no longer be given after she recovers from surgery.
    d. R.M. will now need to have radiation therapy in addition to chemotherapy.

11. R.M. is undergoing a palliative surgical intervention. How will you explain this to R.M. and her family?

12. What additional risks does surgery pose for R.M.?

13. Outline 4 topics to include in her preoperative teaching.

14. Later in your shift, you find R.M.'s daughter sitting in a chair at the end of the hall crying quietly. You pull up a chair and sit. She tells you, "I had always thought mom was going to fight this. It is really just kind of hitting me that she is actually dying. You just think after surgery and all the chemo everything is going to be fine." What is your best response?
    a. "Let's talk about what is going on with your mother's illness."
    b. "Don't worry about her dying now. Focus on getting her through this surgery."
    c. "Your mother is receiving the best care available. Let's talk about her surgery."
    d. "You are being rather pessimistic. You just need to maintain hope for your mother."

9 Cellular Regulation

15. How can you support R.M. and her family at this time?

CASE STUDY OUTCOME

R.M. undergoes the debulking procedure. Because of the presence of multiple small tumors that were not detected on preoperative scanning, the oncologist elects not to place an ostomy. R.M. never fully recovers from surgery and does not resume chemotherapy. She has recurrent bowel obstructions and passes away in hospice care 3 weeks later.

Case Study 115

Name_____ Class/Group_____ Date_____

▶ Scenario

C.O. is a 43-year-old woman who noted a nonpruritic nodular rash on her neck and chest about 6 weeks ago. The rash became generalized, spreading to her head, abdomen, and arms, and was accompanied by polyarticular joint pain and back pain. About 2 weeks ago, she experienced three episodes of epistaxis in 1 day. Over the past week, her gums became swollen and tender and she was severely fatigued. Because of the progression of symptoms, she sought medical attention. Lab work was done, and C.O. was directly admitted to the hematology/oncology unit under the care of a hematologist for diagnostic evaluation. Skin biopsy showed cutaneous leukemic infiltrates, and bone marrow biopsy showed moderately hypercellular marrow and collections of monoblasts. Her lumbar puncture specimen was free of blast cells. The final diagnosis was acute myeloblastic leukemia.

C.O. is to begin remission induction therapy with cytarabine 100 mg/m²/day as a continuous infusion for 7 days and idarubicin 12 mg/m²/day IV push for 3 days. She is scheduled in angiography for placement of a triple-lumen subclavian catheter before beginning her therapy.

Chart View

Laboratory Test Results

Complete Blood Count (CBC)

White blood cells (WBCs)	39,000/mm³ (39 x 10⁹/L)
Monocytes	64%
Lymphocytes	15%
Neutrophils	4%
Blasts	17%
Hemoglobin (Hgb)	10.4 g/dL (104 g/L)
Hematocrit (Hct)	28.7%
Platelets	49,000/mm³ (49 x 10⁹/L)

1. Interpret C.O.'s CBC results. What does the presence of blasts in the differential mean?

9 Cellular Regulation

2. What was the purpose of the bone marrow biopsy?

 3. Considering all the admission data, what potential problem will you be alert for when C.O. returns to the unit after the catheter insertion?

4. What assessments about the central catheter are essential for you to perform?

5. What unique adverse effects are associated with cytarabine and idarubicin?

6. What ongoing assessment will you need to perform to detect these effects?

CASE STUDY PROGRESS

On the ninth day of continuous infusion of cytarabine, the UAP reports C.O.'s vital signs to you.

Chart View

Vital Signs

BP	110/54
Heart rate	115
Respiratory rate	26
Temperature	101.6° F (38.7° C)

7. What other assessments should you make right now and why?

CASE STUDY PROGRESS

Your assessment findings are unremarkable and you notify the intern on call of C.O.'s vital signs. After evaluating C.O., the orders shown in the chart are written.

Chart View

Physician's Orders

Blood cultures now × 2 sites
CBC with differential now
Acetaminophen suppository 650 mg q4-6hr prn
Imipenem/cilastatin sodium 500 mg IV piggyback q8hr
Notify hematologist for temp over 100.0° F (37.8° C)

---

8. Do these orders seem appropriate? Explain.

9. What will your next action be?

Chart View

Laboratory Test Values

WBCs	1200/mm^3 (1.2 x 10^9/L)
Monocytes	25%
Lymphocytes	65%
Neutrophils	5%
Blasts	5%
Bands	0%
Hgb	6.8 g/dL (68 g/L)
Hct	21.3%
Platelets	17,000/mm^3 (17 x 10^9/L)

---

10. What do these lab values indicate about her immune system?

11. Calculate C.O.'s absolute neutrophil count (ANC) and describe its significance.

12. Considering the previous data, what blood products will most likely be given to C.O.?

With continued blood product support and antibiotic coverage, C.O. is able to complete 14 days of therapy and a bone marrow biopsy shows she is in complete remission. HLA typing has been done on all her siblings. Her oldest brother is a perfect HLA match and has agreed to donate bone marrow. C.O. is being discharged with plans to readmit her to the bone marrow transplant unit within the next few weeks.

13. What does "complete remission" mean for C.O., and what effect did it have on the decision to perform a bone marrow transplant?

14. What type of bone marrow transplant will she have? Briefly describe this transplant process.

15. Name 4 priority problems C.O. will face in undergoing a bone marrow transplant. Put a star next to the most important priority

16. What is the **most** important intervention post-transplant?
    a. Giving analgesics for postprocedural pain
    b. Monitoring for signs of infection and bleeding
    c. Weighing her daily and offering small, frequent meals
    d. Offering emotional support to C.O. and her family during recovery

 17. What type of isolation will C.O. need? Outline the guidelines for maintaining this type of isolation.

18. Undergoing a bone marrow transplant is challenging. Describe how you would provide emotional support to C.O. and her family.

19. Name 3 complications C.O. will be at risk for after the transplant.

20. Describe graft-versus-host disease.

21. True or false. If the transplanted cells do not engraft, C.O. will die unless another transplant is tried and successful. Defend your response.

CASE STUDY OUTCOME

C.O. underwent the bone marrow transplant and stayed in the hospital for 8 weeks while her immune system recovered. After her release, she returned to the hospital daily for 1 month and followed neutropenic precautions for the next 3 months. At her 3-year anniversary mark, she and a group of family and friends took part in a half marathon to raise money for the hospital where she had her transplant.

9 Cellular Regulation

Tissue Integrity

Case Study 116

Name_____ Class/Group_____ Date_____

▶ Scenario

You are working in the emergency department (ED) of a community hospital when the ambulance arrives with A.N., a 28-year-old woman who was involved in a house fire. She was sleeping when the fire started and managed to make her way out of the house through thick smoke. The emergency medical system crew started 100% humidified oxygen at 15 L/min per non-rebreather mask and started a 16-gauge IV with lactated Ringer's solution. On arrival in the ED, her vital signs are 100/66, 125, 34, SpO$_2$ 93%. She is alert and oriented x 4 and appears anxious and in pain.

1. Describe the interventions needed to care for A.N. on her arrival in the ED.

2. Because you are concerned about smoke inhalation, what will you assess for in A.N.?

3. As you perform your initial assessment, you note burns on A.N.'s right anterior leg, left anterior and posterior leg, and anterior torso. Shade the affected areas, and then, using the rule of nines, calculate the extent of A.N.'s burn injury.

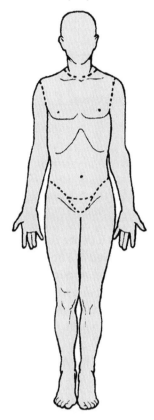

Modified from Ignatavicius DD, Workman ML: Medical-surgical nursing, ed. 6, St. Louis, 2010, Saunders.

4. You suspect that A.N. has deep partial-thickness burns. Which **best** describes this type of burn?
   a. The skin is blackened; the charred skin is insensitive to pain.
   b. The wounds are red, blanch, and have accompanying edema.
   c. The skin is shiny, red, moist, has fluid filled blisters and is painful.
   d. The wounds are dry, waxy white and hard; burned area has insensitivity to pain.

Chart View

Laboratory Test Values	
Hgb	20 g/dL (200 g/L)
Hct	51%
K	4.9 mEq/dL (4.9 mmol/L)
Na	133 mEq/dL (133 mmol/L)
Cl	100 mEq/dL (100 mmol/L)
Glucose	159 mg/dL (8.8 mmol/L)
BUN	28 mg/dL (10.0 mmol/L)
Creatinine	1.0 mg/dL (88.4 mcmol/L)

5. Interpret A.N.'s lab results.

6. A.N. is undergoing burn fluid resuscitation using the standard Baxter (Parkland) formula. She was admitted at 0400. She weighs 154 pounds (70 kg). Calculate her fluid requirements, specify the fluids used in the Baxter (Parkland) formula, specify how much will be given, and indicate what time intervals will be used.

7. A.N. is in severe pain. What is the drug of choice for pain relief after burn injury, and how should it be given?

10 Tissue Integrity

CASE STUDY PROGRESS

A.N. does not show any signs of smoke inhalation injury and is admitted to the medical unit for further treatment. As her nurse, you are concerned about meeting her needs for infection prevention, skin integrity, nutrition, fluids, and psychological support.

8. Because of her significant burn injury, A.N. is at high risk for infection. What measures will you institute to prevent infection?

9. A.N.'s burns are being treated by the open method with topical application of silver sulfadiazine. In caring for A.N., which interventions will you perform? Select all that apply.
   a. Shave all hair within the wound beds
   b. Keep the room temperature at 85° F (29.4° C)
   c. Use clean technique when changing A.N.'s dressings
   d. Monitor the CBC and WBC with differential frequently
   e. Apply a $\frac{1}{16}$-inch (1.5 mm) film of medication, covering entire burn
   f. Do not allow her to bathe for the initial 72 hours after injury

10. A.N. has one area of circumferential burns on her right lower leg. What complication is she in danger of developing? How will you monitor for it?

11. Describe 4 interventions that will help promote A.N.'s peripheral tissue perfusion.

12. A.N. is ordered a special burn diet. She has always gained weight easily and is concerned about the size of the portions. What diet-related teaching will you provide?

13. List 6 interventions you can use to assist in meeting A.N.'s nutrition goals.

14. Tissues under and around A.N.'s burns are severely swollen. She looks at you with tears in her eyes and asks, "Will they stay this way?" What is your answer?

15. A.N. is concerned about visible scars. What will you tell her?

Chart View

Vital Signs

BP	90/50
Heart rate	130
Respiratory rate	24
Temperature	99.0° F (37.2° C)

CASE STUDY PROGRESS

Eighteen hours after the injury, the UAP reports these vital signs and states A.N.'s urine output for the past 2 hours was 40 mL.

16. What do you suspect is occurring, and why does this concern you?

17. What treatment do you expect?

Chart View

Laboratory Test Values

Hgb	24 g/dL (240 g/L)
Hct	59%
K	5.3 mEq/Dl (5.3 mmol/L)
Na	128 mEq/Dl (128 mmol/L)
Cl	92 mEq/Dl (92 mmol/L)
Glucose	122 mg/dL (6.8 mmol/L)
BUN	38 mg/dL (13.6 mmol/L)
Creatinine	1.9 mg/dL (168 mcmol/L)

10 Tissue Integrity

18. The provider increases A.N.'s IV rate and orders a new set of lab work. Compare the current results with those from admission.

19. By the end of your shift, which assessment findings would **best** indicate that A.N. is responding to therapy?
   a. Respiratory rate 22; BP 120/74
   b. BP 120/70; urine output 25 mL/hr for past 4 hours
   c. BP 104/64; urine output 40 mL/hr for past 4 hours
   d. Heart rate 110; urine output 20 mL/hr for past 4 hours

CASE STUDY OUTCOME

Four days after her injury, A.N. begins a formal rehabilitation program and is able to maintain full range of motion and tissue mobility. Her recovery is prolonged by two wound infections, and she does experience some scarring. One year later she is still struggling with adapting to her new body image, but she is finding encouragement from family, friends, and her support group.

Case Study 117

Name_____ Class/Group_____ Date_____

▶ Scenario

You are entering the outpatient clinic room of a new patient, D.G., a 57-year-old man whose reason for being seen is listed as "a sore on lower right calf." He is requesting antibiotics to "help it heal" and a "stronger Lasix to help the swelling go down." He says that the Lasix he is on is not "doing the trick." D.G. tells you he does not remember any specific trauma to the area. He says the sore "just appeared" about 6 weeks ago. He says both his legs have been more swollen recently and elevating them has not helped. Periodically he has noticed a small amount of warm clear or yellow discharge running down his right leg. At first the sore did not hurt, but now he describes it as "on fire" with occasional severe, throbbing pain "that has brought me to tears, which has never happened to me before." He has been unable to sleep at night. Walking has become very difficult, so he prefers to sit as much as possible. His medical history includes osteoarthritis, obesity, and hypertension. His current medications include furosemide, atenolol, ramipril, losartan, ibuprofen, and aspirin. His current weight is 225 pounds (102 kg), and he is 5'10" (178 cm) tall.

1. Describe the pathophysiology of chronic venous insufficiency (CVI).

2. What are common risk factors for CVI? Underline the risk factors D.G. has.

3. Name 3 complications that can occur with CVI.

4. What signs and symptoms typically occur with CVI?

D.G. has an irregularly shaped wound, measuring 5 cm × 8 cm, just above his right medial malleolus. Serosanguinous, yellow, foul-smelling drainage is present in the distal portion of the wound. The surrounding skin is erythematous and warm. The skin of the right leg is dry, dark brown, and thickened from below the right knee to the foot. Pedal pulses are present at 1+ bilaterally. Capillary refill is brisk. There are no signs of neuropathy. Ankle-brachial index (ABI) is .97. VS: 154/98, 92, 16, 100° F (37.8° C).

5. What type of ulcer do you suspect D.G. has and why?

6. How can CVI lead to an ulcer?

7. What signs would alert you to the presence of a possible wound infection? Underline those D.G. has.

8. What does an ABI of .97 indicate?
   a. Diabetic neuropathy
   b. Peripheral arterial disease
   c. Normal arterial circulation
   d. Chronic venous insufficiency

The provider suspects D.G. has an infected venous leg ulcer and admits him to the hospital for wound debridement and IV antibiotic therapy. D.G. is started on pentoxifylline (Trental) 400 mg orally three times daily and morphine sulfate 3 mg IV every 3 hours as needed for pain. After debridement, the wound nurse prescribes a wound care regimen that involves cleansing the ulcer with sterile water, applying an antimicrobial barrier dressing, placing a foam dressing on top, and securing both in place with kling. The last step is to apply a continuous compression wrap.

9. What are 3 goals of care for D.G.?

10. What is the reason for starting D.G. on pentoxifylline?

11. Compression is essential for venous ulcer healing. Describe 3 options for providing compression therapy.

12. Explain the role other interprofessional team members may have in D.G.'s care.

13. Realizing D.G. has special dietary needs, you request a consult with the registered dietitian. Describe an optimal diet for D.G.

14. Identify 4 nursing interventions you will implement to promote venous return.

15. Which intervention is the **most** important in treating a venous leg ulcer?
    a. Keeping the affected leg elevated
    b. Maintaining continuous compression
    c. Performing physical therapy twice daily
    d. Applying the antimicrobial barrier dressing

10 Tissue Integrity

16. D.G. is given a prescription for therapeutic compression stockings with instructions to apply a stocking to his left leg. He will wear both after his wound heals. What teaching do you need to provide D.G. about compression stocking therapy?

17. You determine D.G. understands your instructions about proper foot and leg care when he says: (Select all that apply.)
a. "I will apply Vaseline every day to my legs."
b. "Checking the skin every day for infection is a must."
c. "It is important to be careful to avoid extra skin trauma."
d. "It is best to avoid extremes of hot and cold next to my skin."
e. "I will wash my legs with a mild soap, then dry them carefully."

18. What aspect of D.G.'s care can you delegate to the UAP working with you?
a. Teaching D.G. the signs of a wound infection
b. Explaining the reason for keeping the legs elevated
c. Assisting D.G. with applying compression stockings
d. Evaluating capillary refill and pedal pulses each shift

19. You encourage D.G. to take part in a weight reduction program focusing on diet and exercise. Why would you recommend this to D.G.?

CASE STUDY OUTCOME

After 1 week as an inpatient, D.G. is discharged with home health care to change the wound dressing twice weekly. The drainage had decreased significantly, and the wound appeared less red. D.G. still reports feeling some pain but confirms that it has decreased since he was in the hospital. He is to return in 2 weeks to reassess wound progress and evaluate the effectiveness of compression therapy.

Case Study 118

Name_____ Class/Group_____ Date_____

▶ Scenario

B.M., a 22-year old female, saw her primary health care provider 1 week ago because she had a mole on her right arm "that started changing." For years, the mole was flat and brown; over a period of several weeks recently, B.M. reports that the mole became slightly raised with irregular borders and changed to a blackish color. The provider noted the presence of a hard, non-tender mass in B.M.'s right axillary region. B.M. has a fair complexion, red hair, and blue eyes. She says that as a child, she had a bad sunburn at least once every summer but reports that she now uses sunscreen regularly. B.M. states that an uncle and a few cousins have had skin cancer, but it was "not the bad kind." She has come to the dermatologist's office today for further assessment.

1. What are the risk factors for melanoma? Underline those that B.M. has.

2. What role does exposure to UV radiation play in the development of melanoma?

3. Where are the sites melanoma is commonly found?

4. B.M. said her relatives did not have the "bad kind" of skin cancer. Compared with melanoma, why would basal and squamous cell carcinoma not seem "bad"?

5. Outline the ABCDEs of assessing a potential melanoma lesion.

6. How would you expect B.M.'s lesion to appear?
   a. A small macule with dry, rough scales
   b. A soft, white papule with firm borders
   c. A firm nodule with a central, ulcerated area
   d. An irregularly shaped lesion with a blackish color

7. Draw a normal mole and a malignant melanoma, as they might appear on B.M.

8. The dermatologist believes that if B.M. does have melanoma, it may have already metastasized. Why?

9. B.M. asks about the anesthesia she will receive and if the procedure will hurt. How should you respond?

CASE STUDY PROGRESS

The biopsy confirms the presence of superficial malignant melanoma. B.M. is scheduled for a wide excision of the lesion with grafting.

10. What tests will need to be done to determine whether B.M.'s melanoma has metastasized?

11. Describe the surgical procedure B.M. will undergo.

B.M. undergoes a wide excision as a surgical outpatient of a 3 × 5 mm lesion with a split-thickness skin graft from her right thigh. The procedure goes smoothly, and the dermatologist covers the arm wound with a bulky dressing. There is a pressure dressing sutured underneath holding the graft in place. The thigh wound has a pressure dressing.

12. You find B.M. trying to lift up a corner of the arm dressing. She says that she wants to see what the scar will be like. What do you tell her?

13. True or false. Having a skin graft eliminates scarring.

14. You recognize B.M. may be experiencing some anxiety, which is a common response during this time. How will you provide B.M. emotional support?

15. As you prepare B.M. for discharge, what teaching do you need to provide?

16. Which statements show B.M. understands your discharge instructions about skin care? Select all that apply.
   a. "There will be some swelling and tenderness in both areas."
   b. "I will avoid overusing or overstretching the surgery areas."
   c. "Tomorrow I will remove the bulky dressing and take a bath."
   d. "I can alternate aspirin and acetaminophen to control the pain."
   e. "Apply ice to the site for 15 minutes, four times daily, for discomfort."

10 Tissue Integrity

CASE STUDY PROGRESS

Five days later, B.M. returns to the clinic to have the bulky dressing removed. The final pathology report has returned and confirmed the diagnosis of superficial spreading melanoma, invasive to a Breslow's thickness of 1.8 mm.

17. Describe the clinical use of Breslow's thickness.

18. What ongoing monitoring will B.M. need?

19. Outline the measures you need to teach B.M. to reduce the likelihood of her developing another skin cancer.

CASE STUDY OUTCOME

B.M. underwent excisional biopsy of the axillary lymph node. Fortunately, the lymph node was found to be cancer-free. Imaging showed no lesions and B.M. received a final diagnosis of superficial spreading melanoma, stage 1A. B.M. had follow-up visits every 3 months with the dermatologist and oncologist and, 3 years later, is still cancer-free.

Case Study 119

Name_____ Class/Group_____ Date_____

▶ Scenario

You are a nurse working on the unit and take the following report from the emergency department (ED) nurse: "We have a patient for you: R.L. is an 81-year-old frail woman who has been in a nursing home. Her primary admitting diagnoses are sepsis, pneumonia, and dehydration, and she has a known stage 3 right hip pressure injury. Past medical history includes remote cerebrovascular accident with residual right-sided weakness and paresthesia, remote myocardial infarction, and peripheral vascular disease. She is a full code. Her vital signs are 98/62, 88 and regular, 38 and labored, 100.4° F (38° C). Lab work is pending; she has oxygen at 4 L per nasal cannula and an IV of D5.45 at 100 mL/hr. We just inserted an indwelling catheter. The infectious disease doctor has been notified, and respiratory therapy is with the patient—they are just leaving the ED and should arrive shortly."

1. What major factors increase risk for developing a pressure injury?

2. Each health care setting should have a policy that outlines how to assess patients' risk for developing a pressure injury. What should be included in that assessment?

3. As part of R.L.'s admission assessment, you conduct a skin assessment. What areas of R.L.'s body will you pay particular attention to?

4. What are the advantages of using a validated risk assessment tool to document her skin condition on admission?

5. How often should patients be reassessed for the risk of developing an injury?

During your assessment, you note that R.L. has very dry, thin, almost transparent skin. She has limited mobility from her stroke and is currently bedridden. There are several areas of ecchymosis on her upper extremities. She is alert and oriented to person only. You review the transfer summary from the long-term care facility and note she has a history of urinary and fecal incontinence.

6. Evaluate R.L. with the Norton risk assessment scale.

	Physical Condition		Mental Condition		Activity		Mobility		Incontinence		
Date	Good	4	Alert	4	Ambulant	4	Full	4	Not	4	Total Score
	Fair	3	Apathetic	3	Walk/help	3	Slightly Limited	3	Occasional	3	
	Poor	2	Confused	2	Chair bound	2		2	Usually/urine	2	
	Very bad	1	Stupor	1	Bed rest	1	Very limited Immobile	1	Urinary and fecal	1	

7. Knowing that R.L. is frail, has right-sided weakness, and has a pressure injury, what consultations or referrals could you initiate?

As you are completing R.L.'s assessment, the wound nurse specialist comes in. She knows R.L. from a prior admission; as soon as she received the request for a wound care consultation, she ordered a specialty mattress. She says an air overlay should be delivered to your unit before your shift ends.

8. Why is a specialty mattress used for immobile or compromised patients?

9. Why are patients placed on specialty mattresses still at risk for skin breakdown?

10. Why do the heels have the greatest incidence of breakdown, even when the patient is on a specialty mattress?

11. What intervention can you initiate to protect R.L.'s heels?

12. Compare friction and shear.

13. What risk factor does using a draw sheet prevent or minimize?

10 Tissue Integrity

14. Describe 6 interventions aimed at minimizing friction and shear.

15. Elevated skin temperature and perspiration increase risk for pressure injury. Write 4 specific measures to manage the microclimate.

16. Which instructions will you give to the UAP helping you care for R.L.? Select all that apply.
   a. Assess R.L.'s skin status every shift
   b. Develop an every-2-hour turn schedule
   c. Use the appropriate sheets on the airflow bed
   d. Keep R.L.'s head of bed below a 30-degree angle
   e. Assist with hygiene measures when R.L. is incontinent
   f. Empty and measure output in the urine collection device

17. Write an outcome related to R.L.'s skin integrity.

CASE STUDY PROGRESS

The wound nurse needs to evaluate the preexisting pressure injury. She gently removes the old dressing, using the push-pull method and adhesive remover wipes. After taking off the outside dressing, or the secondary dressing, she pulls out the primary dressing and states that R.L. has a tunneled wound that was "packed too hard."

18. What problems can be created by packing a wound too full?

19. The nurse systematically assesses the injury and confirms the presence of a stage 3 wound with moderate yellow drainage. There is no tissue necrosis or debris. What does it mean to "stage" a wound?

20. What would you expect a stage 3 pressure injury to look like?

21. What is a tunneling wound? What risk factors are associated with tunneling?

22. What are the dimensions of R.L.'s wound?

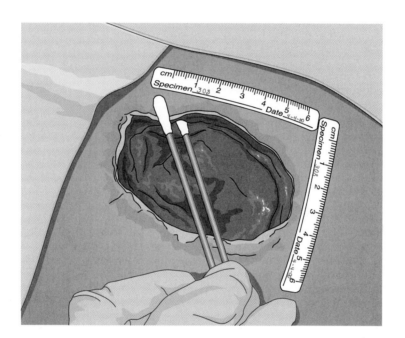

CASE STUDY PROGRESS

After the wound nurse obtains a set of wound cultures, you watch as she packs the wound with gauze. The wound nurse charts the findings and makes formal recommendations for management of the wound to the primary care provider.

23. When collecting a wound culture with a swab, the nurse should culture the
   a. Wound drainage
   b. Healthy-appearing tissue
   c. Most necrotic-appearing tissue
   d. Very outer edges of the wound

 24. Describe the technique for packing a tunneled wound.

25. What factors influence the choice of a wound dressing?

26. What do you feel would be the best choice for dressing R.L.'s wound?

27. What wound documentation is necessary at this time?

28. Complete an example of a documentation entry for R.L.'s wound care.

Wound Location
Pressure Injury Stage
Wound Dimensions
Undermining
Tissue Type
Drainage
Periwound Condition
Cleansing Agents
Dressing Type Applied

CASE STUDY OUTCOME

Despite aggressive treatment, R.L.'s sepsis and pneumonia are overwhelming, and she dies 9 days later from multiple organ failure.

Cognition

Case Study **120**

Name_____ Class/Group_____ Date_____

▶ Scenario

You are the nurse working on the surgical floor. One of your patients, M.M., a 70-year-old man, was transferred in last night from the ICU. He is postop day 3 after a Whipple procedure for pancreatic cancer. M.M. is NPO and has an NG tube to continuous low wall suction, an indwelling urinary catheter, and a triple-lumen subclavian catheter with D_5NS at 75 mL/hr. The abdominal dressing is dry and intact, with 2 Jackson-Pratt drains to bulb suction.

Midway through the morning, M.M.'s daughter comes to the nurses' station and tells you that there is "something wrong" with her father. She said her mother and she just arrived and were speaking with him about his night. He told them he was worried because he saw a nurse wheel his granddaughter down the hall on a stretcher and that from his window, he could see the men on the roof of the building across the street aiming guns at her room and his room.

1. Using the mnemonic "DELIRIUM," what are the possible causes of M.M.'s confusion?

2. What assessment do you need to perform?

You accompany his daughter back to M.M.'s room to perform an assessment. As soon as you enter the room and reintroduce yourself, he yells, "Get down! The men are back on the roof and are aiming this way!"

3. How should you respond to M.M.?

4. You would document M.M.'s report of his seeing the men on the building roof aiming guns at his room as he is displaying:
   a. Mania
   b. Delusions
   c. Hallucinations
   d. Flight of ideas

5. You administer the Confusion Assessment Method (CAM) to M.M., which evaluates for the presence of delirium. Describe the CAM.

6. Besides the symptoms M.M. has, what are other symptoms of delirium?

7. Compared with dementia, which signs are unique to delirium? Select all that apply.
   a. Irritability
   b. Incoherent speech
   c. Visual hallucinations
   d. Long-term memory loss
   e. A slow decline in cognition
   f. Changing levels of consciousness

8. Briefly describe the 3 types of delirium.

9. Which medication from M.M.'s current list is *most* likely to be related to his change in mental status?
   a. Omeprazole 40 mg IV once daily
   b. Enoxaparin 30 mg subcutaneous daily
   c. Ondansetron 4 mg IV every 6 hours as needed
   d. Morphine sulfate 4 mg IV every 3 hours as needed

10. M.M.'s wife states that she has never seen her husband act like this before and she is scared. How would you explain what is happening to his family?

Your assessment findings are as follows: Vital signs 94/72, 109, 32, 100.8° F (38.2° C), Spo_2 89% on room air. You auscultate decreased breath sounds and coarse crackles in the left lower lobe posteriorly. M.M. is alert and oriented to name. He does not answer all your questions and is unable to follow simple instructions. There is minimal eye contact and he continues to look furtively out the window. The rest of his assessment is unremarkable.

11. Score M.M. on the CAM.

12. You believe his delirium may be associated with hypoxia and fever from atelectasis. Using SBAR, outline the report you need to give to the provider.

11 Cognition

CASE STUDY PROGRESS

Hearing your report, the provider orders oxygen therapy, blood cultures, CBC with differential, basic metabolic panel, ECG, and a chest x-ray now and in the morning. The chest x-ray confirms the presence of atelectasis in the left lower lobe. His blood chemistry findings and CBC are all within normal limits except for WBC count, which is elevated at 11600/ mm³ (11.6 x 10⁹/L). The provider orders the following:

Chart View

Medication Orders

Ceftriaxone 1 gram IV q12hr
Albuterol 2.5 mg/ipratropium 250 mcg nebulizer treatment STAT, then q4hr
Acetaminophen 650 mg PO q6hr
Haloperidol 1 mg IV q3hr as needed for agitation

13. What outcome is associated with each of the medications ordered for M.M.?

14. What are the health care team's primary goals for M.M. at this time?

15. Write an outcome statement addressing M.M.'s risk for injury.

16. What is the focus of the ongoing assessment you need to perform?

17. Describe the physical changes you should make to M.M.'s environment to promote safety.

18. Another nurse tells you that you must apply restraints to protect M.M. from injury. How do you respond?

19. What other interventions can you use to promote orientation? Select all that apply.
   a. Place the television on a news channel
   b. Refrain from administering pain medications
   c. Have him wear his hearing aid and eye glasses
   d. Orient M.M. of person, place, and time, as needed
   e. Encourage his family to "go along" with his hallucinations
   f. Reintroduce him to health care providers with each contact

20. How should you communicate with M.M.?

21. Which tasks are appropriate to assign to the UAP assisting you with M.M.'s care? Select all that apply.
   a. Keeping the call light within M.M.'s reach
   b. Ambulating M.M. to the chair and bathroom
   c. Assisting M.M. with performing oral hygiene
   d. Emptying the two Jackson-Pratt drains each shift
   e. Obtaining routine vital signs and M.M.'s daily weight

CASE STUDY OUTCOME

The next day he is less delirious but is not near his baseline mental status. As his respiratory status improves and he resumes a normal diet and ambulates, his orientation improves. By discharge 6 days later, the delirium has resolved.

11 Cognition

Case Study **121**

Name _____ Class/Group _____ Date _____

> ▶ **Scenario**

You are the nurse working in the outpatient clinic. This afternoon, a woman brings in her father, K.B., who is 74 years old. The daughter reports that over the past year she has noticed her father has progressive problems with his mental capacity. These changes have developed gradually but seem to be getting worse. At times, he is alert, and at other times he seems disoriented, depressed, and tearful. He is forgetting things and doing things out of the ordinary, such as placing the milk in the cupboard and sugar in the refrigerator. K.B. reports that he has been having memory problems for the past year and at times has difficulty remembering the names of family members and friends. His neighbor found K.B. down the street 2 days ago, and he did not know where he was. This morning he thought it was nighttime and wondered what his daughter was doing at his house. He could not pour his own coffee, and he seems to be getting more agitated. A review of his medical history is significant for hypercholesterolemia and coronary artery disease.

1. What are some cognitive skills that may decline in an older adult?

2. Physiologic age-related changes in an older adult can influence cognitive functioning. Name and discuss one.

3. For each behavior listed, specify whether it is associated with delirium (DL) or dementia (DM).

_____ a. Gradual and insidious onset
_____ b. Hallucinations or delusions
_____ c. A sudden, acute onset of symptoms
_____ d. Progressive functional impairment
_____ e. Personality changes with emotional lability
_____ f. Incoherent interactions with others
_____ g. Possible wandering behavior
_____ h. Lucid at times, but often worsens at night

4. Based on the information provided by K.B.'s daughter, do you think he is showing signs of delirium or dementia? Explain.

5. You know there are several types of dementia that cause cognitive changes. List 3 of these types of dementia.

6. How does the health care team determine the degree of cognitive impairment?

7. Name 4 common cognitive assessment tools.

CASE STUDY PROGRESS

K.B.'s vital signs are within normal limits. He is pleasant, with coherent speech, although he does not speak unless asked specific questions. General and neurologic assessment findings are normal. On cognitive testing, he scores a 24/30 on the Mini-Mental State Examination, missing 4 points on orientation, 1 point on recall, and 1 point on intersecting pentagon drawing. Further detailed testing confirmed deficits in orientation, memory, and visual-spatial skills. He also had difficulty with the clock drawing test.

11 Cognition

8. Several diagnostic tests are ordered for K.B. From the tests listed, select those which would be used to help diagnose the type of dementia.

_____ Toxicology screen
_____ Electrocardiogram
_____ Electroencephalogram
_____ Complete metabolic panel
_____ Complete blood count with differential
_____ Thyroid function tests
_____ Colonoscopy
_____ Rapid plasma reagin (RPR) test
_____ Serum B_{12} and folate levels
_____ Bleeding times
_____ Liver function tests
_____ Vision and hearing evaluation
_____ Magnetic resonance imaging (MRI)
_____ Urinalysis

CASE STUDY PROGRESS

After reviewing K.B.'s history and diagnostic test results, K.B. is diagnosed with Alzheimer disease (AD). The provider calls a family conference to discuss the implications with K.B. and his family. Fortunately, K.B. has a supportive daughter and 3 sons who live nearby who can function as caregivers.

9. What neuroanatomic changes are seen in persons with AD?

10. How would you explain AD to them?

11. K.B.'s son asks, "How did he get Alzheimer disease? We don't know anyone else who has it." How would you respond?

CASE STUDY PROGRESS

The family decides they will provide 24-hour supervision at home for K.B. using a combination of family, friends, and home health caregivers. K.B. receives a prescription for donepezil orally disintegrating tablet (Aricept ODT) 5 mg daily. As you review the prescription with the group, K.B.'s daughter tells you she is "so happy" because she did not know there were medications that could cure AD.

12. How do you respond?

13. What do you need to teach K.B. and his family about donepezil? Select all that apply.
   a. "The best time to take donepezil is in the morning."
   b. "Swallow each tablet whole. Drink a glass of water afterward."
   c. "Notify the provider if you have trouble urinating or muscle weakness."
   d. "You may have some nausea. Taking the medication with food may help."
   e. "Keep the tablet in the blister pack until you are ready to take the medicine."

 14. Recognizing that safety is a priority for K.B., you prepare a teaching plan aimed at promoting K.B.'s safety for him and his family. List 6 things you will review with them.

15. What interventions can help K.B. maintain his independence? Describe 4.

16. You discuss the importance of considering future planning in terms of advance directives and financial concerns. Why would you discuss this now?

17. What community resources may be available to K.B. and his family?

CASE STUDY OUTCOME

Two years later, K.B. is no longer able to care for himself. He has become increasingly depressed and paranoid, and recently started a fire in the kitchen. His children decide to place him in the Alzheimer unit at a local extended care facility.

11 Cognition

Case Study **122**

Name_____ Class/Group_____ Date_____

▶ **Scenario**

K.B. is a 76-year-old man who has a 2-year history of having Alzheimer disease (AD). He has become increasingly depressed and paranoid, recently started a fire in the kitchen, and yesterday fell down a partial flight of stairs. His children have come to the Alzheimer unit at your extended care facility to discuss the possibility of placing K.B. You assure the family of your experience in addressing the questions and concerns of most people in their situation.

1. AD typically proceeds through 7 general stages. After the family describes K.B.'s behavior, you determine that he is in stage 5 of AD. Place in order the stages of AD, with "1" being stage 1, and "7" being stage 7.
   _____ a.   Memory lapses are beginning to occur, though no one else notices.
   _____ b.   The person cannot respond to the environment or control movements.
   _____ c.   Family and friends begin to notice problems with memory and judgment.
   _____ d.   Personality changes take place and the person needs help with ADLs.
   _____ e.   The person is not yet experiencing any memory problems or impairments.
   _____ f.   Difficulty performing complex tasks and arithmetic becomes obvious.
   _____ g.   The person begins to need help with day-to-day activities.

2. What precipitating factors may have resulted in K.B.'s fall?

CASE STUDY PROGRESS

K.B.'s daughter states, "How are you going to take care of him? He wanders around all night long. He cannot find his way to the bathroom in a house he has lived in for 43 years. He cannot be trusted to be alone anymore; he almost burnt the house down. We're all exhausted, and we can't keep up with this." You acknowledge how tired they must be from trying to keep him safe. You tell the family that Alzheimer units have been created to provide a structured, safe environment.

3. Describe 5 specific nursing interventions that are part of National Patient Safety Goals aimed at minimizing fall risk.

 4. K.B.'s son asks why you can access the unit only through a door that has a keypad control. He wants to know if there are violent patients on the unit. How will you respond?

5. K.B.'s son asks whether his father is going to continue taking the donepezil (Aricept ODT) daily. How would you respond?

6. You relate that care on the unit is delivered by an interprofessional team. In addition to the physician and nursing, name 4 other team members who likely will be involved in K.B.'s care and the role each will have.

7. You try to comfort the family by telling them the problems they are experiencing are common. You explain family support is a major focus of your facility's program. List 4 ways in which K.B.'s family might receive the support they need.

CASE STUDY PROGRESS

K.B.'s family decide to place him in the Alzheimer unit. During his first few days at the facility, he is very restless and agitated, constantly wandering around the unit. He has slept only 2 to 3 hours per night. The UAP reports to you that she just found him sitting on the bathroom floor incontinent of urine.

11 Cognition

8. What factors are likely contributing to K.B.'s wandering and restlessness?

 9. As you develop K.B.'s plan of care, which problem has the highest priority?
   a. Risk for injury
   b. Chronic confusion
   c. Urinary incontinence
   d. Impaired communication

10. What other medications might be prescribed for K.B. and why?

11. True or false? A patient with AD is not able to sleep without drug therapy.

12. Describe 4 interventions that may promote a normal sleep pattern for K.B.

13. Which interventions would help K.B. function at his highest level possible? Select all that apply.
   a. Avoiding unfamiliar situations whenever possible
   b. Maintaining consistency with day-to-day activities
   c. Furnishing the environment with familiar possessions
   d. Reducing environmental stimuli to decrease overstimulation
   e. Having him take part in activities that distract and occupy time
   f. Encouraging him to perform cognitive skills above his level of ability

14. You are concerned K.B. is not able to verbalize his needs. Write an outcome addressing this issue and identify independent nursing actions to promote communication.

11 Cognition

15. Which activities can you delegate to the UAP to promote K.B.'s self-care? Select all that apply.
   a. Assisting him with eating as needed
   b. Helping him with his morning hygienic care
   c. Ambulating him to the bathroom every 2 hours
   d. Assessing K.B.'s self-care needs and ability to perform care
   e. Encouraging K.B. to take part in his care as much as possible

CASE STUDY OUTCOME

After a few weeks, K.B. seems to adjust to being on the unit. He is relatively stable for several months. He passed away 18 months later from pneumonia after experiencing a rapid decline in cognitive function.

Infection and Inflammation

Case Study **123**

Name_____ Class/Group_____ Date_____

▶ **Scenario**

A.P. is an 8-year-old who is sent to the nurse's office because she has had a 2-day history of scratching her head so badly that she complains that her "head hurts." You complete a general examination of A.P.'s head and notice that she has red, irritated areas with several scratch marks; a few open sores; and sesame seed–sized, silvery white and yellow nodules (bugs) that are adhered to many of her hair shafts. You determine that A.P. has pediculosis capitis.

1. What is pediculosis capitis?

2. What will be your next steps in A.P.'s care?

3. What should be included in the educational plans for A.P. and her parents?

4. The parents take A.P. home to treat her. Which statement by A.P.'s mother would help make A.P. the most comfortable during this treatment period? Explain.
   a. "I sure hope this works. I never thought this would happen!"
   b. "Here is the shampoo. Be sure to scrub your head for several minutes."
   c. "It might be best to go ahead and cut your hair. It will grow back quickly."
   d. "We can pretend you're at the beauty parlor! Lean back while I wash your hair."

5. Why would head lice occur in school-aged children?

6. What possible complications can occur as a result of failing to treat head lice?

7. What nursing actions would you take regarding A.P.'s classmates?

8. A.P.'s mother calls you to ask what complications may occur with the head lice infestation. Which answer is correct?
   a. "Head lice are common carriers of impetigo."
   b. "Head lice are not known to transmit disease."
   c. "Head lice may transmit certain viral illnesses."
   d. "It is common to have a ringworm infection after a case of head lice."

Ten days later, A.P.'s mother calls you and states, "I think she has lice again! We worked so hard to get rid of them and clean everything. Is there something else we can use to treat her? What do we do now?"

9. What would you tell A.P.'s mother at this time?

10. List 3 Internet resources A.P.'s mother may find helpful.

11. A.P.'s pediatrician prescribes spinosad (Natroba) at this time. You will provide teaching to A.P.'s mother. Which statements are correct? Select all that apply, and correct the ones that are incorrect.
   a. Apply Natroba to wet hair.
   b. Shake the bottle before using.
   c. Leave it on the scalp without rinsing for 24 hours.
   d. An adult needs to apply the medication to A.P.'s scalp.
   e. A second treatment, if needed, may be applied in 1 week.
   f. After the medication is washed off, use a fine-tooth comb to remove treated lice and nits from the hair and scalp.

CASE STUDY OUTCOME

A.P.'s lice infestation cleared up after 2 treatments with Natroba, and none of her family members or classmates were infested.

12 Infection and Inflammation

Case Study 124

Name_____ Class/Group_____ Date_____

▶ Scenario

T.B. is a 65-year-old retiree who is admitted to your unit from the emergency department (ED). On arrival, you note that he is trembling and nearly doubled over with severe abdominal pain. T.B. indicates that he has severe pain in the right upper quadrant (RUQ) of his abdomen that radiates through to his mid back as a deep, sharp, boring pain. He is more comfortable walking or sitting bent forward rather than lying flat in bed. He admits to having had several similar bouts of abdominal pain in the last month, but "none as bad as this." He feels nauseated but has not vomited, although he did vomit a week ago with a similar episode. T.B. experienced an acute onset of pain after eating fried fish and chips at a fast-food restaurant earlier today. He is not happy to be in the hospital and is grumpy that his daughter insisted on taking him to the ED for evaluation.

After orienting him to the room, you perform your physical assessment. The findings are as follows: He is awake, alert, and oriented × 3, and he moves all extremities well. He is restless, constantly shifting his position, and complains of fatigue. Breath sounds are clear to auscultation. Heart sounds are clear with no murmur or rub noted and with a regular rhythm. His abdomen is flat, slightly rigid, and very tender to palpation throughout, especially in the RUQ; bowel sounds are present. He reports having light-colored stools for 1 week. The patient voids dark amber urine but denies dysuria. Skin and sclera are jaundiced. Admission vital signs are blood pressure 164/100, pulse of 132, respiration 26, temperature of 100° F (37.8° C), Spo_2 96% on 2 L of oxygen by nasal cannula.

1. What structures are located in the RUQ of the abdomen?

2. Which of the previously mentioned organs are typically palpable in the RUQ?

3. As you palpate T.B.'s abdomen, you deeply palpate the costal margin in the RUQ and ask him to take a deep breath. This causes T.B. to stop inspiration abruptly, midway, and exclaim, "Oh, that hurts!" What does this finding indicate? Explain your answer.
   a. Murphy sign
   b. Hepatomegaly
   c. Splenomegaly
   d. Rebound tenderness

T.B.'s abdominal ultrasound demonstrates several retained stones in the common bile duct and a stone-filled gallbladder. T.B. is admitted to your floor, placed on nothing by mouth (NPO) status, and scheduled to undergo endoscopic retrograde cholangiopancreatography (ERCP) that afternoon.

4. Describe an ERCP and its purpose in T.B.'s situation.

CASE STUDY PROGRESS

T.B.'s other lab results are posted, and you review them.

Chart View

Preoperative Laboratory Test Results

WBC	11,900/mm³ (11.9 x 10⁹/L)
Hgb	14.3 g/dL (143 g/L)
Hct	43%
Platelets	250,000/mm³ (250 x 10⁹/L)
ALT	200 units/L
AST	260 units/L
ALP	450 units/L
Total bilirubin	4.8 mg/dL (82 mcmol/L)
PT/INR	11.5 sec/1.0
Amylase	50 units/L
Lipase	23 units/L
Urinalysis	Negative

5. Which results are abnormal, and what do they reflect?

CASE STUDY PROGRESS

T.B. undergoes the ERCP, and stones and bile are released; however, imaging reveals that a stone is still retained within the cystic duct and multiple stones remain within the gallbladder itself. A surgical consultation is obtained, and a laparoscopic cholecystectomy ("lap choley") is planned.

6. Identify at least 4 preoperative orders that will likely need to be completed before T.B. goes to surgery.

12 Infection and Inflammation

7. T.B. is medicated with morphine sulfate 2 mg IV push (IVP) q2hr as needed. After the first dose, he reports that on a scale of 1 to 10, his pain has decreased from a 10 to a 4 within 30 minutes. What other methods could be used to help T.B.'s pain?

8. Which assessment findings are consistent with common bile duct obstruction?

CASE STUDY PROGRESS

T.B. undergoes a successful laparoscopic cholecystectomy the next morning. An intraoperative cholangiogram shows that the ducts are finally cleared of stones at the conclusion of the surgery. When he returns to the nursing unit, his stomach is soft but quite distended. His wife asks you whether anything is wrong.

9. How will you respond to her question?

10. One of the postoperative orders is for imipenem/cilastatin (Primaxin) 500 mg IV now, then q6hr × 2 doses. Before you give the antibiotic, what will you assess?

11. As you review the orders, you note that Primaxin contains cilastatin. What is the purpose of the cilastatin?
   a. It enhances the action of the imipenem.
   b. It reduces the chance of an allergic reaction.
   c. It promotes the renal secretion of the imipenem.
   d. It causes the bacterial cell wall to become unstable.

The next day, you prepare for the first dressing change as ordered by the surgeon. When you remove the tape the next day to change the dressing, you note that the skin is red and blistered underneath. Otherwise, he is doing well; his VS are 128/72, 80, 16, 99.8° F (37.7° C), and Spo_2 of 96% on room air. He even tolerated a light breakfast. To protect the blistered area from further damage, you apply a hydrocolloid dressing to the damaged skin.

12. What has T.B. experienced, and what are the benefits of using a hydrocolloid dressing?

The rest of the day is uneventful, and that afternoon, T.B. is discharged to home.

13. What discharge teaching does T.B. need? List at least 6 points.

14. After providing discharge teaching, you use the Teach-Back technique to assess T.B.'s learning. Which statement by T.B. indicates an adequate understanding of his postoperative care?
a. "I can go back to the gym to work out once I get home."
b. "I will eat a low-fat diet for several weeks after the surgery."
c. "I will leave the bandages on until I see the surgeon in 6 weeks."
d. "I can expect to have abdominal pain and nausea for a few weeks, but it will get better."

At his 6-week follow-up appointment, T.B. reports that he feels "so much better" and has not had any problems with foods. He has lost 10 pounds (4.5 kg) and has taken up nature photography as a hobby.

12 Infection and Inflammation

Case Study **125**

Name_____ Class/Group_____ Date_____

▶ **Scenario**

J.J., a 79-year-old woman with a history of COPD and renal insufficiency, was hospitalized for pneumonia for over a month. While hospitalized, she received intravenous clindamycin and steroids. She was discharged a week ago on oral antibiotics and steroids. This morning, she developed severe, watery diarrhea that has a strong odor and abdominal pain. This evening, her daughter took her to the emergency department because J.J. had become extremely weak and drowsy, with some confusion. Her vital signs are: BP 100/68, P 118, R 24, T 100.5° F (38.1° C). Her daughter stated, "All of a sudden she had terrible diarrhea, about 8 or 9 times, and she said her belly hurt. She hasn't eaten a thing all day, and I could not get her to drink anything." An IV of 0.9% normal saline at 125 mL/hr was started.

Chart View

Physician's Orders
Normal saline IV at 125 mL/hr
Obtain stool specimen for culture, O&P and *C. Diff* PCR assay
CBC, basic metabolic panel
Admit to medical-surgical department
Clear liquids as tolerated
BRP with assistance only

1. Describe the correct way to obtain a stool specimen for these tests.

2. What problem is J.J. most at risk for because of the diarrhea?

3. Which signs and symptoms occur with fluid volume deficit? Select all that apply.
   a. Weakness
   b. Confusion
   c. Decreased pulse
   d. Increased urine output
   e. Dry mucous membranes

The *Clostridium difficile* PCR results are positive. The hospitalist visits J.J. and tells her daughter that J.J. has an antibiotic-associated *C. difficile* infection (CDI).

4. Explain CDI and the significance of the positive *C. diff* PCR result.

5. What likely led J.J. to develop CDI?

6. How is CDI spread to others?

7. Describe the precautions needed for the suspected diagnosis of CDI to prevent the spread of disease.

8. As J.J.'s daughter leaves the room to go home, the nurse notices that she removed the gown and gloves without washing her hands afterward. Which actions by the nurse are appropriate?
   a. Nothing, because the daughter is going home.
   b. Ask the daughter to wash her hands when she gets home.
   c. Remind the daughter to wash her hands immediately with soap and water.
   d. Remind the daughter to wash her hands with the alcohol-based hand cleanser.

CASE STUDY PROGRESS

The hospitalist orders vancomycin, 250 mg PO 4 times a day. When the nurse comes in to give J.J. the first dose, her daughter asks, "If this was caused by an antibiotic, why is she getting another antibiotic now?"

12 Infection and Inflammation

9. What is the nurse's best response to the daughter's question?
   a. "You're right! I'll check with the hospitalist about this."
   b. "The antibiotic will cause the bowel's normal bacteria to grow."
   c. "We need to make sure she does not develop pneumonia again."
   d. "This antibiotic works directly in the bowel to kill the organism that is causing the diarrhea."

10. Which adverse effects are possible with oral vancomycin? Select all that apply.
   a. Nausea
   b. Tachycardia
   c. Nephrotoxicity
   d. Mouth irritation
   e. Red rash on the face, neck, upper torso

11. True or False? Oral vancomycin is poorly absorbed by the GI tract.

12. J.J.'s daughter asks, "Can you give her some medicine to stop the diarrhea?" What is your response?

13. Which nursing action should the charge nurse delegate to the LPN/LVN?
   a. Performing regular assessments of J.J.'s hydration status.
   b. Reviewing J.J.'s medical history for any risk factors for CDI.
   c. Giving the ordered vancomycin 250 mg PO 4 times a day.
   d. Explaining the purpose of the IV fluids to the patient and her family.

Over the next few days, J.J. continues to have frequent diarrhea stools. She is able to take some clear liquids, and she is less confused. She is able to make it to the bathroom for most of her bowel movements, but does have occasional incontinence.

14. List at least 4 problems that are high priorities in J.J.'s continued care.

15. What interventions would you implement to meet the expected outcome of maintaining perineal skin integrity?

16. Fecal microbiota transplantation (FMT) is a possible treatment for CDI. Explain this process.

J.J.'s diarrhea finally stopped after 5 days of treatment, and she started physical therapy (PT) to regain her strength. She was discharged to a skilled care facility to continue PT for strengthening and endurance.

12 Infection and Inflammation

Case Study 126

Name_____ Class/Group _____ Date_____

▶ Scenario

R.O. is a 12-year-old girl who lives with her family on a farm in a rural community. R.O. has 4 siblings who have recently been ill with stomach pains, vomiting, diarrhea, and fever. They were seen by their primary care provider (PCP) and diagnosed with viral gastroenteritis. A week later, R.O. woke up at 0200 crying and telling her mother that her stomach "hurts really bad!" She had an elevated temperature of 37.9° C (100.2° F). R.O. began to vomit over the next few hours, so her parents took her to the local emergency department (ED). R.O.'s vital signs, complete blood count, and complete metabolic panel were normal, so she was hydrated with IV fluids and discharged to home with instructions for her parents to call their PCP or to return to the ED if her condition did not improve or if it worsened. Over the next 2 days, R.O.'s abdominal pain localized to the right lower quadrant, she refused to eat, and she had slight diarrhea. On the third day, she began to have more severe abdominal pain, increased vomiting, and fever that did not respond to acetaminophen. R.O. has returned to the ED. Her VS are 128/78, 130, 28, 39.5° C (103.1° F). R.O. is guarding her lower abdomen, prefers to lie on her side with her legs flexed, and is crying. IV access is established, and morphine sulfate 2 mg IV is administered for pain. R.O.'s white blood count is 12,000 mm³ (12 x 10⁹/L).

1. Which findings are common clinical manifestations of appendicitis? Select all that apply.
   a. Fever
   b. Diarrhea
   c. Vomiting
   d. Arthralgia
   e. Constipation
   f. Diffuse rash
   g. Left lower quadrant abdominal pain

2. Discuss why R.O.'s presenting clinical manifestations make diagnosis more difficult. Identify 2 other possible diagnoses.

An abdominal CT scan confirms that R.O. has appendicitis. The ED physician has written orders.

3. Note whether the orders are appropriate or inappropriate and give a rationale for each response.

Chart View

Emergency Department Orders

1. Make patient NPO
2. Place a peripheral IV and begin D_5 ½ NS at 80 mL/hr
3. Administer Fleet Enema now to rule out impaction
4. Administer morphine sulfate 2 mg IV q2hr for pain
5. Obtain surgical consent from patient
6. Administer cefotaxime (Claforan) IVPB, at 50 mg/kg STAT

4. R.O.'s weight is 42 kg, and her height is 155 cm. Calculate her bolus fluid dose (20 mL/kg) and her maintenance fluid needs once fluid resuscitation has occurred and discuss how these will be met.

12   Infection and Inflammation

5. R.O.'s parents give informed consent, and R.O. assents to the surgery after the procedure is explained to her. Why is it important for R.O. to provide her assent for the procedure?

6. What should be included in the preoperative teaching for R.O. and her parents?

CASE STUDY PROGRESS

R.O. undergoes an appendectomy; the appendix has ruptured. The peritoneum is inflamed and abscesses are seen near the colon and small intestine. R.O. is admitted to the surgical unit from the postanesthesia care unit (PACU). She is NPO and has a nasogastric tube (NGT), Foley catheter, IV line, abdominal dressing, and a Penrose drain.

7. Identify the priority nursing considerations at this time. Select all that apply.
   a. Pain
   b. Wound infection
   c. Skin integrity changes
   d. Potential hypothermia
   e. Cardiac output changes
   f. Reduced bowel function
   g. Changed family processes
   h. Potential fluid and electrolyte imbalance

CASE STUDY PROGRESS

On postoperative day 2, R.O. continues to improve and is tolerating ice chips. Breath sounds are clear, and she is performing her pulmonary hygiene. The NGT has minimal drainage. The Foley catheter and Penrose drain have been removed, and her urine output is adequate. Her IV line is saline-locked. The incision is well approximated with no drainage or redness. Her pain is 4 to 6 of 10 with pain medication every 4 hours.

Later that evening your assessment shows that R.O. is pale and listless; bowel sounds are absent; abdomen is distended and tender to the touch; and the NGT is draining an increased amount of dark, greenish black fluid. Her lung sounds are moist bilaterally, and her temperature has spiked to 40.2° C (104.4° F), O_2 saturation is 97% on room air. She rates her pain at 10 of 10 and is having difficulty taking deep breaths because of the pain, which she says "hurts over my whole stomach."

8. What actions would you take?

9. Using SBAR, what would you communicate to the surgeon?

10. What will you consider as part of your nursing management of R.O.'s pain?

The surgeon assesses R.O. and orders an immediate return to the operating room. R.O. returns to surgery, where she has lysis of adhesions, removal of necrotic bowel, and drainage of an abscess. The surgeon has left her abdominal wound open and has ordered wound packing changes twice daily and abdominal irrigation with normal saline. R.O. cries and becomes agitated when you go to perform the procedure.

11. Which pain and coping concept would you question as you assist R.O. to prepare for the procedure? Explain your answer.
   a. R. may fear loss of control during the dressing change.
   b. R. is concerned about privacy during the dressing change.
   c. Prior coping strategies can be used to prepare for the dressing change.
   d. R. may fear separation from family members during painful experiences.

12. In anticipation of R.O.'s discharge, identify expected outcomes that must be achieved before discharge from the hospital.

After a week, R.O. continues to meet expected outcomes, with her wound healing well. Her discharge to home is planned for the next day. You provide discharge teaching to R.O. and her parents.

13. Using the Teach-Back technique, you ask the parents to reflect back what they have learned. Which statements would indicate that more teaching is required? Explain your answer.
   a. "We need to return if R.O. begins vomiting again or develops a fever."
   b. "R.O. should wait 1 week before returning to her gymnastics program."
   c. "We will keep the incision clean and call if we see redness or drainage."
   d. "R.O. can advance her diet to most of the regular foods she likes to eat."

R.O. is discharged to home with her parents and has an uneventful recovery. She is scheduled for a follow-up visit with the surgeon in 2 weeks.

12 Infection and Inflammation

Case Study 127

Name _____ Class/Group _____ Date _____

▶ Scenario

M.R., who is 81 years old, lives alone in a senior citizens' apartment complex. After she missed several planned holiday activities, and a neighbor knocked on her door to check on her. M.R. answered the door and said that she has had a cold for 4 days and did not want to spread it to others. She said, "It happened so fast, and it just won't go away. It seems to be getting worse no matter what I do." She said she felt very achy and weak, with a headache, and has had no appetite, but did not want to bother her son, who is very busy with his job. M.R.'s neighbor convinced her to call her health care provider (HCP), whose office is in the same building. The nurse at the office asked M.R. to come immediately for a visit. When she arrived at the office, the HCP called for an ambulance to take M.R. to the hospital. You place a mask on M.R. in anticipation that she may have influenza. M.R. has a history of hyperlipidemia and osteoarthritis in her knees.

1. What causes influenza?

2. Listed below are characteristics of the common cold and influenza. Mark with an "I" the ones that are typical to influenza only.
   _____ Abrupt onset
   _____ Gradual onset
   _____ Fever
   _____ Headache
   _____ Exhaustion
   _____ Sore throat, stuffy nose, sneezing
   _____ May be prevented with a vaccine

3. What symptoms indicate that M.R. has influenza? Provide rationale for your answer.

4. Are there any diagnostic tests for influenza? Will they be used for M.R.? Explain.

M.R. is admitted to a general medical unit and placed on droplet precautions. She is instructed to remain on bed rest with bathroom privileges, and "Fall Risk" measures are posted because of her weakness. An IV of D$_5$ ½ NS at 75 mL/hr is started. In addition to her home medication for hyperlipidemia, other orders include acetaminophen, 650 mg PO every 4 hours as needed for pain or for temperature over 101° F (38.3° C). Her vital signs are BP 110/72, P 110, R 13, T 102.4° F (39.1° C). She is told by the admitting HCP that she most likely has the flu.

5. M.R. states, "How can I have the flu? I had a flu shot last year!" What is your response?

6. According to the Centers for Disease Control and Prevention (CDC), when is the flu season and when is the best time to receive the vaccine?

7. Which of these statements about droplet precautions is correct?
   a. These precautions are used to prevent the spread of tuberculosis.
   b. Droplet precautions prevent the spread of pathogens by direct contact.
   c. Droplet precautions are used to protect the patient from pathogens that may be carried by health care workers.
   d. These precautions are used to minimize contact with pathogens that are spread to the respiratory tract through the air.

The HCP also orders oseltamivir (Tamiflu), 75 mg PO twice daily for 5 days. M.R. expresses relief that she is receiving this drug because "it will cure the flu."

8. True or false? Tamiflu cures the flu.

9. Explain the reason for the order for Tamiflu, even though M.R. has had the flu for several days.

10. Which measures will be part of M.R.'s treatment as she recovers from influenza? Select all that apply.
   a. Rest
   b. Hydration
   c. Antibiotics
   d. Analgesics
   e. Low protein diet

11. Which assessment findings if noted with M.R., would continue to concern you? Select all that apply.
   a. Fever
   b. Dyspnea
   c. Confusion
   d. Sore throat
   e. Dry mucous membranes
   f. Diffuse crackles over the lung fields

12. Specify the potential complications that may occur in a person with influenza.

CASE STUDY PROGRESS

At the change of shift, M.R. calls for help to get up to the bathroom. Before the UAP arrived, M.R. decided to get up by herself and fell. The UAP found her in the floor and called for help. M.R. was placed back into the bed and you assess her. M.R. said she did not hit her head and told the nurse she thinks she hurt her left knee. The on-call hospitalist was notified, and an x-ray of the knee showed no break.

 13. What placed M.R. a risk for falls when she was admitted?

14. Name at least 4 measures to prevent future falls.

15. Per the hospital's policy, an incident report will need to be completed after M.R.'s fall. Which statement about an incident report is correct?
   a. It is completed only if the patient is injured.
   b. The nurse will give it to M.R. for her to complete.
   c. It becomes part of M.R.'s permanent medical record.
   d. It will be sent to the Risk Management department after completion.

CASE STUDY OUTCOME

M.R. is discharged back to her apartment, but she still gets easily tired from activity. Over the next few weeks, she gradually returns to her usual activities. At the 6-week checkup, her HCP offers her the flu shot. "It's still wintertime, and even though you've had the flu, this may still offer some immunity against other strains of the flu." M.R. agrees to receive the vaccine. She plans to get the influenza vaccine next year in early September.

12 Infection and Inflammation

Case Study **128**

Name_____ Class/Group_____ Date_____

▶ Scenario

Three-year-old C.E. is admitted to the emergency department fast track clinic. Her mother tells the nurse that C.E. has had a low-grade fever for 2 days and is complaining frequently of ear pain and a sore throat. C.E.'s mother also notes that C.E. has been coughing and is a little hoarse. C.E.'s mother states that C.E.'s appetite has been "off," but she has been drinking and using the bathroom as usual. As you get C.E. settled in the exam room, you suspect C.E. may have otitis media (OM).

1. Place an arrow where you suspect fluid would be found.

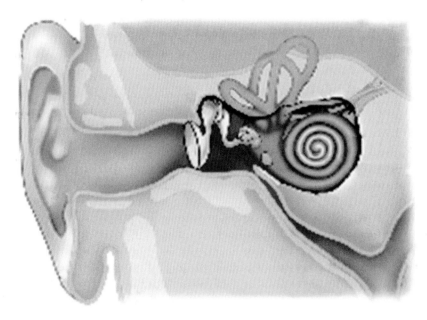

2. What routine information regarding risk factors for OM would you want to obtain from C.E.'s mother?

3. C.E.'s mother asks, "Why does C. keep getting ear infections? Is there something I should do?" Explain the etiology of ear infections.

CASE STUDY PROGRESS

You continue to obtain a history from C.E.'s mother and learn C.E. has had "ear problems" and throat infections since she was a baby. She is in day care each weekday, the father smokes outside of the house, and there is a family history of seasonal allergies. C.E. is allergic to penicillin. Her weight is 14 kg (31 lbs).

4. Describe what you will include in your physical examination and assessment with rationales.

CASE STUDY PROGRESS

The primary care provider (PCP) diagnoses C.E. with bilateral AOM and strep pharyngitis. C.E. is given a prescription for Augmentin 600 mg twice daily PO × 7 days and her mother is instructed to give acetaminophen 240 mg every 4 hours as needed for pain. She is to be discharged to home with instructions to follow up with the ear, nose, and throat (ENT) specialist.

5. You review the orders before completing discharge teaching. What is your first action?

CASE STUDY PROGRESS

C.E.'s mother is given a new prescription for azithromycin (Zithromax) PO 160 mg/day × 5 days. Azithromycin is dispensed as 200 mg/5 mL.

6. Calculate how much azithromycin C.E.'s mother needs to administer to C.E., and mark the amount on the oral syringe below.

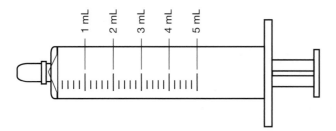

7. Calculate the therapeutic dose/range for each medication and indicate whether the ordered dose is safe and therapeutic.

8. You are providing C.E.'s mother with information on medication administration. You use the Teach-Back technique to assess C.E.'s mother's learning. Which statements by C.E.'s mother indicates need for further teaching? Select all that apply, and explain your answers.
   a. "This medicine can be given with or without food."
   b. "I don't have to finish the medication if she feels better after a few days."
   c. "I will place the correct amount of antibiotic in the ear canal once a day."
   d. "If C. refuses to take her medication, I will tell her it tastes like the candy we get at the movies."
   e. "I will monitor for vomiting, diarrhea, or stomachaches because this might be a side effect of the medication."

9. C.E.'s mother asks when C.E. can return to day care. Which statement is your best response?
   a. "She should be able to return in about a week."
   b. "She can return 48 hours after her last documented normal temperature."
   c. "She can return 24 hours after her last documented normal temperature."
   d. "She can return 24 hours after she starts her antibiotics and is free of fever."

CASE STUDY PROGRESS

C.E.'s mother takes C.E. to an ENT specialist. It is determined that her enlarged tonsils might be contributing to the frequent throat and ear infections, and a tonsillectomy and adenoidectomy (T&A) is scheduled. She is admitted postoperatively for 24-hour observation. After the surgery, the postoperative nurse receives C.E. in the short-stay unit from the postanesthesia care unit (PACU). C.E. is awake and alert, bilateral breath sounds are clear, and her O$_2$ saturation is 98% on room air. She has tolerated sips of clear fluids, and her parents are with her.

10. Which orders would you expect to see postoperatively? Select all that apply, and discuss the rationale for each choice.
   a. Ice collar as tolerated
   b. Vital signs q4hr and prn
   c. Clear liquids; advance to regular toddler diet
   d. Home prescription for amoxicillin (Amoxil) 120 mg PO q8hr
   e. Methylprednisolone (Solu-Medrol) 2.3 mg IV q8hr × 3 doses
   f. Aggressively gargle and swish with water after eating or drinking
   g. Acetaminophen (Tylenol) 210 mg (15 mg/kg) PO q4hr prn for pain
   h. Maintain peripheral IV with D$_5$ ½ NS at 50 mL/hr; saline lock when taking PO well

11. State at least 2 nursing interventions for each of these commonly encountered nursing problems during the postoperative phase of care.
   a. Airway
   b. Pain
   c. Fluid and electrolyte balance
   d. Bleeding risk

12. C.E. is able to verbalize discomfort to you and her mother. Which pain rating scales would be most appropriate? Explain your answer.
   a. 1 to 10 scale
   b. Neonatal Infant Pain Scale (NIPS)
   c. Oucher or Wong Baker FACES Pain Rating Scale
   d. Face, Legs, Activity, Cry, Consolability (FLACC) scale

13. You are reviewing discharge instructions with C.E.'s mother. She asks, "How would I know if we need to come back?" Discuss common findings and when C.E.'s mother would need to seek immediate medical attention for C.E.

CASE STUDY OUTCOME

C.E.'s mother indicates an understanding of discharge instructions and follow-up care. C.E. continues to take oral fluids well, meets discharge criteria, and is discharged to home to follow up with the ENT physician in 2 weeks.

12 Infection and Inflammation

Case Study **129**

Name_____ Class/Group_____ Date_____

▶ Scenario

J.D., age 45, noticed a red spot on his calf after a day of yard work. It did not bother him at first, and he thought it may have been a spider bite. The next morning, he noticed that the spot had grown to the size of a nickel, and it was hardened and very painful. His wife asked him to get it checked, but he said he could take care of it, and tried to pierce it with a pocketknife he had sterilized with a match in an attempt to drain it. Nothing came out when he tried this, so he put some antibacterial ointment over it and covered it with a bandage. Two days later, he realized that the wound was draining yellowish fluid, and the skin around the wound was red and tender. He decides to see his health care provider (HCP), who told J.D. that he had developed cellulitis around the wound, which was infected.

1. What is cellulitis? What contributed to the development of cellulitis in J.D.'s situation?

2. The HCP obtains wound cultures. Which statements reflect the correct technique for obtaining an aerobic wound culture? Select all that apply.
    a. Swab the drainage that is present on the bandage.
    b. Collect from the edges of the wound near the skin.
    c. Label the specimen tube before sending it to the lab.
    d. Collect from an area of fresh drainage from within the wound.
    e. Remove old exudate from the wound before obtaining a specimen.

3. Explain the difference between an aerobic and an anaerobic wound culture.

J.D. is sent home with a prescription for doxycycline capsules. Two days later, the results from the cultures are reported to the HCP. J.D. is asked to go to the hospital for treatment for a MRSA infection.

Chart View

Wound Culture and Sensitivity Report

Staphylococcus aureus (MRSA)	≥100,000 colonies
Amoxicillin	R
Ceftriaxone	R
Ciprofloxacin	R
Clindamycin	R
Doxycycline	R
Levofloxacin	R
Linezolid	S
Trimethoprim-sulfa	R
Vancomycin	R

Anaerobic Culture

No growth after 2 days

4. What is "MRSA," and what are the implications of this infection?

5. Explain the "R" and the "S" results on the culture report. Which drug will be chosen to treat J.D.'s infection, based on the report?

6. Differentiate CA-MRSA and HA-MRSA. Which one does J.D. have?

7. What do you need to assess before beginning antibiotic therapy?

8. Which class of medications, if on J.D.'s list of current medications, would be of concern if taken with linezolid?
   a. Aspirin
   b. Beta blockers
   c. Benzodiazepines
   d. Selective serotonin reuptake inhibitor

CASE STUDY PROGRESS

Contact Precautions are implemented. In addition to intravenous linezolid antibiotic treatment, the HCP performs an incision and drainage procedure. Wound care is ordered every 12 hours with sterile normal saline wet-to-dry dressings.

 9. Does J.D. also need to be on Standard Precautions? Explain your answer.

 10. You are about to enter J.D.'s room to give the IV linezolid. Which measures are appropriate for Contact Precautions for wound MRSA? Select all that apply.
   a. Donning gloves
   b. Wearing a gown
   c. Wearing eye protection
   d. Wearing a mask to prevent inhalation of droplets.
   e. Handwashing before entering and upon leaving the patient's room.

11. In addition to the antibiotic, J.D. receives methylprednisolone, 10 mg IV every 6 hours. What is the purpose of this drug?
   a. For antiinflammatory effects
   b. To make the antibiotic more effective
   c. As a second antibiotic to fight MRSA
   d. To reduce pain during routine wound care

12. What potential complications may occur if this wound is not treated properly?

13. Which nursing actions are appropriate to delegate to the UAP? Select all that apply.
   a. Taking vital signs
   b. Assessment of the wound
   c. Obtaining a wound culture
   d. Teaching about wound care
   e. Changing the sterile dressing
   f. Maintaining contact precautions

14. What will you assess during wound care?

15. What is the most important action you can do to promote comfort when it is time to do a dressing change?

CASE STUDY PROGRESS

After 7 days of IV antibiotic therapy, the wound shows signs of healing, and J.D.'s is prescribed an oral antibiotic for the next 14 days. You are providing teaching about oral antibiotic therapy and wound care.

16. Which statement by J.D. reflects correct understanding of the antibiotic therapy?
   a. "I will finish this prescription of antibiotics."
   b. "I will stop the antibiotic when the wound is healed."
   c. "If I have bad side effects, I will stop taking the antibiotic and let the doctor know at my next visit."
   d. "I will stop taking the antibiotic when the wound is healed, but start again if the infection returns."

17. What teaching will you provide to J.D. to prevent this from happening again?

CASE STUDY OUTCOME

After 2 weeks, J.D.'s wound has almost healed. He completed the full course of antibiotics. At his last visit to his HCP, his wound was noted to be scabbed over and the redness and tenderness surrounding it was almost gone.

12 Infection and Inflammation

Case Study **130**

Name_____ Class/Group_____ Date_____

▶ **Scenario**

P.S., a 76-year-old woman, was brought to the emergency department (ED) by ambulance after her husband found her sitting on the side of the bed, awake but nonverbal. She has a history of chronic atrial fibrillation, osteoarthritis, and hypertension. Her current medications include diltiazem, carvedilol, and dabigatran. Upon arrival to the ED, she was sent for a STAT CT scan, then evaluated by the Stroke Team nurse. Her initial vital signs include BP 110/60, P 158, R 20, T 100.8° F (38.2° C). She weighs 198 pounds (90 kg).

1. Name at least 2 risk factors P.S. has that led to the evaluation for a stroke.

2. What other things will you ask about when completing the history?

CASE STUDY PROGRESS

The CT scan results were normal, and the NIHSS Stroke score was rated as zero. The ED physician orders lab work, which has been drawn. P.S. asks to use the bedpan, and her urine was noted to be dark orange, cloudy, with a strong odor. You perform a point of care urinalysis and, suspecting a urinary tract infection (UTI), send a specimen for culture and sensitivity. A second set of vital signs are recorded: BP 98/58, P 164, R 18, T 101.6° F (38.7° C).

Chart View

Laboratory Test Values

Sodium	150 mEq/L (150 mmol/L)
Potassium	4.8 mEq/L (4.8 mmol/L)
Chloride	100 mEq/L (100 mmol/L)
CO_2	25 mEq/L (25 mmol/L)
Glucose	104 mg/dL (5.8 mmol/L)
BUN	10 mg/dL (3.6 mmol/L)
Creatinine	1.2 mg/dL (106 mcmol/L)
Lactic acid	3.2 mg/dL (3.6 mmol/L)
WBC	18.6 1000/mm³ (18.6 x 10⁹/L)
Hgb	14 g/dL (140 g/L)
Hct	40.9%
Platelet	211,000 /mm³ (211 x 10⁹/L)

3. Which lab results concern you and why?

4. The ED physician suspects that P.S. has sepsis. Explain sepsis.

5. After reviewing P.S.'s assessment, which findings reflect positive SIRS criteria? Select all that apply.
   a. Elevated pulse
   b. Elevated temperature
   c. Elevated sodium level
   d. Decreased blood pressure
   e. Elevated white blood cell count

6. Do any of P.S.'s assessment findings indicate organ dysfunction? Provide rationale.

CASE STUDY PROGRESS

Based on the possible urinary tract infection, positive SIRS criteria, and elevated lactic acid level, P.S. is diagnosed with severe sepsis. The physician gives new orders for ceftriaxone 1 gram every 12 hours IVPB; blood cultures × 2; lactic acid every 4 hours × 2; IV bolus of Normal Saline (NS), 30 mL/kg; and O_2 at 2 L per nasal cannula. She is to be transferred to the progressive care unit.

7. Will you administer the ceftriaxone first, or obtain the lab work first? Provide rationale for your choice.

 8. Calculate the dose of the IV NS bolus.

9. What is the purpose of the fluid bolus?

CASE STUDY PROGRESS

P.S. is transferred to the progressive care unit. Current vital signs are BP 108/72; P 148; R 18; T 100.4° F (38° C). P.S. seems more alert and is asking what has happened. When told that she is in the hospital, she states, "I don't even remember getting here!" You explain to P.S. that she is receiving antibiotics for a serious infection and ask P.S. how long her urine had looked dark and cloudy. P.S. replied, "It's been a week or so. I just didn't want to bother anyone."

10. The nurse discusses with P.S. the importance of reporting the signs and symptoms of a UTI and reviews the importance of proper perineal hygiene. Which statement by P.S. indicates that she understands instructions?
a. "If I think I have a urine infection, I will start an antihistamine."
b. "If I drink enough cranberry juice, I won't get any urine infections."
c. "I will be sure to wipe from back to front when I use the bathroom."
d. "If I think I'm getting another infection, I will call my doctor right away."

11. Which tasks are appropriate to assign to the UAP assisting you with P.S.'s care? Select all that apply.
   a. Take vital signs.
   b. Assist P.S. to walk to the bathroom.
   c. Assess P.S.'s lung and heart sounds.
   d. Provide teaching about her sepsis diagnosis.
   e. Attach P.S. to portable telemetry monitoring.

CASE STUDY PROGRESS

P.S.'s second lactic acid level results are 2.8 mg/dL (3.1 mmol/L), and her vital signs are BP 118/72, P 136, R 18, T 100.2° F (37.9° C). She is awake, alert, and asking for dinner.

12. Interpret her lactic acid level. What does the result indicate?

13. P.S. will stay in the progressive care unit for another 24 hours, then will be transferred to a medical/telemetry unit before she is discharged. During this time, what is your priority action?

CASE STUDY OUTCOME

P.S. is discharged after 3 days in the hospital. At her 1 month follow-up checkup, she tells her provider that she "has not felt strong" since she was hospitalized and hopes to regain her strength soon.

Developmental

Case Study **131**

Name_____ Class/Group_____ Date_____

▶ **Scenario**

P.M. comes to the obstetric (OB) clinic because she has missed 2 menstrual periods and thinks she might be pregnant. She states she is nauseated, especially in the morning, so she completed a home pregnancy test and she reports that the result was positive. As the intake nurse in the clinic, you are responsible for gathering information before she sees the physician.

1. What are the 2 most important questions to ask to determine possible pregnancy?

2. You ask whether she has ever been pregnant, and she tells you she has never been pregnant. How would you record this information?

3. What additional information would be needed to complete the TPAL record?

4. It is important to complete the intake interview. What categories will you address with P.M.?

CASE STUDY PROGRESS

Per the clinic protocol, you obtain the following for her prenatal record: Complete blood count, blood type with Rh factor, urine for urinalysis (protein, glucose, blood), vital signs, height, and weight. In addition, the pregnancy is confirmed with a blood or urine hCG test and an ultrasound. Next, the nurse-midwife performs a physical examination, which includes a pelvic examination. The examination and tests confirm that P.M. is pregnant. P.M. has a gynecoid pelvis by measurement, and the fetus is at approximately 6 weeks' gestation.

Chart View

Vital Signs

Blood pressure	116/74
Heart rate	88
Respiratory rate	16
Temperature	98.9° F (37.2° C)

5. Do any of these vital signs cause concern? What should you do?

6. P.M. tells you that the date of her last menstrual period (LMP) was February 2. How would you calculate her due date? What is her due date?

7. What is the significance of a gynecoid pelvis?

8. What specimens are important to obtain when the pelvic examination is done?

CASE STUDY PROGRESS

Nursing interventions focus on monitoring the mother and fetus for growth and development, and detecting potential complications. Educating P.M. about the importance of proper nutrition, managing the common discomforts of pregnancy, and activities of self-care will help in the wellbeing of her and her baby.

9. A psychological assessment is done to determine P.M.'s feelings and attitudes regarding her pregnancy. How do attitudes, beliefs, and feelings affect pregnancy?

10. P.M. asks you whether there are any foods she should avoid while pregnant. She lists some of her favorite foods. Which foods, if any, should she avoid eating while she is pregnant? Select all that apply.
    a. Sushi
    b. Yogurt
    c. Hot dogs
    d. Deli meat
    e. Cheddar cheese

11. As the nurse, you understand that assessment and teaching are vital in the prenatal period to ensure a positive outcome. What information is important to include at every visit and at specific times during the pregnancy?

12. After her examination, P.M. states that she is worried because her sister had an ectopic pregnancy and had to have surgery. She asks you, "What are the signs of an ectopic pregnancy?" Identify the correct response. Select all that apply.
    a. Nausea
    b. Increased fatigue
    c. Dark red or brown vaginal bleeding
    d. Fullness and tenderness in her abdomen, near the ovaries
    e. Pain, either unilateral, bilateral, or diffuse over the abdomen

13. P.M. asks the nurse about what should be reported to her doctor. List at least 6 of the danger signs during pregnancy.

14. Common changes in the body caused by pregnancy include relaxation of joints, altered center of gravity, syncope, and generalized discomfort. These changes can lead to problems with coordination and balance. After a teaching session about safety measures, you use the Teach-Back technique to assess P.M.'s understanding. Which statement by P.M. indicates a need for more teaching?

a. "I will take rest periods throughout the day."
b. "I will always wear a helmet when riding my bike."
c. "I will avoid activities that cause sudden, jarring moves to my body."
d. "Later in my pregnancy, I won't use a seatbelt in the car because I'll be too big."

15. P.M. asks, "Is a vaginal examination done at every visit?" Select the best response and provide a rationale for your answer.

a. "No, a vaginal examination will not be done again until you go into labor."
b. "No, vaginal examinations are not routinely done until the final weeks of your pregnancy."
c. "Yes, an examination is done with each visit because it offers vital information about the status of the pregnancy."
d. "Yes, an examination is done with each visit because it allows the examiner to note any possible infections that may be developing."

CASE STUDY OUTCOME

P.M. makes an appointment for her next checkup. She is excited and cannot wait to tell her family that she is pregnant.

Case Study **132**

Name_____ Class/Group_____ Date_____

▶ Scenario

You are the charge nurse working in labor and delivery at a local hospital. D.H. arrives, reporting contractions and feeling somewhat uncomfortable. You take her to the triage room to provide privacy, have her change into a gown, and begin your assessment to determine your next course of action.

1. What 4 initial questions will you ask, and why?

2. D.H.'s contractions are 2 to 3 minutes apart and lasting 45 seconds. It is her third pregnancy (gravida 3, para 2-0-0-2). She tells you that she is 39 weeks pregnant and she is due to deliver in 3 days. Before performing a vaginal exam, you would need to ask D.H. addition information. What additional information do you need?

3. What assessment should you make to gain further information from D.H.?

4. On examination, D.H. is 80% effaced and 4 cm dilated. The fetal heart rate (FHR) is 150 and regular. She is admitted to a labor and delivery room on the unit. What nursing measures should be done at this time?

5. As part of your assessment, you review the fetal heart rate strip pictured here. Based on the findings, what is your intervention?

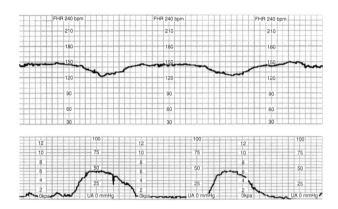

6. Identify the stage of labor D.H. is experiencing

7. List the stages of labor.

8. How long does labor last?

9. D.H. states she is feeling increasing discomfort and asks you whether there is alternative therapy available before taking a medication. List at least 4 alternative methods to assist D.H. with controlling her discomfort.

10. As you assess both D.H. and the fetus during the active stage of labor, you will monitor for potential abnormalities. Identify which potential abnormalities you may encounter in your assessment. Select all that apply.
   a. Unusual bleeding
   b. Sudden, severe pain
   c. Increased maternal fatigue
   d. Brown or greenish amniotic fluid
   e. Decelerations of the fetal heart rate
   f. Contractions that last 40 to 70 seconds

CASE STUDY PROGRESS

Although D.H. continues to use alternative therapies for discomfort, she asks for pain medication and receives a dose of meperidine (Demerol). She is also placed on an oxytocin (Pitocin) infusion.

11. What is the purpose of the oxytocin infusion?
   a. To reduce pain.
   b. To stimulate uterine contractions.
   c. To prevent maternal hypertension.
   d. To increase cervical effacement and dilation.

CASE STUDY PROGRESS

Three hours later, D.H. is lying on her back, and during contractions you notice a few late decelerations of the FHR. You stay with D.H. to monitor her and her fetus and immediately call for someone to notify the primary care provider.

12. Put these actions in order of priority:
   a. Discontinue the oxytocin infusion.
   b. Increase the rate of the maintenance IV fluids.
   c. Turn D.H. onto her left side and elevate her legs.
   d. Administer oxygen at 8 to 10 L/min by nonrebreather face mask.

13. Decelerations occur in an early, variable, or late pattern. What is the significance of these patterns? State what the nurse should do for each type.

13 Developmental

14. As you monitor D.H., you observe for signs of umbilical cord prolapse. Describe what this is and what can happen to the fetus if this occurs.

15. Describe your interventions if you were to note that D.H. has umbilical cord prolapse.

CASE STUDY PROGRESS

The decelerations stop, and the rest of her labor is uneventful. D.H. has an episiotomy to allow more room for the infant to emerge, and she delivers a male infant.

16. What is involved in the immediate care of the newborn?

17. As you assess the newborn, you observe for central nervous system (CNS) depressant effects that might result because the mother received an opioid during labor. What drug would be helpful to reverse signs of CNS depression in the infant?
   a. Nalbuphine
   b. Naloxone (Narcan)
   c. Midazolam (Versed)
   d. Carbamazepine (Tegretol)

18. D.H. has her episiotomy repaired and the placenta delivered. What are the signs that the placenta has released from the uterine wall?

19. What assessments are important for D.H. after delivery?

CASE STUDY OUTCOME

D.H. and her newborn baby boy are taken to the maternity unit. DH begins to breastfeed him and all is well.

Case Study **133**

► **Scenario**

T.N. delivered a healthy male newborn 2 hours ago. She had a midline episiotomy and an epidural block for her labor and delivery. She is now admitted to the postpartum unit.

1. What is important to note in the initial assessment?

2. You find a boggy fundus during your assessment. What corrective measures can be instituted?

3. The patient complains of pain and discomfort in her perineal area. How will you respond?

 4. The nurse reviews the hospital security guidelines with T.N. The nurse points out that her baby has a special identification bracelet that matches a bracelet worn by T.N. and reviews other security procedures. Which statement by T.N. indicates a need for more teaching? Explain your answer.

   a. "Nurses on this unit all wear the same purple uniforms."

   b. "If I have a question about someone's identity, I can ask about it."

   c. "Each staff member who takes my baby somewhere will have a picture identification badge."

   d. "If someone takes my baby for an examination, that person will carry my baby to the examination room."

5. An hour after admission, you recheck T.N.'s perineal pad and notice there is a very small amount of drainage on the pad. What will you do next? Explain your answer.

   a. Ask T.N. to change her perineal pad.

   b. Check her perineal pad again in 1 hour.

   c. Check the pad underneath T.N.'s buttocks.

   d. Document the findings in T.N.'s medical record.

6. That evening, the unlicensed assistive personnel assesses T.N.'s vital signs. Which vital signs would be of concern at this time?

Chart View

Vital Signs

Temperature	99.9° F (37.7° C) oral
Pulse rate	120
Blood pressure	94/50
Respiratory rate	16

7. What will you do next?

8. After your prompt intervention, you need to document what happened. Write an example of a documentation entry describing this event.

9. Two hours later, you perform another perineal pad check and note the findings in the diagram. How will you describe the amount of drainage in your note?
   a. Scant
   b. Light
   c. Heavy
   d. Moderate

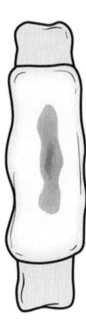

10. T.N.'s condition is stable and you prepare to provide patient teaching. Identify the key points in your patient teaching.

11. T.N. tells you she must go back to work in 6 weeks and is not sure she can continue breastfeeding. What options are available to her?

CASE STUDY OUTCOME

T.N. is seen by a lactation specialist before being discharged home. She plans to consult a lactation support group before returning to work.

13 Developmental

Case Study **134**

Name_____ Class/Group_____ Date_____

▶ **Scenario**

Y.C. was in labor for 12 hours and gave birth vaginally to Baby H, her first child. The nurse will complete the physical assessment and observe for physiologic changes in the newborn's transition from intrauterine to extrauterine life.

1. Name the 3 phases that occur during the newborn transition period and state an approximate time frame for each.

2. Identify the care specific to the first period of reactivity.

3. The sleep phase and second reactive phase might occur in the nursery or while the newborn is with the mother. Identify 8 assessments that the nurse needs to do during the transitional care periods of the decreased responsiveness and second period of reactivity.

4. You are preparing to give the injection of vitamin K (AquaMEPHYTON). The order is to give 0.5 mg subcutaneously on arrival in the nursery. The medication comes in a solution of 1 mg/0.5 mL. Calculate the medication dose you will draw up into the syringe.

5. Erythromycin ointment is instilled in both eyes to prevent which infection?
   a. Gonorrhea
   b. Chlamydia
   c. Herpes simplex virus infection
   d. Human papillomavirus (HPV) infection

6. Once the transitional care and documentation are completed, the infant might be transferred to the normal newborn nursery. The newborn nursery nurse is responsible for what ongoing care of the newborn infant?

13 Developmental

7. The lab performs a direct Coombs test on Baby H. What is the purpose of the direct Coombs test?
   a. It checks the RBCs for anemia.
   b. It is a test for immunity to the hepatitis virus.
   c. It is done to identify the infant's blood type.
   d. It tests for damage to the RBCs from maternal antibodies.

8. True or False? A phenylketonuria (PKU) blood test can be done any time before an infant is discharged to home. If false, explain your rationale.

CASE STUDY PROGRESS

Y.C. has decided to breastfeed her infant. She asks for assistance.

9. Identify 6 important points to include in your teaching plan.

10. Y.C. calls you to tell you that her baby seems too sleepy and is not feeding well. What will your next action be?

You are meeting with Y.C. to review discharge instructions.

11. Baby H.'s mother asks you about cord care and circumcision care for her infant. Your teaching instructions would include:

12. Y.C. asks you how she can keep her infant from catching a cold or some other type of infection. What is the most important measure to teach her?

13. After discharge, it is important for Baby H. to receive follow-up care. What information will you give to Y.C. to help her understand the importance of regular visits to the pediatrician?

 14. You realize Y.C. needs information about safety issues before being discharged. After a review of safety issues, you use the Teach-Back technique to assess her understanding. Which statement by Y.C. indicates that she needs further instruction?
a. "I will not drink hot coffee while holding my baby."
b. "I will check the bath water temperature before bathing him."
c. "I have a car seat and will use it for my baby every time we use the car."
d. "I can leave him on the infant table for just a few moments while he is a newborn."

CASE STUDY OUTCOME

Baby H. is discharged to home with his parents and will be seeing a pediatrician in the next 2 weeks for his follow up care.

Case Study **135**

Name_____   Class/Group_____   Date_____

▶ Scenario

P.T. is a married 30-year-old gravida 4, para 1-2-0-3 at 28 weeks' gestation. She arrives in the labor and delivery unit reporting lower back pain and frequency of urination. She states that she feels occasional uterine cramping and does not believe that her membranes have ruptured.

1. You are the charge nurse and admit P.T. to the unit. Based on her symptoms you suspect she may be experiencing signs of:

2. You need additional information from P.T. to direct your nursing interventions. What important questions do you need to ask P.T. at this time?

3. Identify the priority nursing interventions you would implement before calling the health care provider?

4. Early recognition of preterm labor is essential for a successful outcome. Explain the signs and symptoms of preterm labor.

5. What possible problems might be going on with P.T. that you should consider?

CASE STUDY PROGRESS

P.T.'s history reveals that she had 1 preterm delivery 4 years ago at 31 weeks' gestation. The newborn girl was in the neonatal intensive care unit (NICU) for 3 weeks and discharged without sequelae. The second preterm newborn, a boy, was delivered 2 years ago at 35 weeks' gestation and spent 4 days in the hospital before discharge. She has no other risk factors for preterm labor. Vital signs are normal. Her vaginal examination findings indicate her cervix to be long, closed, and thick with membranes intact. Abdominal examination revealed that the abdomen was nontender, with fundal height at 29 cm, and the fetus in a vertex presentation.

6. While you are waiting for lab results, what therapeutic measures do you consider?

7. The provider orders a loading dose of indomethacin (Indocin) 50 mg PO now, followed by 50 mg PO every 6 hours for up to 48 hours. Explain the purpose of the indomethacin.

8. Lifestyle modifications are required for P.T. because of the symptoms of preterm labor. Which activities would you discuss with P.T.?

13 Developmental

CASE STUDY PROGRESS

While waiting for lab results, you consider that if P.T. is actually experiencing preterm labor, she would receive antenatal glucocorticoids.

9. What is the reason for giving antenatal glucocorticoids for preterm labor?
   a. To soften the cervix
   b. To stop uterine contractions
   c. To prevent maternal infection
   d. To accelerate fetal lung maturity

10. How long do these drugs take to become effective?

11. Which situations are considered contraindications to antenatal glucocorticoids when a woman is in preterm labor? Select all that apply.
    a. Cord prolapse
    b. Chorioamnionitis
    c. Abruptio placentae
    d. Presence of twin fetuses
    e. Cervical dilation of 2.5 cm

CASE STUDY PROGRESS

Two hours later, the lab results indicate a urinary tract infection (UTI). The contraction monitor indicates infrequent, mild contractions. Her physician discharges her to home on an antibiotic for the UTI.

12. What follow-up measures should be considered in providing P.T. with discharge instructions?

CASE STUDY OUTCOME

P.T. completes the antibiotic that was prescribed for the UTI, and 2 weeks later her urine tests were negative for an infection. She has no further complications and delivers a healthy baby girl at 38 weeks.

Case Study 136

Name_____ Class/Group_____ Date_____

▶ Scenario

J.F. is an 18-year-old woman, gravida 1 para 0, at 38 weeks' gestation. She felt fine until 2 days ago, when she noticed swelling in her hands, feet, and face. She states she has a frontal headache, which started yesterday and has not been relieved by acetaminophen or coffee. She says she feels irritable and does not want the "overhead lights on." Her physician is admitting her for induction of labor. You begin to assess her.

Chart View

Assessment

Vital signs: BP 152/84; HR 88
Oral temperature: 98.8° F (37.1° C)
Weight: 186 lb (84.4 kg); height: 5 ft, 4 in (163 cm)
Edema: Noted in hands, feet, and face
Deep tendon reflexes (DTRs) +2, no clonus
Urine dipstick reveals proteinuria +3

1. Based on J.F.'s assessment data, what do you think the possible cause is at this time?

2. As you assess J.F. for edema in her ankles, you note that she is closest to letter B in the figure below, with edema at about 4 mm. How would you document this edema?

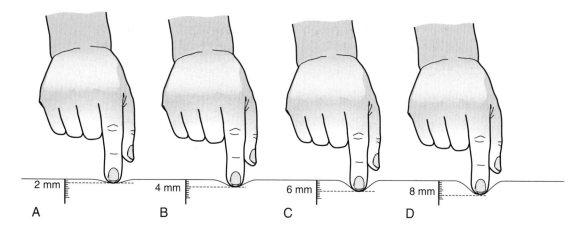

2 mm A   4 mm B   6 mm C   8 mm D

3. During your assessment, you note that her deep tendon reflexes (DTRs) are more brisk than expected or slightly hyperactive. How would you rate this DTR assessment?
   a. 1+
   b. 2+
   c. 3+
   d. 4+

4. You check her medical record and note that she has gained 8 pounds since her last visit, 1 week ago. What other assessment questions should you ask her at this time?

5. What information should you obtain from her obstetric record?

6. What lab values should be considered at this time?

7. Name at least 3 possible maternal and 3 possible fetal complications with J.F.'s potential diagnosis.

8. What risk factors does J.F. have that cause her to be at risk for this condition? Select all that apply.
   a. Obesity
   b. Nulliparity
   c. Coffee drinker
   d. Single-fetus pregnancy
   e. Age younger than 40 years

9. Based on your nursing assessment, identify 8 nursing interventions that you would implement to help J.F with her signs and symptoms.

CASE STUDY PROGRESS

The physician orders a magnesium sulfate infusion. You prepare the infusion and explain to J.F. what you are doing.

10. J.F. asks you, "Why am I getting magnesium now?" Explain your answer.

11. As you monitor J.F., you observe for signs of magnesium sulfate toxicity. What are potential signs of magnesium sulfate toxicity? Select all that apply.
    a. Oliguria
    b. Absent DTRs
    c. Muscle rigidity
    d. Severe hypotension
    e. Increased respiratory rate

12. Is there an antidote for magnesium sulfate?

CASE STUDY PROGRESS

An oxytocin infusion has been ordered by the physician and is being given intravenously in increments to achieve an adequate contraction pattern. You notice on the fetal monitor strip that J.F. is experiencing 7 uterine contractions in a 10-minute period over a 30-minute window, with late decelerations noted on the fetal monitor.

13. Explain what is happening at this time.

14. What are your priority interventions?

15. After your prompt intervention, J.F.'s tachysystole resolves. Write an example of a documentation entry describing this event.

CASE STUDY PROGRESS

J.F. progresses in labor, and at 4-cm dilation her membranes spontaneously rupture. The small amount of amniotic fluid is green.

16. What does the green amniotic fluid indicate? What are the risks?

CASE STUDY PROGRESS

Four hours later, J.F. delivers a 6-pound, 8-ounce (2948 grams) boy, with Apgar scores of 6 and 7.

17. What are your responsibilities at this time?

CASE STUDY OUTCOME

J.F. is hospitalized for 5 days. By the time of discharge, her BP was within normal limits and her edema had subsided. Her baby boy experienced no problems.

Reproductive

Case Study 137

Name _____ Class/Group _____ Date _____

▶ **Scenario**

L.B. and her husband, J.B., come to the clinic, saying they want to become pregnant. L.B. is 29 years old and a self-employed photographer. J.B. is 31 years old and a dispatcher with a local oil and gas company. They have been married for 4 years and have been trying to become pregnant for just over 2 years. L.B. has not been pregnant previously; J.B. says he has never gotten a girl pregnant "that he knows of."

1. Is this couple infertile? Defend your response.

2. What type of infertility does the couple have, primary or secondary?

3. What are the common causes of male infertility?

4. What are the common causes of female infertility?

5. Describe the reproductive and sexual history you need to obtain from the couple.

6. In addition to performing a general physical examination, what lab tests do you expect the provider to order?

CASE STUDY PROGRESS

Chart View

General Assessment

L.B.
29 years old
BMI 26.1
Reproductive structures normal
Slightly irregular menses with a cycle of
   28–35 days
Nonsmoker; nondrinker

J.B.
31 years old
BMI 27.4
Reproductive structures normal
No problems with erection or ejaculation
Nonsmoker; drinks 1–2 alcoholic beverages
   weekly

Both report their spouse has been their only sexual partner for the past 6 years. They engage in intercourse an average of 2 to 3 times per week and deny any sexual problems. L.B. had been using oral contraceptive pills for about 4 years prior to their attempting to conceive. She says her menses were regular before using the oral contraceptives, but once she stopped using them, regular menses did not resume. Both deny any history of urinary tract and sexually transmitted infections. Their general physical assessments are unremarkable except for their BMIs. Neither engages in any regular physical exercise. The provider orders an ultrasound for L.B. and lab testing for both. L.B. is to begin performing basal body temperature (BBT) charting in conjunction with using an ovulation kit.

7. J.B. needs a semen analysis. What instructions will you give him about specimen collection? Select all that apply.
   a. Keep the container in an insulated bag with ice.
   b. Bring the specimen to the office within 8 hours.
   c. Place the specimen in a clean container for transport.
   d. He can collect the specimen in a sterile, nonlubricated condom.
   e. He should not have sex or ejaculate for 2 to 5 days before the procedure.

8. What information is obtained from a semen analysis?

9. The provider orders follicle stimulating hormone (FSH), estradiol, and progesterone levels for L.B.; a luteinizing hormone (LH) level for J.B.; and TSH levels for both. When will you schedule these tests?

10. What is the purpose of BBT charting?

11. What teaching will you provide L.B. on how to perform BBT charting?

12. Outline the teaching you will provide L.B. on how to use an ovulation kit.

13. Because lifestyle and sexual practices can affect fertility, what do you encourage the couple to do to enhance their ability to conceive? Select all that apply.
a. Relax in a hot tub daily before going to bed.
b. Avoid the use of artificial lubricants during sex.
c. Have them drink alcohol before sex to help relax.
d. Eat a healthy diet with plenty of fruits and vegetables.
e. Use strategies that are usually helpful in reducing stress.
f. Engage in moderate exercise for 30 minutes, 3 to 4 times per week.

14 Reproductive

14. As you are finishing the appointment, L.B. begins to cry and says, "I can't believe this is happening to us when all of my friends are just popping out babies." How do you respond?

Chart View

Laboratory Results

L.B.
Progesterone low
Estradiol normal
FSH normal
TSH normal
Pelvic ultrasound normal

J.B.
Testosterone normal
LH normal
TSH normal
Seminal parameters normal

J.B.'s semen analysis reveals no apparent problem. L.B. appears to be ovulating normally. BBT charting captures a change in temperature, and ovulation testing reveals an LH surge. The provider suspects L.B. may have a luteal phase defect because her progesterone levels are low after ovulation. The provider decides to order an hysterosalpingogram (HSG) for L.B.

15. How will you describe a HSG to the couple?

16. You tell L.B. that it is important for her to call the office when her menstrual cycle starts so the HSG can be scheduled between days 7 and 10 of her cycle. It is important they abstain from sex between the first day of her cycle until after the test. L.B. asks why. What do you tell her?

The HSG was normal, with no blockage to the fallopian tubes. The provider speaks with the couple about starting L.B. on clomiphene (Clomid) and progesterone vaginal suppositories, starting 2 days after ovulation.

17. What is the expected outcome associated with each of these medications?

18. You determine that L.B. understands your teaching about clomiphene therapy when she says: (Select all that apply.)
   a. "I do not need to use the LH testing kits anymore."
   b. "There is a higher risk of my having twins, or more."
   c. "I will take this medicine orally for 5 days each month."
   d. "I may experience some flushing and breast tenderness."
   e. "My husband will need to learn to give me daily injections."

On the fourth round of clomiphene, L.B. and J.B. were successful in becoming pregnant. She delivered an 8 pound, 7-ounce (3827 grams) baby boy vaginally at 38 weeks after having an induced labor because of mild preeclampsia.

Case Study **138**

Name _____ Class/Group _____ Date _____

▶ Scenario

J.H., a 53-year-old man, comes to the primary care provider's office for his annual physical. He has a history of familial hypercholesteremia for which he takes atorvastatin. His only other medication is a once daily, low dose aspirin. During the initial intake, he tells you his greatest concern is that he cannot get an erection. He states, "my wife and I have only had sex a few times in the past 6 months!"

1. What is the best response to J.H.'s concern?
   a. "Let's talk more about your concern and what is going on."
   b. "Have you discussed with your wife how important sex is to her?"
   c. "Don't worry, we can start you on medications that will help you have sex again."
   d. "That sounds normal. Couples tend to have sex less often the longer they are married."

2. Describe the history you need to obtain from J.H.

3. What are the primary risk factors for ED?

CASE STUDY PROGRESS

J.H. says the quality of his erections and the ability to keep an erection has been worsening over the past year. When he does have an erection sufficient for intercourse, he says it is less firm but ejaculatory function and sensations are normal. There are no morning or nocturnal erections. He denies any problems with libido or history of trauma, STIs, or UTIs.

4. What should be included in J.H.'s physical assessment?

CASE STUDY PROGRESS

J.H. is 6 ft, 3 in (190.5 cm) and weighs 250 lb (113 kg). His physical assessment is otherwise unremarkable. He has a normal, circumcised penis without any discharge or lesions. His testes are bilaterally descended, with normal size and texture. Perianal sensations are intact. The digital rectal exam completed by the provider shows no prostate enlargement or nodules. His femoral and pedal pulses are all 2+. His VS are 140/80, 90, 16, 97.7° F (36.5° C).

5. What lab tests do you expect the provider will order and why?

6. What other diagnostic tests may be done to evaluate ED?

7. While waiting on the results of lab work, the provider decides to start J.H. on sildenafil (Viagra) 50 mg orally once daily as needed, 30 minutes to 1 hour before sexual activity. How does sildenafil work?

 8. You review J.H.'s medical record to verify that it is safe for him to take sildenafil. What may preclude J.H. from taking sildenafil?

9. You teach J.H. about which common side effects of sildenafil? Select all that apply.
   a. Flushing
   b. Headache
   c. Dizziness
   d. Sleepiness
   e. Constipation
   f. Hypertension

10. What teaching will you provide J.H. about the safe use of sildenafil?

11. After teaching J.H. about the safe use of sildenafil, you determine your teaching has been effective if he says:
   a. "I should contact my provider if I have any vision loss."
   b. "We can have sex all night because my erections will last 3 to 4 hours."
   c. "Having a few beers before will help the medication work more quickly."
   d. "I can take two in 1 day on special occasions if I don't have any chest pain."

12. Describe 4 other treatments options for ED.

13. Describe the counseling you will provide to J.H. to help him cope with the psychosocial implications of ED.

CASE STUDY PROGRESS

Chart View

Laboratory Test Results (Fasting)

Total cholesterol	189 mg/dL (4.9 mmol/L)
HDL	28 mg/dL (0.7 mmol/L)
LDL	112 mg/dL (2.9 mmol/L)
Triglycerides	270 mg/dL (3.1 mmol/L)
Glucose	108 mg/dL (6.0 mmol/L)
Total testosterone	673 ng/dL (23.3 nmol/L)
TSH	1.04 mU/L

14. Which, if any, of J.H.'s lab results concern you and why?

15. The provider adds metformin 500 mg orally twice daily to J.H.'s medication regimen. Why?

16. A teaching plan for J.H. should include which intervention? Give your rationale.
   a. Removing all sugars from his diet
   b. Exploring lower stress career options
   c. Following a liquid meal replacement diet
   d. Exercising 60 minutes, 4 to 5 times per week

CASE STUDY PROGRESS

A few days later J.H. calls into the office and asks if the provider can write a different prescription. He tells you that although the drug did work, filling the 5-pill prescription cost $336 and he "won't be having too much sex – I can't afford to at those prices!" He says a friend of his told him to get 100 mg pills, which only cost a few dollars more, and cut them in half.

17. How will you handle J.H.'s request?

 18. What will you tell J.H. is the safest way to split a pill?

CASE STUDY OUTCOME

With diet and exercise, J.H. loses 25 pounds (11 kg) over the next several months. However, he still requires sildenafil to achieve an adequate erection but is satisfied with the results of therapy and has continued its use.

14 Reproductive

Case Study **139**

Name_____ Class/Group_____ Date_____

▶ **Scenario**

You are working in a busy obstetrics/gynecology (OB/GYN) office. The last patient of the day is P.B., a 27-year-old who is being married in 2 weeks. She wants to use birth control but is not sure what to choose. Her fiancé and she are both in graduate school and have limited health insurance, so she is anxious not to become pregnant right away. She asks you to review the various methods and help her explore what is best for her.

1. What factors influence the choice of the most appropriate method of birth control?

2. What past medical information will you need to obtain from P.B. and why?

3. What lifestyle information will help you aid P.B. in choosing a birth control method?

4. P.B. asks you about the effectiveness rating of available birth control methods. Describe the term *efficacy.*

5. What factors influence how effective a contraceptive method is?

6. Match the available contraceptive methods according to their efficacy ratings:

____ 1. Cervical cap	A. Most effective, more than 99%
____ 2. IUD	B. Highly effective, 88%–97%
____ 3. Male and female condoms	C. Moderately effective, less than 85%
____ 4. Combination oral contraceptives	
____ 5. Hormone implants	
____ 6. Sterilization	
____ 7. Withdrawal	
____ 8. Transdermal contraceptive patch	
____ 9. Natural family planning	
____ 10. Hormone injections	

14 Reproductive

7. P.B. asks you to review the main advantages and disadvantages of the hormonal birth control methods first.

Method	Advantages	Disadvantages
Oral contraceptives		
Transdermal patch		
Hormone injections		
Hormone implants		
Vaginal ring		

8. After reviewing the hormonal methods, you choose to discuss intrauterine devices. How would you describe the copper and levonorgestrel (Mirena) IUD systems to P.B.?

9. Next, you steer the conversation to barrier methods. What will you share with P.B. about the use of a diaphragm or cervical cap and condoms?

10. The *major* advantage of using a condom for birth control is that condoms:
   a. Do not require monthly injections
   b. Are easy to obtain and inexpensive
   c. Reduce the risk for acquiring infections
   d. Come in assorted styles, shapes, and textures

11. Describe what you would tell P.B. about the natural family planning method.

12. P.B. wants to know about the associated costs with each method because she is on a tight budget. How would you respond?

13. She asks you which method you would pick. What do you tell her?

CASE STUDY PROGRESS

P.B. comes back in a week and tells you that she can get a low-cost oral contraceptive (OC) through a local store. You convey this information to the nurse practitioner, who examines P.B. and writes a prescription for a biphasic 28-day pill pack containing ethinyl estradiol and norethindrone. You are asked to discuss the use of the OC pill with P.B.

14. Explain how biphasic OC pills work.

15. When should P.B. take her first OC?

14 Reproductive

16. You tell P.B. that is does not matter what time of day she takes the OC, just that she takes it at the same time each day. Describe 3 suggestions you can offer to help her remember to take her pill.

17. What should you tell her about missed pills?

18. How will you prepare P.B. for possible side effects?

19. Using the acronym *ACHES*, what symptoms should you teach P.B. to report?

20. Are there any other key points you should review?

21. A few months later, P.B. calls the clinic because she missed a dose of her first week of OC the prior day and cannot remember what you told her. What will you tell her? Select all that apply.
a. "Throw that pill away. Restart taking your pills tomorrow."
b. "It's okay; you're still protected from pregnancy if you take two now."
c. "You should use a backup form of contraception for the next 7 days."
d. "Please make an appointment so we can insert a temporary intrauterine device."
e. "Don't take any more pills. Begin a new pack when you start your next menses."
f. "Take the missed pill now, along with today's pill, then resume the pack tomorrow."

CASE STUDY OUTCOME

P.B. uses OC without experiencing a pregnancy. She stops 4 years later, and her husband and she conceive their first child 6 months later.

Case Study **140**

Name_____ Class/Group_____ Date_____

▶ Scenario

R.Z., a 34-year-old man, presents to the urgent care clinic reporting dysuria and a purulent urethral discharge for 3 days.

1. What key sexual and health history questions do you need to ask R.Z.?

CASE STUDY PROGRESS

R.Z. says he is married and has unprotected vaginal intercourse with his wife 1 or 2 times per week, the last time being 4 days ago. He believes his wife is asymptomatic. He goes on to tell you that while on a trip to a business conference 10 days ago, he "had way too much to drink" and had a one-time sexual encounter with a work associate. They had unprotected oral and vaginal sex. He says he has not "had anything like this before."

2. What should be included in R.Z.'s physical assessment?

3. R.Z.'s physical examination is unremarkable except for the genital examination. The urethral meatus is red with a mucopurulent discharge. Given his symptoms and findings, what differential diagnoses do you consider?

4. What diagnostic tests do you expect the provider to order and why?

CASE STUDY PROGRESS

Chart View

Laboratory Test Results

Pharyngeal culture	Negative *Neisseria gonorrhoeae*
Urethral culture	Positive *N. gonorrhoeae*
	Negative *Chlamydia trachomatis*
	Negative *Trichomonas vaginalis*
RPR	Nonreactive
HIV Antibody Test	Negative

5. Based on the assessment and diagnostic test results, what problem does R.Z. have?

6. What are your overall goals of nursing care for R.Z.?

7. How is this problem treated?

8. The provider orders ceftriaxone 250 mg IM. How many milliliters will you give for this dose? Mark the syringe with your answer. Round to the tenth.

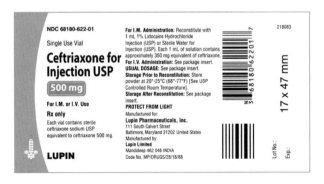

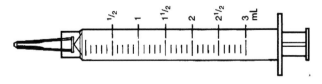

From Gray Morris D. (2010). Calculate with confidence (5th ed.). 5, St. Louis, MO: Mosby.

9. Where is the best place to inject the ceftriaxone?

10. What teaching will you provide R.Z. to promote successful treatment?

11. What complications may R.Z. develop if treatment is not successful?

12. R.Z. says he is not going to tell his wife, because "she is going to kill me," or his work associate, because he is embarrassed. What are the possible complications in women if this STI remains untreated?

13. What symptoms do women with this STI commonly experience?

14. R.Z. asks if you are going to tell anyone about his infection. How do you respond?

15. What implications might this diagnosis have for R.Z. and his wife?

16. What advice do you offer R.Z. about telling both women?

17. R.Z. pauses for a moment, then asks if it is possible for someone from the health department to tell his work associate. How do you respond?

18. Which additional instructions will you include in your discharge teaching?
   a. "Make sure you do not have sexual intercourse for 21 days."
   b. "It is important to wash your hands frequently so you don't spread the infection."
   c. "You will need to come back for a follow-up appointment if the drainage does not stop."
   d. "If you do have sexual intercourse in the next 7 days, have your partner douche afterward."

19. R.Z. asks what he could do to prevent getting another infection. You determine he understands your teaching when he states:
   a. "I will not have sex with women I do not know."
   b. "Using a spermicidal cream will decrease my risk."
   c. "I will use a fresh condom each time I have intercourse."
   d. "If I don't see any signs of infection, then that partner is safe."

CASE STUDY OUTCOME

R.Z. does return to the clinic for the follow-up visit and his symptoms resolved with the prescribed treatment. He states his wife also developed the infection. R.Z. is currently staying with his brother until his wife "cools off" and they "work some things out." He says that they will be starting marital counseling the following week.

14 Reproductive

Case Study **141**

Name_____ Class/Group_____ Date_____

▶ Scenario

You are working as the triage nurse in the emergency department (ED) when a woman arrives with heavy vaginal bleeding and extreme pain. S.K. is single, 47 years of age, and has been bleeding for 24 hours, soaking one pad per hour. She works in a law firm as a paralegal and was embarrassed yesterday when she leaked around her pad and stained a chair in the conference room. She has 2 sexual partners currently and has been relying on condoms for birth control. She thinks her last menstrual period was 2 months ago, but they have been irregular, and she is not sure. She has had some occasional spotting during the past 6 months. She says she is afraid because of the amount of bleeding in the past 24 hours.

1. Identify 3 conditions that would require emergency care and could prove life-threatening.

2. She asks you, "Could I be pregnant?" How will you respond?

3. You ask her how she would feel if she was pregnant, and she says, "It would ruin my life." She states she is a single mother with 2 children in high school. What can you tell her to help her with her obvious distress?

4. Describe the assessment needed to determine what might be occurring with S.K.

5. What is your priority concern as you care for S.K.?

Chart View

Laboratory Test Results

Hgb	12.2 g/dL (122 g/L)
Hct	44%
RBCs	4.2 dL
hCG	Negative
Vital Signs	
BP	110/68
Heart rate	88
Respiratory rate	22

---

6. Interpret S.K.'s lab results and vital signs.

7. S.K. is obviously relieved about not being pregnant, but she expresses fear the bleeding could be caused by cancer. What will you tell her to reassure her?

CASE STUDY PROGRESS

You determine that S.K. is stable at the present; she is not diaphoretic or pale. The provider orders an ultrasound to evaluate possible causes of her bleeding. Shortly after she returns from the ultrasound, her BP drops to 90/42, and she complains of considerable cramping.

Physician's Orders

Infuse 1 L of D_5 LR over 4 hours
Meperidine 5 mg IV now

 8. Before administering the meperidine, what will you ask her?

 9. What precautions do you need to take to safely administer meperidine? Select all that apply.
   a. Administer the medication undiluted
   b. Have oxygen equipment and naloxone at her bedside
   c. Administer the dose over a minimum of 4 to 5 minutes
   d. Place her in semi-Fowler position with her head to the side
   e. Monitor S.K.'s respiratory status every 15 minutes for 1 hour after

10. You are preparing to infuse the D_5 LR. The available IV tubing supplies 15 gtt/mL. At how many drops per minute will you regulate the infusion?

CASE STUDY PROGRESS

Thirty minutes later the UAP reports S.K.'s vital signs are 90/64, 118, 8, 97.6° F (36.4° C), and Spo_2 84% on room air.

 11. What is your immediate concern and why?

12. What actions will you initiate?

14 Reproductive

CASE STUDY PROGRESS

With treatment, S.K. stabilizes within an hour. You give her a nonopioid analgesic for pain and continue to monitor her status. The ultrasound results arrive and show there are no polyps or fibroids. The endometrial lining is thick, even after 24 hours of bleeding.

13. What is the most likely cause of S.K.'s bleeding and why?

14. S.K. asks if there is any way to stop the bleeding. How will you respond?

CASE STUDY PROGRESS

You continue to monitor S.K. for the next few hours. Her respiratory status remains stable, and she is feeling more comfortable. The provider prescribes oral contraceptive pills to control the bleeding. He tells her to take 1 pill 4 times a day for the next 5 days or until her bleeding stops. Once the bleeding has stopped, she should continue taking 1 pill per day, for the rest of the cycle, then continue to use the pills for at least 3 cycles. She will need to follow up with her OB/GYN.

15. What risk factors will you ask her about because she is starting oral contraceptives?

16. What warning signs and symptoms do you need to teach her as she starts oral contraceptives?

17. Which statements indicate S.K. understands the discharge instructions? Select all that apply.
   a. "I can take 325 mg of aspirin every 6 hours for the cramping pain."
   b. "I will try to eat more beans and spinach over the next several days."
   c. "I will call if I continue to have heavy bleeding, soaking a pad an hour."
   d. "I will avoid sexual intercourse until the bleeding has completely stopped."
   e. "If I get dizzy or feel my heart beating funny, I will come back to the emergency room."

CASE STUDY OUTCOME

The oral contraceptives lessen but do not completely alleviate her bleeding. Her next 3 cycles last 7 days, with heavy flows and moderate cramping. She undergoes an endometrial ablation and has a significant reduction in symptoms that lasts until she completes menopause.

Case Study **142**

Name_____   Class/Group_____   Date_____

▶ **Scenario**

You are the nurse in a walk-in clinic. A.P. is being seen this morning for a 2-day history of diffuse, severe abdominal pain. She has some nausea; she denies vaginal bleeding or discharge. A.P. reports having unprotected sex with a few partners recently who "might have" had penile discharge. Her last menstrual period ended 3 days ago. She has no known drug allergies and denies prior medical or psychiatric problems. Vital signs are 108/60, 110, 20, 100.6° F (38.1° C). Physical examination reveals her abdomen is very tender. The slightest touch of her abdomen causes her to wince with pain. Bowel sounds are normal. Pelvic examination reveals purulent material pooled in the vaginal vault, which appears to be coming from the cervix. A sample of the vaginal drainage is obtained and sent for culture. The result of a pregnancy test is negative; a rapid diagnostic test for chlamydial infection has a positive result.

1. Which assessment findings are significant and why?

2. What medical interventions can you expect?

3. What are the risk factors for chlamydia?

4. Describe the common symptoms of chlamydia infection in men and women.

5. What are the consequences of an untreated chlamydia infection in women?

6. How will you offer emotional support to A.P.?

CASE STUDY PROGRESS

The provider has 2 options of treating A.P. The first option is doxycycline 100 mg orally twice a day for 7 days. The second option is a one-time dose of azithromycin 1 gram orally, which would be given at the clinic.

7. Which choice is best for A.P.? Explain your reasoning.

8. You tell A.P. that chlamydial infection is a sexually transmitted infection (STI) that must be reported to the health department. What is the purpose of reporting the infection, and what actions will the health department take?

9. A.P. says she does not understand why her partners must be told about the infection. How will you respond?

10. Based on the information A.P. has given you, you decide that she is at risk for other STIs and unplanned pregnancy. Based on the "5 Ps," what risk assessment questions do you need to ask A.P.?

11. You ask whether someone has talked with A.P. about "safe sex." She laughs. Undaunted, you ask if she would be willing for you to discuss the use of condoms with her sexual partners. She tells you that she is already careful; if she does not "know the guy," then she uses a condom. How are you going to respond?

12. You ask A.P. whether she has been tested for HIV. She says no, she does not know anyone with acquired immunodeficiency syndrome (AIDS) and she only has sex with "100% straight guys." Now what are you going to say?

13. You ask her whether she would like to be tested for HIV. You tell her the test will not cost her anything, only she will know the results, no one else, and test results are completely confidential. She agrees to the test. What counseling will you provide A.P.?

14. You make an appointment for A.P. to return to the clinic in 1 week for her HIV test results. Describe the instructions you will give to A.P. before she leaves the clinic.

CASE STUDY PROGRESS

A.P. returns to the clinic in 1 week for her HIV test results, which are negative. Her culture results confirm the diagnosis of chlamydial infection.

15. What are your primary nursing concerns right now?

14 Reproductive

16. A.P. has completed the course of antibiotic therapy and is not experiencing any symptoms. After counseling her on ways to reduce her risk for acquiring another STI, you determine A.P. understood your teaching about safe sexual practices if she says she will: (Select all that apply.)
   a. Have her partner wear a new condom with each sexual encounter
   b. Not worry about contacting an STI if the man says he has few partners
   c. Apply a new application of spermicidal jelly before each sexual encounter
   d. Douche with an over-the-counter solution within 4 hours of having intercourse
   e. Inspect the genitalia of her partner before intercourse or other contact with perianal area

CASE STUDY OUTCOME

A.P. returns to the clinic a few months later with symptoms of another STI and is diagnosed with both chlamydia and gonorrhea. Treatment of both infections is started, and you again review measures to prevent acquiring an STI. You report the STIs to the health department. A.P. does not return to your clinic for follow-up.

Case Study 143

Name_____ Class/Group_____ Date_____

▶ Scenario

T.C. is a 49-year-old woman who underwent a vaginal hysterectomy and right salpingo-oophorectomy for abdominal pain and endometriosis. Intraoperatively, she had an intra-abdominal hemorrhage, requiring transfusion with 3 units of packed red blood cells (RBCs). T.C. is now being admitted to your unit from the postanesthesia care unit (PACU).

T.C.'s vital signs are 130/70, 94, 16, 99.7° F (37.6° C). Respirations are shallow and her Spo_2 is 93% with oxygen at 2 L by nasal cannula. She is easily aroused and oriented to place and person. She dozes between verbal requests. She has a low-midline abdominal dressing that is dry and intact, and a Jackson-Pratt drain that is fully compressed and has a scant amount of bright red blood. Her indwelling urinary catheter has clear yellow urine. She is receiving an IV of 1000 mL D5.45NS at 100 mL/hr in her left forearm, with no swelling or redness. T.C. is receiving IV morphine sulfate for pain control through a patient-controlled analgesia (PCA) pump. The settings are dose 2 mg, lock-out interval 20 minutes, 4-hour maximum dose of 30 mg. When aroused, she says that her pain is an 8 on a scale of 1 to 10.

1. What concerns you most right now about T.C. and why?

2. Identify 3 factors likely affecting T.C.'s respiratory status.

3. Name 5 interventions you need to implement to promote T.C.'s respiratory status.

CASE STUDY PROGRESS

The unit is busy, and you are concerned about monitoring T.C. carefully enough. Your present patient load is 6; of these, 2 patients are newly postoperative and 1 is getting ready for discharge. You have one experienced UAP to help you. You are concerned T.C.'s respiratory status may further decline.

4. Formulate a plan for the UAP and you to care for T.C. during your shift.

5. Which of T.C.'s vital sign values would be most important for the UAP to report to you at once?
   a. Heart rate of 100
   b. Temperature of 100° F (37.8° C)
   c. Respiratory rate of 9
   d. Blood pressure of 160/80

6. Name 3 outcomes you expect for T.C. because of your interventions.

CASE STUDY PROGRESS

Throughout the first postoperative day, balancing T.C.'s need for pain medication and depression of her respiratory status is difficult.

7. Discuss how PCA devices are used for controlling pain.

 8. During the first 24 hours, T.C. has 122 PCA demands and 31 doses delivered. How many total milligrams of morphine sulfate did she receive?

 9. What adjustments could be made to her plan of care to better control her pain?

10. What other measures can you use to manage T.C.'s pain more effectively?

11. How do you best evaluate the effectiveness of the PCA therapy?
   a. Assess the time interval between doses received
   b. Have T.C. state her pain level on a scale of 1 to 10
   c. Determine how many doses of morphine T.C. received
   d. Appraise whether T.C. understands the purpose of PCA therapy

CASE STUDY PROGRESS

The surgeon adjusts T.C.'s pain management regimen. By the end of the second postoperative day, her pain is better controlled, although she is still complaining of moderate incisional pain. She can ambulate in her room with help, voided after the indwelling catheter was removed, and tolerates oral fluids without nausea. As you perform your shift assessment, you note the abdominal dressing is saturated with blood.

12. What 2 assessments do you need to make and why?

13. How should her wound appear at this time?

14. When you remove the dressing, you note a large amount of bloody drainage coming from the distal end of the wound. What other assessments do you need to obtain?

15. Her assessment findings are unremarkable, and you place a new sterile dressing on the wound. What will you do next?

CASE STUDY PROGRESS

The surgeon comes, and after examining T.C. thinks she could have some internal bleeding. He takes her back to surgery, where he isolates an area where the sutures have broken and cauterizes the affected vessels. T.C. returns to the unit, and her condition is quickly stabilized. The next evening you overhear T.C. and her husband saying they are very dissatisfied with the care provided by the surgeon. The couple believes the surgeon mismanaged T.C.'s care. They are discussing the possibility of getting an attorney. They ask you what you think.

16. What do you do and why?

17. You state, "Tell me what's going on with you right now. Maybe I can help you be more comfortable." What would be the benefit of taking this approach?

18. What referrals might be beneficial?

CASE STUDY OUTCOME

The rest of T.C.'s recovery is uneventful, and she requires no further surgeries. Her husband and she meet with a social worker and representative from the hospital. Together, they are able to work through the couple's concerns.

Mood, Stress, and Addiction

Case Study 144

Name_____ Class/Group_____ Date_____

▶ **Scenario**

You are working the day shift on a medical inpatient unit. You are discussing discharge instructions with J.B., an 86-year-old man who was admitted for mitral valve repair. His serum blood glucose is 250 mg/dL (13.9 mmol/L) and increasing for the past several months. During this admission, his dosage of insulin was adjusted and he was given additional education in managing his diet. While you are giving these instructions, J.B. tells you his wife died 9 months ago. He becomes tearful when telling you about his loss and the loneliness he has been feeling. J.B. states he just doesn't feel good lately, feels sad most of the time. J.B. also expresses his lack of involvement in his normal activities. He has few friends left in the community because most of them have passed away. He has a daughter in town, but she is busy with her work and grandchildren. He tells you he has been feeling "depressed" the last few months with thoughts of suicide.

1. What further assessment data is needed to determine the seriousness of J.B.'s thoughts of suicide?

2. What characteristics of J.B. put him at high risk for suicide?

3. Which psychiatric disorders can result in suicidal ideations or gestures? Name at least 3.

4. People with a physical illness, often have trouble sleeping, experience a change in appetite, reduce their level of activity, and have thoughts of death. How can you tell the difference between old age with illness and depression?

5. List 5 of the most common signs of depression in the older adult.

CASE STUDY PROGRESS

You use the SAD PERSONS scale to assess J.B.'s potential for suicide and find that he is at a 4 on the 10-point scale. J.B. tells you he has general thoughts of suicide, but has not really thought about how he would do it.

6. What important questions about suicide must the nurse ask J.B. at this time?

You recall that there are 2 types of suicide methods based on lethality: higher risk or hard methods and lower risk or soft methods.

7. Which of these would be considered soft methods of suicide? Select all that apply.
   a. Hanging
   b. Using a gun
   c. Ingesting pills
   d. Inhaling natural gas
   e. Slashing one's wrist
   f. Poisoning with carbon monoxide

CASE STUDY PROGRESS

You decide to notify J.B.'s physician about your findings. The attending physician calls in a psychiatrist to evaluate J.B. In addition, Suicide Precautions are ordered.

8. Which interventions are part of Suicide Precautions? Select all that apply.
   a. Document his behavior every shift.
   b. He is not permitted to leave his room.
   c. No glass or metal dishes or utensils with meals.
   d. Observe him swallow each dose of oral medication.
   e. One-to-one observation and interaction 24 hours per day.

9. Identify 2 treatments that are available for depression.

10. Would J.B. be a candidate for electroconvulsive therapy (ECT)? Why or why not?

CASE STUDY PROGRESS

The psychiatrist on call evaluates J.B. and writes an order for escitalopram (Lexapro) 10 mg/day at bedtime. J.B. is scheduled to see the psychiatrist the day after he is discharged from the hospital.

11. What special instructions will you give him regarding the Lexapro? Select all that apply.
   a. There are no known food interactions.
   b. Taking a glass of wine at bedtime will help him go to sleep.
   c. The full effects of the medication might not be seen for 4 to 6 weeks.
   d. The medication may cause nausea, dry mouth, sedation, and insomnia.
   e. The herbal product St. John's wort will enhance the action of the Lexapro.

CASE STUDY PROGRESS

J.B.'s daughter visits him in the hospital. She is shocked to hear that her father is lonely, depressed, and thought about suicide. The daughter discusses with you how she will do all she can to help him when he goes home.

12. What important information needs to be conveyed to J.B.'s daughter about the first few weeks of therapy with the SSRI?

CASE STUDY OUTCOME

J.B. is discharged to home with a psychiatric home health nurse scheduled to visit him twice a week for 4 weeks. J.B.'s daughter also plans to check in on him daily and makes an effort to include him in more family activities. He also is considering a move to an assisted living facility.

15 Mood, Stress, and Addiction

Case Study **145**

Name _____ Class/Group _____ Date _____

▶ **Scenario**

You are the registered nurse case manager in an outpatient mental health clinic. S.T. is here today for her outpatient mental health appointment. She was diagnosed with bipolar disorder type II 2 years ago, and has been stable for the past year. Her last episode was one of mania that required hospitalization. S.T. is 29 years old, married, with two children aged 2 and 4. She reports that her mood is better than it has been in a long time and she has lots of energy. When asked whether she thinks this is a recurrence of mania, she says *no,* she thinks that things are just finally getting better.

1. It is common for patients with bipolar illness to deny the onset of mania because it feels good. What other information would be important to ask S.T.?

2. What other information would help determine whether S.T. is experiencing the onset of a manic or hypomanic episode?

3. Bipolar disorder is a disorder of mood, characterized by episodes of depression, mania, or hypomania. What symptoms might you see if S.T. is experiencing mania?

4. How is hypomania different from mania?

CASE STUDY PROGRESS

Lithium (Eskalith) is a mood stabilizer commonly used to treat bipolar disorders. S.T. has been taking lithium for a year.

5. When S.T. started her initial lithium dose, she would have been cautioned to report side effects. Which are common side effects of lithium? Select all that apply.
   a. Thirst
   b. Nausea
   c. Tremor
   d. Dizziness
   e. Constipation

6. Lithium toxicity can occur in patients taking lithium. What are the symptoms of early lithium toxicity? Select all that apply.
   a. Dyspnea
   b. Diarrhea
   c. Lethargy
   d. Vomiting
   e. Insomnia

7. S.T.'s maintenance lithium level results are reported as 1.0 mEq/L (1.0 mmol/L). Interpret these results.

8. List additional lab examinations that should be routinely performed while S.T. is taking lithium.

9. Explain the instructions you would give S.T. concerning lithium therapy

10. Aside from lithium, list other medications that are used to treat bipolar disorder:

11. You assess S.T.'s understanding of her Lithium drug treatment using the Teach-Back technique. Identify the statement by S.T. revealing a need for further education?
  a. "I take the lithium tablets with meals."
  b. "I need to be careful because lithium is addictive."
  c. "I will call my doctor if I have severe vomiting or diarrhea."
  d. "I will keep my appointments to have my drug levels checked."

12. Given her history of bipolar disorder type II, what should you teach S.T. to minimize mood swings?

CASE STUDY OUTCOME

S.T. is told that her lithium level is within normal limits and states, "I feel better than I've felt in ages!" She expresses hope that this will last a long time.

Case Study **146**

Name_____ Class/Group_____ Date_____

▶ **Scenario**

You are working on an inpatient psychiatric unit and need to do an initial assessment of R.B., who has just been admitted. He has a diagnosis of schizophrenia, paranoid type. He is 22 years old and has been attending the local university and living at home with his parents. R.B. has always been a good student and has been socially active. Last semester his grades began declining. He became very withdrawn and spends most of his time alone in his room. His personal self-care has deteriorated as he can go days without bathing. Prior to admission, R.B. spent several weeks in seclusion. He refused to join family gatherings, isolated himself, and closed the blinds. Within the past 2 days he refused to eat, stating, "They have contaminated the food." As you approach R.B., you note that he appears to be talking to himself. When you talk to him, he looks around and answers in a whisper but gives you little information. He states, "They are watching me and told me not to cooperate."

1. Identify at least 3 negative symptoms of schizophrenia that R.B. might be experiencing.

2. Identify at least 2 positive symptoms of schizophrenia that R.B. might be experiencing.

3. Give the definition of each of the following types of delusional thinking:
   a. Grandeur
   b. Persecutory/Paranoid
   c. Thought insertion
   d. Ideas of reference
   e. Somatic delusions

4. What symptoms indicate that R.B. has paranoid schizophrenia?

5. Why is it important to know R.B.'s history before he is diagnosed with schizophrenia?

6. What diagnostic screenings are important in evaluating R.B.?

7. What are the most important initial interventions for treating R.B.?

CASE STUDY PROGRESS

The psychiatrist evaluates R.B. by conducting a mental status assessment and orders antipsychotic medications with close monitoring in the inpatient setting.

8. Identify the class of antipsychotic medications considered as first-line therapy for schizophrenia?

9. R.B. will need to be monitored closely. How will this be done?

10. Identify 5 types of psychosocial treatments that may be used to treat R.B.'s schizophrenia?

CASE STUDY PROGRESS

R.B. is started on olanzapine (Zyprexa). You inform R.B. and his family about the common side effects of the second-generation antipsychotics.

11. What are the common side effects of second-generation antipsychotics such as olanzapine (Zyprexa)? Select all that apply.
   a. Nausea
   b. Dry mouth
   c. Drowsiness
   d. Palpitations
   e. Weight gain
   f. Tardive dyskinesia

12. Which condition is a risk associated with second-generation antipsychotics, such as olanzapine?
   a. Metabolic syndrome
   b. Prolonged QT interval
   c. Anticholinergic toxicity
   d. Neuroleptic malignant syndrome

CASE STUDY PROGRESS

As you go in to give R.B. his medication, he speaks to you in a hushed tone. "Is that a bird?" Before you can say anything, he asks, "Do you see that bird over my bed? She is telling me not to leave this room. If I move she will swoop down and try to peck at my eyes. Be careful!"

15 Mood, Stress, and Addiction

13. Is he experiencing a delusion or a hallucination? Explain your answer.

14. Identify the appropriate nursing response you would state to R.B. Select all that apply.
   a. "There is no bird over your bed."
   b. "Tell me more about what you are seeing."
   c. "I'll come back to talk to you when you are settled down."
   d. "The voice you are hearing is part of your illness. It can't hurt you."
   e. "I don't see a bird over your head. I can understand how that would be upsetting to you."

CASE STUDY OUTCOME

After 2 weeks of inpatient therapy, R.B. is discharged back to his parents' home and is enrolled in a day treatment program. He and his parents attend family therapy sessions twice a month. He hopes to move to a halfway house in the community.

Case Study **147**

Name_____ Class/Group_____ Date_____

You are on duty in the emergency department (ED) when a "code blue" is called. As the code nurse, you grab the crash cart and rush to the code, which is in the employee lounge of the operating room. On the couch, you find a nurse, Z.H., unconscious, dusky, and barely breathing; she has a palpable pulse.

1. What immediate assessment of Z.H. do you need to perform?

2. What intervention has the greatest priority?
   a. Obtaining a STAT toxicology screen
   b. Connecting her to the portable ECG monitor
   c. Establishing an IV line with 0.9% normal saline
   d. Supporting respirations by manually ventilating her

3. What assessment finding would lead you to suspect that Z.H. had an opioid overdose? Explain your answer.
   a. Hypertension
   b. Fever and tachycardia
   c. Constricted pupils and bradypnea
   d. Diaphoresis and cool, clammy skin

4. Z.H.'s respirations are shallow with a rate of 8. The respiratory therapist intubates her and continues to ventilate her manually. An IV line is established. You attach ECG leads to her chest and find the results shown in the figure. What is your interpretation of Z.H.'s rhythm?

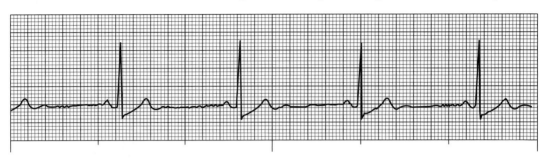

CASE STUDY PROGRESS

Z.H. is given an ampule of 50 mL $D_{50}W$ and 0.4 mg naloxone IV push. Her respirations improve slightly, and her pulse increases to 56. She is transported to the ED.

5. Describe the purpose of administering the combination of $D_{50}W$ and naloxone.

6. What treatment will Z.H. require in the ED?

7. Within 5 minutes of receiving the naloxone, Z.H. is starting to respond. Why do you need to continue to observe her closely? Select all that apply.
   a. Opioid dosage may exceed that of the naloxone.
   b. Z.H. may develop pulmonary edema after receiving naloxone.
   c. A common adverse effect of naloxone is the onset of atrial fibrillation.
   d. The risk for developing diabetic ketoacidosis is high after receiving naloxone and $D_{50}W$.
   e. Rapidly reversing the effects of the drug overdose will cause a rebound decline in level of consciousness.

8. State the onset and duration times for IV naloxone.

9. Z.H. begins to lose consciousness again, and the physician orders an additional dose of naloxone, this time 0.6 mg IV STAT. The vial in the accompanying illustration is available. How many milliliters will Z.H. receive?

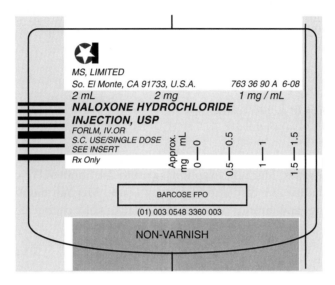

CASE STUDY PROGRESS

After the additional dose of naloxone, Z.H.'s level of consciousness and respiratory effort significantly improve, allowing her to be extubated.

10. What information do you need to obtain from Z.H.?

11. In response to your questions, Z.H, states she "periodically" used fentanyl from the hospital for several months. How does the Health Insurance Portability and Accountability Act (HIPAA) apply given that Z.H. is a nurse?

12. Explain the meaning of a chemically impaired nurse?

13. One of Z.H.'s colleagues, Meghan, telephones you to ask about Z.H's condition. You convey that you cannot discuss her case due to privacy issues. Meghan mentions to you that Z.H's behavior was strange and erratic. What are the behaviors of a chemically impaired nurse?

14. State 4 problems associated with impaired nurses who are practicing.

15. Z.H. asks what is going to happen to her career. What are the regulatory issues related to impaired nurses that will guide your response?

16. Z.H. then asks you to call a friend to come stay with her. What information would you give her friend over the phone?

17. The friend asks you what is wrong. How do you respond?

Once stabilized, Z.H. is admitted to the chemical dependency unit. She successfully completes a rehabilitation treatment program and continues to practice as a nurse. She is now serving as a sponsor for another nurse undergoing treatment for chemical dependency.

15 Mood, Stress, and Addiction

Case Study **148**

Name_____ Class/Group_____ Date_____

> ▶ **Scenario**

You are working the afternoon shift in an inpatient psychiatric unit. The patients are in the day room watching a movie when suddenly someone starts yelling. You and other staff members rush to the day room to find J.J., a 48-year-old male patient, crouched in the corner behind a chair, yelling at the other patients, "Get down. Get down quick." You and the other staff are able to calm J.J. and the other patients and take J.J. to his room. He apologizes for his outburst and explains to you that the movie brought back memories of his experiences in the Gulf War. He had forgotten where he was and thought he was in combat again. He describes to you in detail the memory he had of being ambushed by the enemy and watching several of his comrades be killed. You review J.J.'s chart and note that he was a Gulf War veteran admitted with posttraumatic stress disorder (PTSD).

1. What are common causes of PTSD? What is the most likely cause of J.J.'s condition?

2. List 3 criteria that must be present for a diagnosis of PTSD.

3. Describe the difference between PTSD and acute stress disorder.

4. Which symptom(s) of PTSD did J.J. most likely experience?

5. What therapeutic measures can be done to help J.J. during your shift this afternoon?

While you are in J.J.'s room, he states that he would like to rest for a while, and he requests something to "calm his nerves." You check his Medication Administration Record (MAR) and review the PRN (as needed) medications listed.

Chart View

PRN Medications

Acetaminophen (Tylenol) 650 mg PO every 6 hours prn for pain or fever
Alprazolam (Niravam) orally dissolving tablet, 0.5 mg by mouth every 4 hours prn for anxiety
Zolpidem (Ambien CR) extended release, 12.5 mg PO at bedtime prn for sleep

6. Which medication is most appropriate to give at this time? Explain.

7. What are the adverse effects of long-term use of benzodiazepine anxiolytics?

8. You decide to notify J.J.'s physician about his reaction to the movie. The physician writes an order to start paroxetine (Paxil). How does this medication differ from alprazolam?

9. Which of these are potential side effects of paroxetine (Paxil)? Select all that apply.
   a. Nausea
   b. Tinnitus
   c. Headache
   d. Constipation
   e. Sexual dysfunction

In addition to medications, J.J. has expressed interest about relaxation therapy. He understands it may help with his anxiety and would like to know more about it.

10. What would you discuss with J.J. about relaxation therapy?

11. The physician writes an order for Eye Movement and Desensitization Reprocessing (EMDR) therapy. Explain this type of therapy.

12. List other supportive treatment modalities you may refer J.J. to after his hospitalization to help treat his PTSD and related problems?

Over the next 2 weeks, J.J. participates in individual and group therapy sessions. He mentions to you that he is able to come to terms with his fears and experiences that occurred during the Gulf war. He tells you that he feels "encouraged" and wants to help others with the same problems.

Case Study **149**

Name_____ Class/Group_____ Date_____

▶ **Scenario**

J.G., a 49-year-old man, was assessed in the emergency department (ED) 4 days ago. He was diagnosed with alcohol intoxication, and released after 8 hours to his brother's care. He was readmitted to the ED 12 hours ago with a gastrointestinal (GI) bleed and is being transferred to the intensive care unit (ICU). His diagnosis is upper GI bleed and alcohol intoxication.

You are assigned to J.G. for the remainder of your shift. According to the ED notes, his admission vital signs (VS) were 84/56, 110, 26, and he was vomiting bright red blood. He was given IV fluids and transfused 6 units of packed red blood cells (PRBCs) in the ED. On initial assessment, you note that J.G.'s VS are 102.2° F (39° C), 174/98, 110, 24. He has a slight tremor in his hands, is diaphoretic, and he appears anxious. He reports a headache and appears flushed. No report of vomiting, frank red blood or melena in the stools, according to the chart, for the past 5 hours. In response to your questions, J.G. denies he has an alcohol problem but later on admits to drinking approximately a fifth of vodka daily for the past 2 months. He admits to having seizures while withdrawing from alcohol in the past. He tells you that he "just can't help it" and has strong urges to drink, but that he never means "to drink very much." He has had trouble keeping a job over the past several months.

Chart View

Admission Laboratory Work

Hgb	10.9 g/dL (109 g/L)
Hct	23%
ALT (formerly SGPT)	69 units/L
AST (formerly SGOT)	111 units/L
GGT	75 units/L
ETOH	291 mg/dL (63 mmol/L)
aPTT	35 seconds
PT/INR	12 seconds/1.0
Hepatitis C Screening	Negative

1. Which data from your assessment of J.G. are of concern to you?

2. What do the admission lab results indicate?

3. Which of the previous lab results specifically reflects chronic alcohol ingestion?

4. What are the 2 most likely causes of J.G.'s symptoms?

5. What is the most likely time frame for someone to have withdrawal symptoms after abrupt cessation of alcohol?

CASE STUDY PROGRESS

You discuss with J.G. and his brother about the history of his alcohol use. You conclude J.G. may be demonstrating behaviors of alcohol use disorder.

6. List the criteria for alcohol use disorder as outlined in the *Diagnostic and Statistical Manual of Mental Disorders,* Fifth Edition (DSM-V) and put an asterisk or star next to the ones J.G. demonstrates.

7. Based on the DSM-V criteria, how would you rate the severity of J.G.'s alcohol use? Explain your decision.
   a. No problem
   b. Mild
   c. Moderate
   d. Severe

8. What would be helpful for J.G.'s physician to know regarding J.G.'s substance use history?

CASE STUDY PROGRESS

J.G.'s physician arrives in the ICU and discusses with you the possibility of J.G. manifesting signs of alcohol withdrawal delirium. The physician writes several medication orders.

9. What medications are commonly prescribed for patients withdrawing from alcohol? Select all that apply.
   a. Thiamine, a B vitamin
   b. Beta blockers, such as propranolol
   c. Naltrexone (Revia), an opioid-reversal agent
   d. Benzodiazepines, such as lorazepam (Ativan)
   e. Clonidine (Catapres), an alpha-adrenergic blocker
   f. Acamprosate (Campral), an alcohol deterrent agent
   g. Antiepileptic drugs, such as carbamazepine (Tegretol)

10. Explain the rationale for each of the drugs used during acute alcohol withdrawal.

11. What chronic health problems are associated with alcoholism?

12. What lab tests might the physician order to assess for nutritional deficiencies or other medical problems J.G. is experiencing?

J.G. experiences alcohol withdrawal delirium that lasts for 36 hours before subsiding. He did not experience any seizures this time. As his medical condition stabilizes, he is transferred out of the ICU to the hospital's psychiatric unit. He tells you that he is "ready to go home" and does not want to "touch another drink" but admits that he needs help.

13. What medications might be prescribed to J.G. to assist him with sobriety? What would you discuss with J.G. concerning the treatment regimen, side effects and precautions of his medications?

14. What types of information and referrals will be discussed with J.G. before his discharge from the hospital?

15. J.G. is referred to the local Alcoholics Anonymous (AA) program. What strategy can be implemented to increase his likelihood of attendance at these meetings?

J.G.'s AA sponsor met with him while J.G. was still in the hospital, and the meeting went well. The day after his discharge from the hospital, J.G. attends his first AA meeting with his sponsor.

Case Study **150**

Name_____ Class/Group_____ Date_____

▶ Scenario

It is 1000 hours in the emergency department (ED) when the ambulance brings in G.G., a 35-year-old man who is having difficulty breathing. He complains of chest pain, tightness in the chest, dizziness, palpitations, nausea, paresthesia, and feelings of impending doom. He states, "I don't think I'm going to make it. I must be having a heart attack." He is diaphoretic and trembling. His vital signs are 184/92, 104, 28, 98.4° F (36.9° C). These symptoms began at work during a meeting at approximately 0920 and became progressively worse. A co-worker called 911 and stayed with him until the first responder arrived. The patient has no apparent history of cardiac problems.

1. What are your initial interventions?

CASE STUDY PROGRESS

Following the full medical workup, including testing to rule out MI, pulmonary embolism, and thyroid disorders, it is determined that G.G.'s condition is stable. His shortness of breath and anxiety resolve after he is given lorazepam (Ativan) 1 mg IV push (IVP). The lab work and ECG results are all within normal parameters, and there is no evidence of any physical disorder. A diagnosis of panic attack is made. G.G. admits to having had 3 similar episodes in the past 2 weeks; however, they were not nearly as severe or long-lasting.

2. Based on the evidence in this case, list the signs and symptoms associated with the diagnosis of panic attack.

3. G.G. asks whether there is something wrong with his memory because he has been having trouble remembering things. What effect does panic disorder have on memory?

CASE STUDY PROGRESS

G.G. shares with the ED staff that he has been under severe stress at work and home. He tells them he is going through a divorce, he lost a child last summer in a motor vehicle accident, and his company is downsizing. He will probably be out of a job soon. He hasn't been sleeping well for the past couple of months and has lost about 20 pounds (9 kg).

4. Identify 5 triggers that may be associated with panic attacks.

5. Explain the differences between panic attacks and panic disorders according to the *Diagnostic and Statistical Manual of Mental Disorders,* Fifth Edition (DSM-V).

6. Has G.G. had an expected or unexpected panic attack? Explain your answer.

7. What are possible symptoms of a panic attack? Select all that apply.
   a. Sweating
   b. Drowsiness
   c. Palpitations
   d. Hallucinations
   e. Feelings of choking
   f. Feelings of unreality

CASE STUDY PROGRESS

G.G.'s condition is stable and the ED physician discusses what has happened with G.G. The physician provides G.G. a prescription for alprazolam (Xanax) 0.5 mg tid for 1 week and a referral to see his primary care physician for further treatment and evaluation.

8. Explain the rationale for prescribing Xanax for only 1 week.

9. For each class of medications used to treat panic attacks, what will your patient teaching include?

CASE STUDY PROGRESS

G.G. tells you about his worries with his job and all that has happened to him in the past year. He tells you that he appreciates you listening to him and expresses fear that the panic attacks will return.

10. Identify 5 non-pharmacological techniques you will explore with G.G. to help manage his expressed fear of panic attacks.

11. What actions or interventions are most indicated in the treatment of panic disorder?

CASE STUDY OUTCOME

G.G. makes an appointment with his company's Employee Assistance Program to take advantage of the resources offered for counseling to help him work with his coping strategies. In addition, his primary care physician starts him on a low dose of an SSRI. After a few months, G.G.'s experiences fewer panic attacks, and he joined a yoga class to help manage his stress.